Generating
Middle Range Theory

Sister Callista Roy, PhD, RN, FAAN, professor, William F. Connell School of Nursing, Boston College, has been involved in nursing education for 46 years. Her numerous faculty appointments include positions at Mount St. Mary's College, where she also served as department chair (1971–1982); at the University of Portland, Oregon, where she helped to initiate a master's program; and at the University of San Francisco. At the Connell School of Nursing, Dr. Roy was part of the team that initiated a PhD program in nursing that graduated 161 PhD alumni in the first 21 years. Other visiting faculty appointments include La Sabana University, Colombia; University Autonoma de Nuevo Leon, Mexico; St. Mary's College, Kurume, Japan; University of Lund, Sweden; and University of Conception, Chile. Dr. Roy served on the board of the International Network for Doctoral Education from 2003 to 2006. She is faculty senior nurse scientist at the Yvonne L. Munn Center for Nursing Research at Massachusetts General Hospital and was a charter member of the Nursing Research Study Section, Division of Research Grants, and National Institutes of Health. Dr. Roy is best known for developing the Roy adaptation model of nursing and leadership for knowledge-based practice. She has lectured in 36 countries on 5 continents. As early as 1987, an estimated 10,000 nurses had studied in schools where the curricula used the Roy adaptation model and the impact of the model on practice continues as health care agencies use it in designing strategies for Magnet status. Dr. Roy has 136 publications to her credit, 11 of which are books, including *Nursing Knowledge Development and Clinical Practice* (2006), with book translations in 12 languages. Her published analyses of 163 studies based on the Roy model provided a blueprint for theory-based scholarship in nursing. Dr. Roy has received 42 research and training grants. She holds several teaching awards; five honorary doctorates; national awards from Sigma Theta Tau International, the National League for Nursing, and NANDA; was appointed a Living Legend of the American Academy of Nursing and of the Massachusetts Association of Registered Nurses; as well as receiving Massachusetts State House recognition for her volunteer work with women in prison. She is a Sister of St. Joseph of Carondelet.

Generating
Middle Range Theory

From Evidence to Practice

Sister Callista Roy, PhD, RN, FAAN
With the Roy Adaptation Association

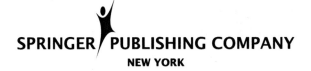

SPRINGER PUBLISHING COMPANY
NEW YORK

Springer Publishing Company, LLC
11 West 42nd Street
New York, NY 10036
www.springerpub.com

Acquisitions Editor: Joseph Morita
Composition: diacriTech

ISBN: 978-0-8261-1009-1
e-book ISBN: 978-0-8261-1005-3

Faculty Guide ISBN: 978-0-8261-9632-3
Video Introductions ISBN: 978-0-8261-9633-0

Qualified instructors may request the Faculty Guide and Video Introductions by emailing textbook@springerpub.com

13 14 15 16 17 / 5 4 3 2 1

The author and the publisher of this Work have made every effort to use sources believed to be reliable to provide information that is accurate and compatible with the standards generally accepted at the time of publication. The author and publisher shall not be liable for any special, consequential, or exemplary damages resulting, in whole or in part, from the readers' use of, or reliance on, the information contained in this book. The publisher has no responsibility for the persistence or accuracy of URLs for external or third-party Internet websites referred to in this publication and does not guarantee that any content on such websites is, or will remain, accurate or appropriate.

Library of Congress Cataloging-in-Publication Data

Roy, Callista.
  Generating middle range theory: from evidence to practice / Callista Roy
with the Roy Adaptation Association.
    p. ; cm.
  Includes bibliographical references and index.
  ISBN 978-0-8261-1009-1—ISBN 978-0-8261-1005-3 (e-book)
  I. Roy Adaptation Association. II. Title.
  [DNLM: 1. Nursing Theory. 2. Adaptation, Physiological. 3. Adaptation,
Psychological. 4. Models, Nursing. 5. Nursing Research—methods. WY 86]
  RT84.5
  610.7301—dc23
                                                    2013017219

Special discounts on bulk quantities of our books are available to corporations, professional associations, pharmaceutical companies, health care organizations, and other qualifying groups. If you are interested in a custom book, including chapters from more than one of our titles, we can provide that service as well.

For details, please contact:
Special Sales Department, Springer Publishing Company, LLC
11 West 42nd Street, 15th Floor, New York, NY 10036-8002
Phone: 877-687-7476 or 212-431-4370; Fax: 212-941-7842
E-mail: sales@springerpub.com

Printed in the United States of America by Gasch Printing.

Dedicated to the loving memory of Susan Pollock, PhD, RN, FAAN, an exceptional scholar who brought us together, initiated this work, and began the Roy Adaptation Association—our mentor, our colleague, our friend

Contents

Contributors

AUTHORS, ROY ADAPTATION ASSOCIATION BOARD MEMBERS, AND FELLOWS

Alexandra Bennett-Roach
Graduate Student
Doctor of Nursing Science Program
The Graduate Center
The City University of New York
New York, New York

Ellen B. Buckner, DSN, RN, CNE
Professor of Nursing at the College of Nursing
University of South Alabama
Mobile, Alabama

Marjorie C. Dobratz, DNSc, RN
Professor, Nursing Program
University of Washington Tacoma
Tacoma, Washington

Keville Frederickson, EdD, RN, FAAN
Professor and Director of Research and Scholarship
Department of Nursing
Lehman College
Bronx, New York
Executive Officer, Doctor of Nursing Science Program
The Graduate Center
The City University of New York
New York, New York

Ann Harrington
Undergraduate Research Fellow
Connell School of Nursing
Boston College
Chestnut Hill, Massachusetts

Susan J. Hayden, PhD, RN
Assistant Professor
University of South Alabama, College of Nursing
Mobile, Alabama

Kathryn Lauchner, PhD, RN
Professor of Nursing
Austin Community College
Austin, Texas

Carolyn Padovano, PhD, RN
Director of Health IT
Center for the Advancement of Health IT
Social, Statistical & Environmental Sciences
RTI International
Washington, DC

Sister Callista Roy, PhD, RN, FAAN
Professor and Nurse Theorist
Connell School of Nursing
Boston College
Chestnut Hill, Massachusetts

Martha V. Whetsell, PhD, RN
Associate Professor of Nursing
Lehman College
Bronx, New York
Doctor of Nursing Science Program
The Graduate Center
The City University of New York
New York, New York

Research Reviewers

ROY ADAPTATION ASSOCIATION BOARD MEMBERS

Stacey H. Barone, PhD, RN, CNS
Associate Clinical Professor
Connell School of Nursing
Boston College
Chestnut Hill, Massachusetts

Debra R. Hanna, PhD, RN, CNRN
Associate Professor of Nursing
Molloy College
Rockville Centre, New York

Pamela M. Senesac, PhD, SM, RN
Senior Director, Performance Improvement Commonwealth Medicine
University of Massachusetts Medical School
Shrewsbury, Massachusetts

CONNELL SCHOOL OF NURSING, BOSTON COLLEGE—RESEARCH FELLOWS

Clare Butt, PhD, RN
Ann Harrington
Beth Harvey
Elizabeth Johnson, BS, RN
Elizabeth Long, BS, RN

RAZI SCHOOL OF NURSING AND MIDWIFERY

Mansooreh A. Forouzi, MSc

Preface

This book stems from significant trends established in nursing, yet it may be the first of its kind. Knowledge for nursing practice is an abiding need to meet the social mandate of nursing. All professions respond to needs in society from their own specific knowledge base. The profession is accountable for developing knowledge and for implementing it in practice. Theoretical and research knowledge in nursing are growing at a rapid pace. Funding for nursing research, the focus on evidence-based practice, and middle range theory (MRT) are significant movements that aim to close the gap between developing nursing knowledge and the changing demands in nursing practice. A gap between knowledge and practice limits the impact of nursing care. Given the significant advantage of having a reservoir of 15 years of research based on one theoretical model and having already published a review of the first 25 years of research based on this model, the Executive Board members of the Roy Adaptation Association (RAA) took on the challenge of developing and illustrating an innovative way to close the gap between knowledge and practice. The unique approach being offered is generating MRTs from 172 studies based on the Roy adaptation model and using the research evidence from the studies within the MRTs to provide evidence for practice. With a focus on creative ways to apply this knowledge to practice illustrated throughout the book, this cumulative knowledge can change practice and affect policies for practice.

The authors assert that this approach to knowledge can be helpful to beginning students, students in advanced practice, those studying for the DNP and for the PhD, as well as nurses in practice, particularly those working to attain the accreditation of Magnet status for their institutions. Nurse scholars using these approaches in isolation will welcome this new combination of knowledge development strategies. To bring theory and research to the practice level is a significant skill for all nurses. The approach provided here is easy to understand. The usefulness of research of all designs, both qualitative and quantitative, can be readily understood. Further, the relevance of research findings to practice can be explored for any setting. Similarly, creating MRT is demystified as concepts are identified from multiple research projects. The simple concepts are linked in statements and in pictorial schemas so that relationships are apparent. Each MRT has a compelling exemplar for practice. The author then specifically establishes the evidence-based practice for the MRT and relates this to Roy's levels of readiness for practice. An added bonus is two approaches to studying and showing how theory and research are used globally, one for Latin American countries and the other for sampling the globe.

The book is organized into five parts, each with an introduction. Part I sets the stage for this project and in Chapter 1, we describe knowledge that has been created and why we propose an alternative approach. Chapter 2 outlines the processes that make up the approach. In Part II the research projects are described in tables and text. The organization is to help the reader see the contribution of many research designs. Chapter 3 is on qualitative research and introduces this topic, then presents the studies by types of qualitative designs. Chapter 4 covers the descriptive quantitative studies and organizes them by clusters of concepts of the Roy adaptation model. Chapter 5 contains studies that aim to explain, predict, and proscribe, all organized by clusters of model concepts. The final chapter on quantitative studies, Chapter 6, describes the intervention studies clustered by related concepts.

In Part III the five MRTs are generated: coping (Chapter 7); adapting to life events (Chapter 8); adapting to loss (Chapter 9); adapting to chronic health conditions (Chapter 10); and adapting families (Chapter 11). Each chapter follows the 6-step process laid out in Chapter 2 and focuses on how the MRT can affect practice. Part IV (Chapter 12) details the important step of putting together the MRTs derived from research with the evidence that supports them and showing their readiness for practice now and in the future. Part V (Chapter 13) samples the theory and research around the globe. The appendix of instruments and measurements used in the studies will be particularly useful for researchers in identifying how other scholars have measured concepts of the model. We are pleased to offer to educators in health care and academic settings two kinds of teaching tools online. The sections of the book are introduced in videos featuring the theorist, and a study guide by an RAA educator provides discussion questions at varying levels of complexity. **These can be found at the Springer Publishing Company website at textbook@springerpub.com.**

We hope that this effort will lead to similar new approaches to accumulating knowledge for practice, closing the gap between knowledge and practice, and linking the strengths of theory and research to lead change in practice that provides access to quality care for all.

Sister Callista Roy, PhD, RN, FAAN, and
The Executive Board of the Roy Adaptation Association

Acknowledgments

A project of this scope has relied on the contributions of many people to whom we are indebted for making it possible to bring this product to our readers. First, we thank the hundreds of researchers who published their work and gave us the great gift of developing nursing knowledge, each of which is valuable in itself, but together provided the rich data bank we could draw on. Our gratitude goes out to the team of reviewers and authors who worked together for 2 years to design the project, identify, and locate copies of the studies, evaluate the work and prepare it for its place in the publication. We have summarized their roles in two categories, but all contributed in ways large and small from going to the office of Springer Publishing Company in New York to talk about our proposal to the final formatting of references. In the early stages of developing the manuscript, Dr. Pamela Grace, a colleague at Boston College, read sections of the work and provided insightful critique that contributed significantly to the clarity of presenting middle range theories. We thank the authors in particular as crucial to the project. They understood the whole and patiently dealt with changing directions as each part of the project evolved, building on another section that also was going through updating. We are particularly grateful for the expertise, consistent loyalty, and good nature of Emily Keen, the executive director of the Roy Adaptation Association (RAA) who created a real-time collaborative editing website for common use that was invaluable from the beginning to end of the work. Emily facilitated communication among all involved in many additional ways, and took on the detailed task of repeatedly reconciling the lists of studies with the tables created by the authors and of chapter content with reference lists. We thank the Sisters of St. Joseph of Carondelet, Los Angeles Province, who provide a restricted gift to fund Emily's work with the RAA organization and as an editorial and staff assistant with Sister Callista Roy.

A general message of gratitude is extended globally to all those who have stimulated and contributed to the development of the Roy adaptation model, which is the basis for the research, theory building, and evidence for practice of this text. Former and current faculty from Mount St. Mary's College have had a special role in this development and in welcoming the RAA for conferences. Faculty and students around the globe and nurses in practice have all provided insightful observations, support and questions that encourage this ongoing work.

We appreciate the staff at Springer Publishing Company who have been attentive to detail from the beginning. Early on, Allan Graubard, then executive editor, met with us and provided wise feedback to shape the project as well as later reading and more constructive feedback on selected chapters, which contributed greatly to the quality of the entire project. Joseph Morita, senior acquisitions editor, ably took over the review and preparation of the project for publication and it was then shepherded through the editorial process by Chris Teja, assistant editor, who guided and supported us throughout the process. We are grateful for the significant work of Rose Mary Piscitelli, Senior Editor in the Production Department, who took charge of turning the project into a book. We are appreciative of the interest of the publisher for nursing at Springer, Margaret Zuccarini, who not only kept our project on track, but also took a personal interest in the details of the publication.

Sister Callista Roy, PhD, RN, FAAN, with the Roy Adaptation
Association Executive Board

I

Introduction

*A*s a practice discipline, nursing will continue to develop knowledge to meet the changing health needs of society. A substantial issue in accomplishing this goal is to close the gap between knowledge developed by both theory and research and implementation in practice. This book takes a unique approach to cumulative nursing knowledge development for practice. The purpose of Part I is to set the stage for this project. One chapter provides a background of how knowledge for practice has been created offering a proposal for adding an alternative approach. Another chapter outlines a series of processes that make up that approach.

To orient the reader to a unique approach to developing knowledge for practice in Chapter 1, the author provides an overview of the factors that have affected nursing as a discipline in developing knowledge for practice. The author narrates nursing's rich history and heritage of multiple contributions to the significant growth in nursing knowledge during the 20th century and the beginning decades of the 21st century. The point is made that the significance of knowledge development to date is not debated. However, nurses still face a challenge in taking the lead in advancing a health agenda and thereby closing the gap between our knowledge and impact on practice. We need to make developments in nursing science visible and effective. The aim is to critically review how the discipline of nursing provides evidence and ways used to close the gap between theory and research and knowledge used in practice. The author acknowledges current great achievements of knowledge impacting practice. The significant programs of the National Institute of Nursing Research program on translational research and the evidence-based practice (EBP) movement are discussed. Each is also critiqued for the limitations that allow for another approach.

The content and process of middle range theory are offered as a way to bridge the gap between theory and research and evidence for high-quality practice. A six-step process for developing middle range theory is described. The author outlines a new definition for EBP that allows for three levels of readiness for application in practice: support for implementation, need for review by clinical nurse specialists to confirm readiness, and need for replication of studies. The reader is introduced to the processes that will be used to link middle range theories derived from the research studies to a new perspective on EBP.

In Chapter 2 the author describes the details of how 200 studies based on one theoretical model provide the research findings in multiple clinical areas to generate middle range theory and provide evidence for practice. A number of issues that were dealt with in the processes for description and critical analysis of the research are described. Three primary concerns are identified and discussed: (1) how to identify studies with potential for use in this development of knowledge that is evidence based, (2) how to describe and critically analyze each study to identify the strengths of the evidence, and finally (3) how the studies are organized and presented so they can be used in the generation of middle range theory and evidence for practice. The rest of the project as described in the following chapters stands on these foundational chapters of Part I.

1

Overview of Processes for Creating Knowledge for Practice

SISTER CALLISTA ROY

Nurses in practice face great challenges and opportunities in the early decades of the 21st century. In the United States health care finance dominates the scene, leaving every health care provider facing obstacles to providing safe and high-quality care. Nurses comprise the largest number of health care providers, numbering approximately 3.1 million (AACN, 2012). Nursing has gone through a great growth period in knowledge development and in expanding roles in the past few decades. Increasing education and resources for research have contributed to building knowledge and nurses at all levels have expanded their roles to take more responsibility for the quality of patient care. At the same time, nurses confront the demand to keep ahead of changes in society. As a profession nursing has a social mandate to contribute to the good of society through knowledge-based practice. As a practice discipline, nursing will maintain the priority of quality of care for all people, yet find new ways to meet changing health needs (Meleis, 2007). To meet these needs we recognize that our world is in transition—with changes on multiple levels. Demographics show increased diversity of ethnicities and cultures and an aging population in most developed countries. We are affected by global migration and the globalization of the world's economy, with increasing discrepancies between the rich and the poor both within and among countries. Nurses are dealing also with changes in science and technology such as genetics and information technology.

The past 30 years of growth in nursing knowledge has been shaped by the discipline's values and goals and was designed to improve quality of care and health of individuals, families, communities, and society. Still many authors noted that we have a gap between knowledge development and knowledge used in practice. McEwen recognized that after repeated calls to integrate theory, research, and practice, "the interaction remains fragmented or unrecognized" (2007, p. 416). More recently, Im and Chang (2012) explored trends in nursing theories and identified integration to practice as one of six major themes, but interpreted the data as only the beginning of long overdue efforts to link theory to practice as a basis for nursing care.

In this chapter the author examines the strategies used to develop knowledge for practice. The factors that influence nursing knowledge development are outlined to provide a background to critique approaches taken to close the gaps among theory and research and knowledge used in nursing practice. This critique includes funded translational research and the evidence-based practice (EBP) movement. The content and process of generating middle range theory (MRT) from a set of related studies is offered as a significant way to bridge this knowledge–practice gap. The relevance of MRTs supported by findings from 172 studies using the same conceptual framework is explored as a way of accumulating knowledge to be used as evidence for practice. A distinctive definition of EBP (Roy, 2009) that allows for three levels of readiness for application in practice is described: support for implementation, need for review by advanced practice nurse specialists to confirm readiness, and need for replication of studies.

FACTORS INFLUENCING KNOWLEDGE DEVELOPMENT

The development of knowledge for nursing practice has a rich history that includes the evolution of specific strategies. In a summary of the state-of-the art of nursing knowledge (Roy & Jones, 2007), Roy outlined the key influences on nursing knowledge development in the United States in the last century. These influences came from the growth in nursing education, early scholars, as well as publications and major conferences. These efforts combined to mature the discipline in the 20th century, with clarification of the theoretical focus of nursing as holistic persons with processes and patterns for environmental integration to attain health (Donaldson & Crowley, 1978). From the productive work of the end of the 20th century arose the foci for knowledge as well as development of nursing practice to be used in the 21st century.

Nursing Education

The educational pathway to growth in nursing knowledge was significant, though perhaps not always consistent and direct. The University of Minnesota and Teachers College at Columbia University began granting baccalaureate degrees in the early 1900s, and by 1949 there were 55 programs for degree students in schools owned and operated by a university or college. Rapid growth of baccalaureate programs followed the Brown report (1948), which recommended that schools of nursing be established in universities and colleges, comparable in number to existing medical schools, that they have adequate facilities and faculty, and be well-distributed to serve the needs of the country. Nursing had the opportunity to become an academic discipline and nurse scholars challenged the profession to define its own knowledge base. One nurse leader of influence wrote, "Certainly no profession can long exist without making explicit its theoretical bases for practice so that this knowledge can be communicated, tested, and expanded" (Johnson, 1959).

In the 1950s as noted there was a period of rapid growth of baccalaureate programs in the United States. Colleges and universities established generic programs with a nursing major built on liberal arts and sciences. Applicants met university requirements and graduated with a degree and the preparation to take examinations to become a nurse registered by the state. This growth continued and today there are more than 700 baccalaureate programs in the United States. This was also a period of growth for master's education, with programs maturing from 1964 to 1975. From that time until the present, the age of specialization in master's education, including graduate education for the role of the nurse practitioner, was born. Today there are 300 accredited master's degree programs with an emphasis on advanced practice.

The growth in nursing education hastened the development of nursing knowledge as faculty organized nursing knowledge to be taught in university programs at the undergraduate and graduate levels. This led to identifying the knowledge needed; nurse scholars would add more focused nursing knowledge to educational programs that began with curricula heavily based on biological and behavioral sciences. This need for knowledge from a nursing perspective added momentum to the influences of the people, publications, and conferences of this era. Although academic nursing grew and stimulated growth in nursing knowledge for practice, it must be noted that until the 1960s, diploma programs were the major source of graduates prepared for registration as nurses. These programs held great prominence in the 1950s and 1960s, with approximately 818 diploma schools in the United States in 1963 (American Nurses Association [ANA], 1966). Further, an experiment with 2-year programs in community colleges began in the 1970s. As diploma programs began closing, the explosive growth of the associate degree nursing (ADN) programs was hastened by factors such as a nursing shortage, an increase in federal financial assistance for nursing education, and new concerns about equal access to education and health care (Smith, 2009).

The reality is that to this day all state boards of nursing require each nursing graduate to pass the National Council Licensure Examination (NCLEX), developed by the National Council of State Boards of Nursing (NCSBN) as the standardized exam that determines whether or not a candidate is prepared for entry-level nursing practice. This includes nurses with education in diploma programs, associate degrees, and baccalaureate degrees. As early as 1965 the American Nurses Association Committee on Education issued a statement that was adopted by the Board of Directors and became the "position paper" recommending that the minimum preparation for beginning professional nursing practice should be at the baccalaureate level (ANA, 1965). The ANA committee on education noted in particular the changes in nursing practice at that time, including "major theoretical formulations, scientific discoveries, technological innovations, and the development of radical new treatments" (p. 107). Thus began 40 years of debate and efforts within the profession to establish the minimum level of education for entry into practice. In 2000, 29.6% of nurses in practice received their basic education in diploma programs and the percent educated with associate degrees increased to 40.3 (Nelson, 2002). In a 2009 paper on policy related to entry into practice, Smith concluded, "Considering the accelerated pace of todays' educational, technological, and social changes, it is imperative that the educational foundation on which our profession is based remains in step with these changes. Now more than ever, we must rededicate ourselves to making the initial entry proposal a reality" (Smith, 2009, n.p.).

Although some energy has been expended without positive results on the entry-into-practice issue, at the same time this very concern possibly added momentum to the development of doctoral education in nursing in the 1970s and 1980s. Well-prepared faculty for baccalaureate and master's nursing education became a priority. Historically, Teachers College at Columbia University offered the EdD for nurses in 1933 and New York University followed in 1934. The first PhD degree for nurses was started by the University of Pittsburgh in 1954, with both University of California at San Francisco and Catholic University offering the Doctor of Nursing Science (DNSc) in the 1960s. By the 1970s most new doctoral programs in nursing offered the PhD degree. According to the American Association of Colleges of Nursing (AACN), 30 new PhD programs were added in the 1980s and 26 in the 1990s. Many DNSc programs have converted to the PhD. By 2009 there were 120 PhD programs in nursing that offered the research doctorate. The research doctorate is intended to prepare students to use intellectual inquiry to pursue knowledge and carry out independent research (AACN, 2001).

The PhD programs in nursing are effective approaches to knowledge development for practice because the students admitted to these programs raise significant questions from practice and are socialized into nursing as a scholarly profession with knowledge based on theory and research. The curricula of the PhD programs provides students with a focus for knowledge development and methods for theory development and for research. Each year approximately 600 PhD dissertations in nursing are filed, making available new knowledge, most of which is focused on nursing practice. As PhD graduates, these nurses become committed scholars intent on continuing to develop knowledge and translate the new knowledge into practice.

By 2004 there were changes in advanced practice that led to the AACN position statement calling for educating advanced practice registered nurses (APRNs) and other nurses seeking top clinical positions in Doctor of Nursing Practice (DNP) programs (AACN, 2004). The AACN identified that many factors emerged to build momentum for this change in nursing education at the graduate level, including: "the rapid expansion of knowledge underlying practice; increased complexity of patient care; national concerns about the quality of care and patient safety; shortages of nursing personnel which demands a higher level of preparation for leaders who can design and assess care; shortages of doctorally prepared nursing faculty, and increasing educational expectations for the preparation of other health professionals" (AACN, 2012). Proponents of the movement noted that often advanced practice nurses such as nurse practitioners, clinical nurse specialists, and more specialized programs like nurse midwives and nurse anesthetists are prepared in master's degree programs, which sometimes carry a credit load equivalent to the clinical doctoral degrees in the other health professions. The curriculum for DNP programs build on what is taught in master's degree programs and added content in key areas such as EBP, quality improvement, and systems thinking. In 2012 the AACN reported that there were 217 DNP programs (www.aacn.nche.edu). It remains to be seen whether the DNP movement will actualize the much anticipated bridging of the gap between nursing knowledge and nursing practice.

Theoretical Scholars in Nursing

Leading textbooks on nursing theory and knowledge development outline the key scholars in nursing who influenced the pathway to knowledge development in the discipline. Each version that outlines the scholars varies by the purpose of the publication and the viewpoint of the author. Our purpose in this chapter is to acknowledge major theoretical scholars in nursing with an emphasis on the continued efforts to relate knowledge development to nursing practice.

Peplau (1952) introduced a new way of thinking about nursing practice as an interpersonal relationship with the patient that is focused on growth of the personality of the individual. Peplau contributed greatly to nursing organizations as both president and executive director of the ANA. Contributions that stand out relate to nursing practice, for example, Peplau was on the team that wrote the first ANA Nursing's Social Policy Statement in 1980. She made significant contributions to psychiatric nursing as a specialty, establishing the first master's degree focused on the nurse–patient psychodynamic relationship. Practice principles that she promoted in her writing and the hundreds of workshops she gave around the country included:

1. The nurse being able to understand one's own behavior to help others identify felt difficulties, and to apply principles of human relations to the problems that arise at all levels of the experience.
2. The goal of nursing is the forward movement of personality of the person.
3. The process involves four overlapping phases from orientation to resolution.
4. Nurses take on six different roles, including resource person and teacher.

The influence of another major scholar, Henderson, was felt both nationally and internationally. Her definition of nursing, written in 1966, stated: "The unique function of the nurse is to assist the individual (sick or well), in the performance of those activities contributing to health or its recovery (or to peaceful death) that he would perform unaided if he had the necessary strength, will, or knowledge. And to do this in such a way as to help him gain independence as rapidly as possible" (Henderson, 1991, p. 21). The definition used in her textbook was adopted by the International Council of Nurses and translated into 20 languages. Henderson categorized nursing activities into 14 components, based on human needs. Examples are: "Breathe normally; eat and drink adequately"; and "communicate with others in expressing emotions, needs, fears, or opinions."

Johnson was influential as a speaker, author, teacher, and mentor. As a frequent speaker Johnson's conviction about the need for nursing science influenced other thinkers. For example, she served on an alumnae panel with Rogers at Vanderbilt and this marked a turning point in Rogers' writings. Johnson developed the first nursing model-based curriculum in the 1960s using her human behavioral systems model. Later she offered the first graduate course on nursing models in the 1970s. Johnson was on the faculty at University of California at Los Angeles from 1949 to 1978 and taught or worked with other scholars such as Meleis, Mishel, Roy, Gebbie, and Neuman. In a classic publication in 1974 Johnson laid out three paths to knowledge development: the laissez-faire alternative, or follow the path of medicine, or build the conceptual system of nursing based on the goal of nursing practice. Her belief in defining the goal of nursing practice as the basis for building nursing knowledge had influence in the profession for many years.

During this era two key studies were published that identified the core concepts of nursing. One was based on a review of baccalaureate nursing programs and described the major concepts central to the conceptual models and frameworks used for nursing curricula. Yura and Torres (1975) found that four central concepts emerged, that is, person, society, health, and nursing. These concepts were supported by the discipline for some time and were called nursing's metaparadigm, although minor variations were introduced. The second was based on scholarly discussions on the definition of the discipline and of nursing science by Crowley and Donaldson. This work developed into a scholarly paper for the keynote address at the 10th Communicating Nursing Research of the Western Council on Higher Education for Nursing (WICHEN) and was included in their 1977 proceedings. The paper was published in *Nursing Outlook* in 1978 and listed the core themes of nursing that Donaldson and Crowley derived as:

- Concern with the principles and laws that govern the life processes
- Concern with the patterning of human behavior in interaction with the environment
- Concern with the processes by which positive changes in health status are affected

More recently, a paper describing the concepts of a central unifying focus of nursing has categorized nursing concepts as: facilitating humanization, meaning, choice, quality of life and healing in living and dying (Willis, Grace, & Roy, 2008). These updated concepts have been widely quoted (Meleis, 2007; Reed & Shearer, in press; Walker & Avant, 2011). It remains to be seen whether or not this version of articulating the central unifying focus of nursing will be productive in leading knowledge development and implementation in nursing.

Other major theoretical scholars, known as the Grand Theorists of the 1970s, are listed in Box 1.1 along with the earliest date and focus of their work. In considering the focus of each theorist and that of those discussed earlier, Peplau, Henderson, and Johnson, one notices a strong focus on the person as the focus of knowledge development in nursing. Each theorist was conceptualizing the recipient of nursing care. Sometimes theorists have been criticized as being separated from nursing practice and using mainly deductive theorizing. However, knowing these women and their work personally, I take the stance that their thinking was rooted

---

BOX 1.1
THEORY DEVELOPMENT—1970s, MAJOR GRAND THEORIES

- Myra Levine—Energy Conservation, 1967
- Martha Rogers—Person–Environment Energy Fields, 1970
- Dorothea Orem—Self Care, 1971
- Imogene King—Theory of Goal Attainment, 1971
- Callista Roy—Adaptation Model, 1970
- Betty Neuman—Systems Approach, 1974
- Paterson and Zderad—Humanistic Nursing, 1976
- Margaret Newman—Health as Expanding Consciousness, 1976

---

in nursing practice and aimed at understanding people and how nurses could promote their growth and health.

Although not distinctly separated, there was a group of theoretical scholars known as the Grand Theorists of the 1980s as listed in Box 1.2. Johnson and Rogers are listed first because their work had been widely known through their speaking and handouts. However, the second edition of Riehl and Roy (1980) provided the opportunity to convince both scholars to write a chapter on their theory. Rogers brought a new view of the major concepts of nursing by noting how modern physics did not separate person and environment and using other principles of homeodynamics such as resonancy, helicy, and integrality. Newman, Parse, Fitzpatrick, and Watson began their work based on ideas from Rogers. Leininger, Sisca, and Erickson focused on the role of nursing. Roper, Logan, and Tierney were like the earlier theorists and emphasized the person and how each one lives, but as theorists from the United Kingdom they wanted their work to be distinct from the theorists from the United States.

Also in the 1980s a number of theorists and other authors focused specifically on caring as a core concept of nursing. Leininger did extensive research on cultural care, universals, and diversity. Watson looked further into caring as the essence of practice and a moral ideal; Benner wrote about the relations of caring, stress, coping, health, and caring practices. It was about the same time that other theorists focused on the philosophical perspectives of person with the following emphases:

- Orem concentrated on the person as free agent, emphasizing human choice
- Roy looked at the purposefulness of humankind and a shared common purposefulness
- Newman focused on the pattern of the whole and expanding consciousness

---

BOX 1.2
THEORY DEVELOPMENT—1980s, MAJOR GRAND THEORISTS

- Dorothy Johnson—Behavioral Systems
- Martha Rogers—Person, Environment Systems
- Madeline Leininger—Transcultural Nursing
- Jean Watson—Caring Science
- Joan Riehl Sisca—Interaction Model
- Rosemarie Parse—Person–Living–Health
- Joyce Fitzpatrick—Life Perspective Rhythm
- Helen Erickson—Modeling and Role Modeling
- Nancy Roper, Winifred Logan, and Alison Tierney—Model of Living as Model for Nursing

---

In the 1970s nurses debated about whether we need one nursing theory or many. However, from the later 1970s to the end of the century the usefulness of theories in practice, education, and research encouraged pluralism. The work of the scholars mentioned and their colleagues resulted in significant changes in thinking about nursing as a scholarly discipline and knowledge for practice. By the end of the 20th century, we saw the maturing of the discipline with a clarifying of the theoretical focus of nurses as holistic persons. Nursing has a plurality of grand theories and in the 1990s began developing MRTs, as discussed below. The mutual impact of theory and education led to articulating and testing of theories in practice and research.

From the beginning of the 21st century and beyond, there was a movement to reach beyond pluralism to identify the commonalities of the discipline perspective at higher levels of abstraction. The holism of the person could be identified by characteristics commonly shared by nurses, including persons and environment are systems, persons have purposefulness as individuals and groups, parts are manifestations of the pattern of the whole, persons have consciousness and choice, and persons are interdependent. Similarly, in the 21st century, commonalities of nursing as transforming relationships emerged, including nurses as facilitators of well-being who use knowledge and values in a caring relationship; the nurse uses one's whole self in the process of human to human interaction, mutuality, and encounter; nursing relationships include giving and receiving and involve respect, acceptance, and openness (Box 1.3).

The focus of knowledge development around commonalities of the discipline made unique contributions to knowledge for practice. This development was one way to preserve the lasting effects of the grand theories of nursing, many of which were rooted in practice. The commonalities

---

BOX 1.3
COMMONALITIES OF NURSING FOR THE 21ST CENTURY

1. The holism of the person:
   • Persons and environment are systems
   • Persons have purposefulness as individuals and groups
   • Parts are manifestations of the pattern of the whole
   • Persons have consciousness and choice
   • Persons are interdependent
2. Nursing involves transforming relationships
   • Nurses facilitate well-being using knowledge and values in a caring relationship
   • Nurses use their whole selves in the process of human to human interaction, mutuality, and encounter
   • Nursing relationships include giving and receiving and involve respect, acceptance, and openness

---

were useful for further theoretical and philosophical developments focused on a person-oriented discipline. This focus helped to articulate a research agenda and the terminology became the common parlance for describing practice.

Research Resources

Theory and research go together, yet in knowledge development for nursing practice they are not always at the same pace for a variety of reasons. As nursing developed an academic discipline to educate nurses in colleges and universities, there was a need for theoretical knowledge as well as knowledge that was supported by research. Along with theories that defined nursing, theories from other disciplines with more established research were combined in nursing education. Still, nurse scholars recognized the need to increase the cadre of nurse researchers that would confirm theories and test knowledge for practice.

Funding for independent research took time to develop. The first nursing grant for research was $600 given to Alice Crist Malone by Sigma Theta Tau in 1936. Government grants focused mainly on nursing organizations and the nursing workforce in the 1940s and 1950s. The American Nurse's Foundation, founded in 1955, received and administered funds for nursing research. Walter Reed Army Institute of Research in 1957 established a Department of Nursing Research with a particular focus on clinical nursing research. Also in the late 1950s the regional nursing research organizations began to be established. The organizations initially did not fund research but were active in promoting research as a way to spread findings from research. Later these organizations would take on the role of offering both research grants and awards for research. The ANA began holding nursing research conferences in 1965 and in 1970 established the ANA Commission on Nursing Research. This commission established the Council of Nurse Researchers in 1972, which was a major vehicle for promoting nursing research for many years.

Although educational studies were conducted in the 1950s and 1960s, nursing leaders began to express concern about the lack of research in nursing practice. Nursing regional organizations and the ANA Commission on Nursing Research began to set priorities for research that focused on clinical topics for practice. With the increasing number of studies, *Nursing Research* was published in 1952. Nursing research skills began to improve in nursing in the 1970s and the number of nurses with earned doctorates increased (Polit & Beck, 2012). Several more journals were established in the 1970s, including *Advances in Nursing Science*, *Research in Nursing & Health*, and *Western Journal of Nursing Research*. Sigma Theta Tau, the International Honor Society for Nursing, sponsored national and international as well as chapter research conferences. The organization's journal (*Image*, which became the *Journal of Nursing Scholarship*) became a premier nursing research journal. Clinical nursing research became a focus in the 1980s and 1990s with a variety of clinical nursing journals increasingly publishing research related to clinical specialties. Many nurses received master's and doctoral degrees in the 1980s and 1990s and postdoctoral education was encouraged.

Federal involvement in nursing research began with the establishment of the Division of Nursing within the Office of the Surgeon General, Public Health Service in 1946. Funding for individual nursing research began in 1956 when the United States Public Health Service (USPHS) awarded nearly $500,000 to researchers for projects in nursing in the first year. At the same time federal support for doctoral fellows became available from the Division of Nursing Resources of the USPHS. This division and some institutes within the National Institutes of Health (NIH) for many years funded nursing research. However, a notable statistic quoted by Burns and Grove (2009) is that although federal funds for nursing research increased significantly to more than $39 million awarded from 1955 to 1976, the funding was not comparable to the $493 million in federal research funds received by those doing medical research in 1974 alone.

Another priority for the 1980s and 1990s was to increase funding for nursing research. The National Center for Nursing Research (NCNR) was established within NIH in 1985, and in 1993 became the National Institute of Nursing Research (NINR). The story of establishing the NINR included years of hard work, divisions among nurses, political setbacks, including two presidential vetoes by Ronald Reagan. When Congress voted to override the veto, the center was established in 1986 and nursing seized the political victory to become key members of the NIH. Not initially welcomed at NIH, the NINR had an acting director appointed from among the other health scientists, Dr. Doris H. Merritt. By June of 1987 Ada Sue Hinshaw, PhD, RN, became the first permanent director and served until 1994. Hinshaw (with Heinrich, 2011) authored a book chapter on the establishment of NINR as a case study in changing health science policy. Also, to celebrate the 25th anniversary of nursing at NIH, the first nursing history book was published (Cantelon, 2010); this book provides significant details partially taken from oral history interviews of Merritt, Hinshaw, and the current director, Patricia Grady, PhD, RN. Grady's words in the preface provide a fitting summary of nursing science of this era.

At no time has the nursing profession been transformed more dramatically than in the past thirty years. Behind that revolution, literally millions of nurses have constituted a team of committed actors: clinicians, professional nursing organizations, schools of nursing, and the National Institute of Nursing Research (NINR). Their creativity and cooperation, coupled with the strong support of Congress, fashioned a different nursing profession and moved it beyond procedure to promise, beyond implementation to innovation, and into the mainstream science at the National Institutes of Health (NIH). (Grady, 2010a)

CHALLENGE OF NURSING KNOWLEDGE REACHING PRACTICE

Given the rich heritage of what might be considered a rapid development of knowledge for nursing practice by nurses with increased levels of education, theoretical scholars, and nurse researchers, one might expect outstanding successes for knowledge in nursing practice. Still scholars agree, including Roy and Jones (2007), that the value of knowledge development to date is not debated. Rather what remains a challenge is for nursing to take the lead in advancing a health agenda. The challenge is to make developments in nursing science visible to all.

The approaches used to decrease the gap between knowledge and practice have been significant but many issues remain. Two of these approaches will be highlighted and also critiqued to determine remains to be done. The NINR emphasis on translational research and the EBP movement are two major efforts to bring knowledge to practice. These movements can be examined to show their major contributions along with remaining questions.

NINR Translational Research

Translational research in general refers to the application of knowledge derived from basic health care research to interventions that improve health. In 2006 the NIH initiated a new approach to make translational research a priority by funding a Clinical and Translational Science Award (CTSA) program. By 2010 there were 46 member institutions in 26 states with the goal of 60 research centers when fully funded. Specifically, translational research aims to close the gap and improve quality "by improving access, reorganizing and coordinating system care, helping clinicians and patients to exchange behaviors, make more informed choices, providing reminders and point-of-care decision support tools, and strengthening patient-clinician relationship" (Wolfe, 2008, p. 211). These centers share a vision: (1) to accelerate translational research into treatment for patients to engage local communities in research and (2) to train a new generation of clinical and translational researchers.

In an article on translational research and nursing science, P. Grady (2010b), the director of NINR, emphasized that the perspective of nurse scientists is vital to identifying the most effective strategies to accelerate translational research. She noted that nurse scientists have expertise in research about how individuals respond to illness or adapt to changes. They used data and observations from clinical settings and design and developed basic and applied research. One example Grady provided is positive results from a study of a nurse-led intervention for patients diagnosed with post-stroke depression. The intervention included stroke rehabilitation nurses teaching coping and problem-solving skills and helping participants identify taking part with others in social events and in physical activity.

A detailed example of what is called "from bedside to bench to practice" is given in a description of a series NINR-funded clinical and laboratory studies on improved outcomes for patients who receive tube feedings (Metheny, 2011). New tests were developed to evaluate correct tube placement of gastric versus small bowel. The investigators also identified bedside tests used in the past to detect aspiration during tube feedings as well as a series of studies to attempt to determine effective methods to detect aspiration and reduce aspiration risk. An animal model was used to compare aspiration detection methods. A descriptive clinical study of aspiration was followed by a study of interventions to reduce aspiration. Of particular note is how this research has been translated into practice. By influencing health care policy the research led to improved outcomes for patients who receive tube feedings. Three major policy statements or recommendations, including the American Society for Parenteral and Enteral Nutrition's enteral nutrition practice recommendations (Bankhead et al., 2009), cited findings of this research. In addition at least nine textbooks in nursing and medicine cite publications of this NINR-funded research.

NINH translational research is a promising movement. However, some observations show certain limitations. The studies affecting practice date from 1990 to 2008 and the policy statements are from 2003, 2005, and 2009. The research had a depth of experience that took an extraordinary amount of time and resources. Second, it is recognized that this is a significant clinical issue, yet it is only one of hundreds of potentially dangerous situations faced by large numbers of patients. This interpretation is supported by the observation that although the Institute of Medicine published *Crossing the Quality Chasm* (2001), there is little evidence that the challenges to quality have changed much in the intervening years. For example, one type of challenge is overuse, that is, the application of health care services where the potential for harm exceeds the potential for benefit. Yet nurses deal with the ethical issues every day of futile treatment causing suffering to patients. It seems reasonable to take the stand that as the approach of translational research continues to grow, it is relevant to look for other approaches to develop knowledge and translate that knowledge into practice.

Evidence-Based Movement

Research utilization was the term used in the 1980s and 1990s to deal with concerns about the limited use of research in providing nursing care. Projects on research utilization were conducted by numerous hospitals and professional organizations. The projects were institutional attempts to create changes in practice based on research findings. It was during the 1990s (Polit & Beck, 2012) that research utilization was superseded by the movement for EBP. The history of the EBP movement and some EBP models are discussed in Chapter 13. What is covered here is a synopsis of EBP for the purpose of providing a critique.

EBP is described as a problem-solving approach to the delivery of health care that integrates the best evidence from well-designed studies and patient care data and combines it with patient preferences and values and nurse expertise (Melnyk, Fineout-Overholt, Stillwell, & Williamson, 2010). Commonalities of models for EBP include synthesis of evidence, implementation in practice, evaluation of impact on patient care, and consideration of the context or setting. EBP relies on systematic review of the literature on a selected clinical issue. *Systematic review* refers to an analysis of all available literature, consideration of the evidence, and a judgment of the effectiveness of using the best practices reflected in the literature. Often systematic reviews are conducted by teams of researchers and they take long periods of time. However, students and nurses in practice often need to search for evidence on a current issue and can use an approach to meet their needs even if it is not as rigorous as a systematic review (Pearson, Vaughan, & Fitzgerald, 2005).

Supporters of the EBP movement note that its significance lies in providing a higher quality of care, improving patient outcomes at reduced costs and providing greater nurse satisfaction. A second major advantage of EBP is that it offers a framework for lifelong learning for nurses to seek new knowledge to solve problems in an era of rapidly developing clinical changes. Basing practice on the best available evidence is highly valued by health professionals. The approaches of EBP are increasingly used particularly in the United Kingdom, where it began, and in Australia, both of which have developed considerable infrastructure to help with using EBP especially for nurses. There is growing awareness and use of EBP in the United States.

Some professionals are concerned that in efforts to perfect EBP, the advantages of EBP may be exaggerated, and clinical judgment and patient input may be given less attention. Critics note that EBP gives priority to empiric approaches to knowledge without a way of integrating other ways of knowing. Baumann (2010) noted that the limitations of EBP are not routinely discussed. The author raises a number of questions: (1) Is the current evidence base complete and unbiased and can it ever be? (2) Is EBP sufficient to guide clinical decision making? (3) Is it able to be holistic? (4) Does it neglect primary prevention? (5) Does it adequately contribute to the development of theory and science? (6) Does it help develop nursing? (7) Does it respect human dignity, complexity, freedom, and mystery? Pearson et al. (2005) noted that of equal importance to research-generated evidence is the view that it is more important that practice be well grounded in theory. Given this view and the questions and concerns raised, one could propose that additional approaches can be generated to develop knowledge that is basic and useful for nursing practice.

ALTERNATIVE PROPOSED FOR KNOWLEDGE FOR PRACTICE

Given the significance of developing and implementing knowledge for practice and the limitations of current approaches, the project staff developed the content and process of generating MRT from a set of related studies as a significant way to bridge the knowledge-to-practice gap. Providing an alternative makes it possible to have choices among ways to develop and implement knowledge in practice or to complement approaches. MRT supported by studies using the same conceptual framework is explored as a way of cumulating knowledge to be used as evidence for practice. As noted, both a theory basis and research are important for practice, thus this approach can be expected to make an important contribution. This approach can be duplicated by other reservoirs of studies based on conceptual frameworks or grand theories. A major advantage is uniting the strengths of theory and of research as a basis for practice. At the same time the selected research has been strengthened by accumulating studies based on similar concepts, the concepts of the grand theory. However, what is needed further to reach practice is to capitalize on the benefits of MRTs that are closer to practice.

Rationale and Background on MRT Development

MRT has been credited with providing a significant milestone, marking considerable progress in knowledge development beginning in 1991 to 1995 (Meleis, 2007). The significance of MRT lies in its very characteristics. MRTs are closer to practice because they use fewer concepts at a level of abstraction lower than the grand theories. In this way they can be used in given practice settings yet some can generalize across populations and settings. Some examples of MRT theories that are useful across practice settings are Meleis's theory of experiencing transitions (Meleis, Sawyer, Im, Messias, & Schumacher, 2000) and the theory on uncertainty in illness by Mishel (1990). An example of a more situation-specific MRT is provided by the work of Good (1998), who derived a theory of pain as a balance between analgesia and side effects.

MRT is particularly useful in today's focus on interdisciplinary teams to meet health care needs for two reasons: (1) MRT articulates the focus of nursing to contribute to interdisciplinary dialogue and (2) such theories also help identify knowledge needed from many disciplines. Consider that because MRT helps to answer questions about the overall mission, goals and nature of the discipline of nursing it differentiates nursing's contributions from that of other disciplines. For example, an obstetrician sees the delivery of a baby as a medical event, whereas nursing sees the event as a life transition for a mother and family. Meleis noted that MRT can have a transformational effect on the entire discipline of nursing. Development of theories at the middle range can be considered a clear indication that nursing as a discipline has undergone a turning point toward producing more accessible and functional theories that guide productive research programs and provide theory and research-based evidence for practice.

The connection of MRT to research is important to knowledge development and providing evidence for practice. MRT provides key concepts and the relationships among concepts that are theoretically sound. In addition, the concepts translate to measurable variables. The relationships among the variables can be tested in research. Thus some authors noted that MRT can be used to derive research that provides evidence for practice. The findings of research that test MRT provide evidence for the relational statements of the theory. The statements with the supporting evidence can be used to derive nursing approaches to practice, as in the example of the MRT of the peaceful end of life described on page 20-21. The use of MRT as a basis for research leads to confirming knowledge for practice. The simplicity of the theories promotes their translation to practice. The circular relationship of theory to research to practice that applies to all theory is particularly evident in MRT. An example of this cycle is the work by Kolcaba (1994). With clinical changes such as hospice and long-term care, the significance of comfort came to the fore of nursing concepts. Kolcaba first clarified the concept and developed relational statements or propositions. The theory was tested in a number of research projects. From these, specific recommendations for practice were promoted, such as guided imagery to promote comfort for women with early breast cancer who were receiving radiation therapy.

The theory, research, practice cycle also implies the several ways that MRTs are developed. MRT can be derived from theory, research, or practice. Deriving MRT from theory takes two possible forms. MRTs are derived from grand theories or they can combine existing nursing and non-nursing theories. Box 1.4 lists some examples of MRT derived from grand theories,

---

BOX 1.4
MIDDLE RANGE THEORIES DERIVED FROM GRAND THEORIES

- Theory of coping and adaptation processing—Roy Adaptation Model
- Theory of shared identify of groups
- Theory of moral distress
- Urine-control theory

- Theory of home care effectiveness
- Theory of perception of dissonant pattern—Rogers's Person–Environment Theory
- Theory of restorative subsystem—Johnson's Behavioral Systems Model
- Theory of therapeutic intention—Levine's Energy Conservation Framework

also called models and frameworks (McEwen & Wills, 2011; Roy, 2011). Each of these MRTs focuses on specific concepts of the grand theory and further develops the ideas to create an understanding of the relationships of concepts within a more narrow range. For example, one author took only the restorative subsystem (Grubbs, 1980) of Johnson's eight behavioral subsystems. Another theorized with Rogers's work only on the patterns that are dissonant and how they are perceived. These few examples illustrate one approach to MRT, that is, taking established concepts from a grand theory and using these as the basis for creating a theory that is closer to practice and that can be tested in research. The option of combining nursing and non-nursing is exemplified by Pender's work (1996). In developing a MRT of health promotion, the theorist used behavioral science theories, such as expectancy value theory and social cognitive theory, along with a nursing perspective. Broad theories, whether grand nursing theories or theories about people from related disciplines, are rich sources for creating MRT. When these theories are distilled to key related concepts they can be more readily applied to practice.

There are a number of ways that research is used to create MRT but perhaps the most widely known and used is the grounded theory approach, a well-developed qualitative research method. Developed over time by Strauss and colleagues at the University of California at San Francisco, grounded theory is an inductive process that works from specific empirical observations to generalizations about the data. The researcher is immersed in the clinical data of the project and generates new theoretical insights. The philosophical basis for grounded theory is symbolic interactionism, which explores how people define reality and how their beliefs are related to their actions. Reality is created by attaching meaning to situations. Meanings are shared in interactions. Interactions are the focus of observations in grounded theory. In the analysis process, the categories and properties emerge, develop in abstraction, and become related. The accumulating interrelations form the central grounded theory, which, because of the richness in interpreting meanings, identifies new concepts, patterns, processes, and explanations. An example of using grounded theory to create MRT is the work by Hamilton and Bowers (2007) to develop the theory of genetic vulnerability.

One way that MRT is derived from practice is to use practice guidelines or standards of care. McEwen and Wills (2011) noted that this approach is not used often, but they did find a few examples. In the exemplar they provide, the authors discuss how Rutland and Moore (1998) developed the theory of the peaceful end of life from standards of care of terminally ill patients. In the first step of the process of developing the theory the authors defined the theory's assumptions based on the standards of care.

In the second step they performed what they called a statement synthesis in which five outcome criteria were developed. The outcome criteria were those factors that contributed to a peaceful end of life. These five outcomes were: not being in pain, experience of comfort, experience of dignity and respect, being at peace, and closeness to significant others and persons who care. In step 3 conceptual definitions were written for each outcome criteria. Step 4 included defining relational statements between the outcome indicators and nursing interventions, that is, prescriptors were added to facilitate the outcomes expected. Theory synthesis in step 5 combined the relational statements into an integrated theory that was represented in a schematic diagram of the relationships in the theory.

Process for Using RAM Research to Generate MRT and Evidence

The team considered their understanding of the importance and place of knowledge development as described previously and concerns to make greater strides in today's health care to have nursing knowledge influence practice. A remarkable opportunity was presented as the Roy Adaptation Association Executive Board started a scheduled update of the review of research based on the Roy model. Given the significant cycle of theory, research, and practice it seemed a timely task to extend the review to include generating MRT, providing evidence for practice from the studies. Based on this work it would then be possible to provide recommendations that would contribute toward having nursing knowledge take the lead in advancing a health agenda as called for by nurse leaders.

Based on this conviction, the team began to outline an alternative process for developing knowledge for practice. The outline for this project included six steps. The large database of studies based on the Roy adaptation model was collected and analyzed. Initial screening identified three basic facts about each document retrieved. The work had to be (1) published research, including dissertations and theses; (2) retrievable in English; and (3) used the Roy adaptation model. The accepted works were submitted for analysis. A description of each study was created in a common format. Each study was evaluated by criteria for quality of quantitative or qualitative research, respectively. This process is described in greater detail in Chapter 2.

Given the pool of studies analyzed by a larger team, four authors took on the task of organizing major topics for MRT development. This involved using the purposes/aims of the studies to group those that addressed similar topics. Four foci for adapting were identified and a broad category of general coping was added. The MRTs to be created are general coping, adapting to life events, adapting to loss, adapting in chronic conditions, and adapting families. The creating of the broad categories was influenced admittedly by the interests and background of the theorist, Roy, as the project director. Similarly, the steps of the process outlined depended on the unique experience and understandings of the theorist, including literature reviewed. The process also included dialogue with the other scholars whose assignments were in their particular areas of expertise and those who worked on the analysis who had insights into the areas of strength within the large body of research.

With the topics selected, the team worked on proposing the process for using the Roy adaptation model's research for developing MRT and providing evidence for practice. The six steps outlined in Box 1.5 were derived as the process for generating MRTs from the research. These steps were aligned with previous related work and seemed to meet the needs of the project. First each assigned author selected studies that were clustered together by similarities of content. There was obvious overlap but decisions were made to keep the integrity of each particular MRT in progress. The authors describe the basis for the decisions of study selections as step 1 within each chapter of Part III. In step 2 major concepts were identified using the studies as observations. Several approaches were tried, but the one that worked for all chapters was to use a generic systems model as Roy describes. The stimuli affect the coping strategies that lead to adaptive outcomes.

Sometimes step 3 could be combined with step 2 because as concepts were identified the level of generality became an issue. The authors worked to get them at the MRT level. The concepts had to be discrete and observable, but at a level of abstraction for this project that could be generalized

---

BOX 1.5
HOW MIDDLE RANGE THEORIES ARE GENERATED FROM RELATED RESEARCH STUDIES

1. Studies are selected that cluster together by similarities.
2. The studies are used as observations, are classified, and major concepts identified.
3. The concepts are discrete and observable, but at a level of abstraction that can be generalized across clinical situations.
4. The concepts are used to draw a pictorial schema of the interrelated concepts.
5. The identified concepts are interrelated in theoretical statements or propositions.
6. The findings from the research are used to provide evidence to support the new MRT.

across clinical situations. For step 4 the concepts were used to draw a pictorial schema of the interrelated concepts, and in step 5 the interrelated concepts were spelled out in theoretical statements or propositions. Again, the sequence of the author's approaches may vary, but the steps were all completed and are labeled consistently, using the same numbers for the sake of the reader following the process. Similarly, each chapter completed step 6 by identifying the findings from the research that provided evidence to support the new MRT, although the evidence may have been integrated into a previous section.

The purpose of creating the MRTs is to impact practice. The six-step process provided the syntheses of evidence for Chapter 13 to show how the work can be used as EBP. The definition of EBP that Roy (2009) introduced provides for looking at three possible levels of readiness to implement in practice. Category 1 proposes that certain evidence is ready for practice. The criteria are that a proposition is supported by more than one study; the support noted is unequivocal support and there is a low risk, but a high clinical need. Category 2 requires that advanced practice specialists examine the evidence to see whether it is ready for practice. This category is used when a proposition is supported, but the generalizability is not clear or the risk is not clear, but there is a high clinical need. The final category means that the work is not ready to be used as evidence for practice. This is used when the evidence shows mixed support for propositions, generalizability is unclear, and/or there is high risk. In the review of 163 studies based on the RAM from 1970 to 1994 published by the same group (Boston-Based Adaptation Research in Nursing Society [BBARNS], 1999) using these criteria, 52% studies had high potential for implementation in practice. Other studies were recommended for further clinical evaluation or for additional testing. In this book the determination was not made based on individual studies, but rather based on the evidence for the MRT as further explained and illustrated in Chapter 13. In addition, each chapter proposes ways that the knowledge created can impact changes in practice and/or policy.

CONCLUSION

This chapter introduces the important topic of nursing knowledge for practice. The historical background provided a basis for examining current issues in the gap between nursing knowledge and implementation in practice. After exploring major movements to close this gap, some remaining questions led to proposing a unique approach to relating theory to practice by way of research. A fresh approach to processes for knowledge development links theory, research, and practice in new ways as an attempt to impact changes in practice.

REFERENCES

American Association of Colleges of Nursing. (2001). *Indicators of quality in research-focused doctoral programs in nursing.* Washington, DC: Author.

American Association of Colleges of Nursing. (2004). *AACN position statement on the practice doctorate in nursing.* Washington, DC: Author.

American Association of Colleges of Nursing (AACN). (2012a). *Nursing fact sheet.* Washington, DC: Author.

American Association of Colleges of Nursing (AACN). (2012b). *DNP fact sheet.* Washington, DC: Author.

American Nurses Association. (1965). Education for nursing. *American Journal of Nursing, 65*(12), 106–111.

American Nurses Association. (1966). *Facts about nursing.* New York, NY: Author.

Bankhead, R., Boullata, J., Brantley, S., Corkins, M., Guenter, P., Krenitsky, J., ... A.S.P.E.N. Board of Directors. (2009). A.S.P.E.N. enteral nutrition practice recommendations. *Journal of Parental and Enteral Nutrition, 33*(2), 122–167.

Bauman, S. (2010). The limitations of evidence-based practice. *Nursing Science Quarterly, 23*(3), 226–230.

Boston-Based Adaptation Research in Nursing Society. (1999). *Roy adaptation model-based research: 25 years of contributions to nursing science.* Indianapolis, IN: Sigma Theta Tau International Center Nursing Press.

Brown, E. L. (1948). *Nursing for the future.* New York, NY: Russell Sage Foundation.

Burns, N., & Grove, S. (2009). *The practice of nursing research: Appraisal, synthesis and generation of evidence* (6th ed.). St. Louis, MO: Saunders Elsevier.

Cantelon, P. (2010). *NINR: Bringing science to life.* Bethesda, MD: National Institute of Nursing Research.

Donaldson, S., & Crowley, D. (1978). The discipline of nursing. *Nursing Outlook, 26,* 113–120.

Good, M. (1998). A middle range theory of acute pain management use in research. *Nursing Outlook, 46*(3), 120–124.

Grady, P. (2010a). *Preface to NINR: Bringing science to life.* Bethesda, MD: National Institute of Nursing Research.

Grady, P. (2010b). Translational research and nurse scientists. *Nursing Outlook, 58*(1), 164-166.

Grubbs, J. (1980). An interpretation of the Johnson behavioral system model for nursing practice. In J. P. Riehl & C. Roy (Eds.), *Conceptual models for nursing practice* (2nd ed., pp. 217–254). New York, NY: Appleton-Century-Crofts.

Hamilton, R., & Bowers, B. (2007). The theory of genetic vulnerability: A Roy model exemplar. *Nursing Science Quarterly, 20*(3), 254–255.

Henderson, V. (1991). *The nature of nursing: Reflections after 25 years.* New York, NY: National League for Nursing Press.

Hinshaw, A. S., & Hienrich, J. (2011). Changing health science policy: The establishment of the National Institute of Nursing Research at the National Institutes of Health. In A. Hinshaw & P. Grady (Eds.), *Shaping health policy through nursing research.* New York, NY: Springer Publishing Company.

Im, E., & Chang, S. (2012). Current trends in nursing theories. *Journal of Nursing Scholarship, 44*(2), 156–164.

Institute of Medicine. (2001). *Crossing the quality chasm: A new health system for the 21st century.* Washington, DC: National Academy of Sciences.

Johnson, D. (1974). Development of theory: A requisite for nursing as a primary health profession. *Nursing Research, 23*(5), 372–377.

Johnson, D. E. (1959). The nature of a science of nursing. *Nursing Outlook, 7*, 291–294.

Kolcaba, K. (1994). A theory of holistic comfort for nursing. *Journal of Advanced Nursing, 19*, 1178–1184.

McEwen, M., & Wills, E. M. (2011). *Theoretical basis for nursing* (3rd ed.). Philadelphia, PA: Lippincott Williams & Wilkins.

Meleis, A. I. (2007). *Theoretical nursing: Development and progress* (4th ed.). New York, NY: Lippincott, Williams, & Wilkins.

Meleis, A. I., Sawyer, L. M., Im, E., Messias, D., & Schumacher, K. (2000). Experiencing transitions: An emerging middle range theory. *Advances in Nursing Science, 23*(1), 12–28.

Melnyk, B., Fineout-Overholt, E., Stillwell, S., & Williamson, K. (2010). Evidence-based practice: Step by step: The seven steps of evidence-based practice. *American Journal of Nursing, 110*(1), 51–53.

Metheny, N. (2011). Turning tube feeding off while repositioning patients in bed. *Critical Care Nursing, 4*(2), 96–97.

Mishel, M. H. (1990). Reconceptualization of the uncertainty in illness theory. *Image: Journal of Nursing Scholarship, 22*(4), 256–262.

Nelson, M. (2002). Education for professional nursing practice: Looking backward into the future. *Online Journal of Issues in Nursing, 7*(3).

Pearson, A., Vaughan, B., & Fitzgerald, M. (2005). *Nursing models for practice* (3rd ed.). London: Butterworth Heinemann.

Pender, N. J. (1996). *Health promotion in nursing practice* (3rd ed.). Stamford, CT: Appleton & Lange.

Peplau, H. (1952). *Interpersonal relations in nursing.* New York, NY: Putnam's Sons.

Polit, D., & Beck, C. T. (2012). *Nursing research: Generating and assessing evidence for practice* (9th ed.). Philadelphia, PA: Lippincott Williams & Wilkins.

Reed, P. G., & Shearer, N. C. (2013). *Perspectives on nursing theory* (6th ed.). Philadelphia, PA: Wolters Kluwer/Lippincott Williams & Wilkins.

Riehl, J. P., & Roy, C. (1980). *Conceptual models for nursing practice* (2nd ed.). New York: Appleton-Century-Crofts.

Roy, C. (2009). *The Roy adaptation model* (3rd ed.). Upper Saddle River, NJ: Prentice Hall Health.

Roy, C. (2011). Research based on the Roy adaptation model: Last 25 years. *Nursing Science Quarterly, 24*(4), 312–320.

Roy, C., & Jones, D. (2007). *Nursing knowledge development and clinical practice.* New York, NY: Springer Publishing Company.

Rutland, C., & Moore, S. (1998). Theory construction based on standards of care: A proposed theory of the peaceful end of life. *Nursing Outlook, 46*(4), 169–175.

Smith, T. (2009). A policy perspective on the entry into practice issue. *OJIN: The Online Journal of Issues in Nursing, 15*(1).

Walker, L. O., & Avant, K. C. (2011). *Strategies for theory construction in nursing* (5th ed.). Norwalk, CT: Appleton & Lange.

Willis, D., Grace, P., & Roy, C. (2008). A central unifying focus for the discipline: Facilitating humanization, meaning, choice, quality of life and dying. *Advances in Nursing Science, 31*(1). Retrieved from www.advancesinnursingscience.com

Wolfe, S. H. (2008). The meaning of translational research and why it matters. *Journal of the American Medical Association, 299*(2), 211–213.

Yura, H., & Torres, G. (1975). *Todays's conceptual frameworks with the baccalaureate nursing programs* (National League for Nursing Publication No. 15-1558, 17–75). New York, NY: National League for Nursing.

2

Processes for Description and Critical Analysis of Research

SISTER CALLISTA ROY

Research data is significant to the major focus of this book, generating middle range theory and providing evidence for practice. To prepare the data for use in knowledge development the project team developed a number of processes. In this chapter we describe these processes and share with the reader how a large group of studies were analyzed, evaluated, and organized for presentation. The purpose of the chapter is to describe each process of preparing the research data for use in knowledge generation and to show how these processes build toward the goal of creating cumulative knowledge for nursing practice. The specific aims are to (a) describe the search for relevant literature; (b) demonstrate strategies for screening and describing studies; (c) illustrate the processes for evaluating studies, including establishing interrater reliability; (d) show the results of the selection and evaluation processes; and (e) explain how studies were organized into major categories and then subcategories to present in Part II.

SEARCH FOR RELEVANT RESEARCH

Literature reviews are the mainstay of an initial strategy for knowledge development. Finding out what is already known on a topic is crucial to moving the knowledge forward. Such reviews will vary by the specific purpose of the review. The purpose of this review was stated clearly as locating research published in English that used the Roy adaptation model (RAM) as the framework for the study. The theorist was assigned undergraduate research fellows at Boston College who conducted the initial reviews with the guidance of a knowledgeable nursing-reference librarian. Major online data bases included: CINAHL, MEDLINE, PubMed, ProQuest, ERIC, and PsycINFO. Key search words were: RAM and research. Of the 350 citations recovered for years 1995–2010, initial hand searches of the abstracts of each publication by the research fellows directed by the theorist led to deleting 150 studies as either not a primary research study, as not based on the RAM, or a duplicate. The research fellows then located electronic copies of full texts of the publications, including dissertations, and posted each on a real-time collaborative editing web site. Approximately 200 studies were available for further screening and review. The project team decided early in the work to include dissertation and thesis research that was available because they wanted to be inclusive. Further, given the educational purpose of dissertations and theses, the quality would be supervised and the use of conceptual frameworks was likely to be explicit.

STRATEGIES FOR SCREENING AND DESCRIBING STUDIES

The executive board of the Roy Adaptation Association met twice face to face in the planning phases of the project and once in the writing phase. These meetings were supplemented by conference calls, e-mail communication, and a real-time collaborative editing web site for common use. At the first meeting the members reviewed forms for description and evaluation of research used in an earlier related work (Boston-Based Adaptation Research in Nursing Society [BBARNS], 1999). Significant updating was done to the process and the forms used.

The screening process involved two steps by project team members reviewing the full-text versions of the research. The use of the RAM was important to the premise that multiple investigators were using common concepts and the work could be cumulative. The first step in screening was to verify that the RAM was used as a framework for the research. This meant that the author(s) of the research report made explicit links to the model generally in three ways, that is, in establishing the purpose of the study; in the design, including variables; and in discussing the findings. One link could be implicit, but none could be absent.

Second, this full-text review provided the opportunity to confirm that the report was about research. Fine distinctions were made between research and project evaluation. In general the purpose stated by the author provided the key to this distinction. That is, wording that related to knowledge development, understanding adaptation of people, their coping with changing situations or interventions to promote adaptation was confirmed as research. When the screening was completed the assigned team member proceeded to describe the study.

The forms used to describe and evaluate the studies were made to serve the purposes of the current project. The description process is described here and the evaluation process will follow. The description forms were designed to provide the authors with key information about each study as well as having the full text available on the shared worksite. The key information was provided in standard format. The form used for description was a table that included rows for each study with columns listing: Author(s) and date, purpose, sample, design, measurement and instruments, and findings. Of significance for use of this form was a glossary to describe the research design using standard terms. Box 2.1 includes the definition of terms used to describe the designs. Early examination of the studies indicated the expanding breadth and depth of methods used in model-based research and the team deemed it significant that all reviewers used common terms.

BOX 2.1
GLOSSARY OF TERMS USED TO DESCRIBE RESEARCH DESIGN

Quantitative

Descriptive
- Correlational interrelationships among variables
- Comparative cohort study

Explain–Predict–Prescribe
- Linear multivariate model testing
- Regression analysis
- Path analysis
- Structural equation modeling

Intervention
- Single group pretest and posttest
- Nonequivalent control group and intervention group, may be posttest only
- Repeated measures—between subjects and within subjects
- Experimental, randomly assigned control and experimental groups
- Action research

(continued)

BOX 2.1
GLOSSARY OF TERMS USED TO DESCRIBE RESEARCH DESIGN
(CONTINUED)

Qualitative

Content Analysis
- Conventional—categories flow from data
- Directed—use categories of framework to validate or extend
- Summative—latent interpretation of terms

Grounded theory—Glaser and Strauss
Ethnography—analyze emic (insider view) and etic (outsider—researcher view)

Phenomenology
- Descriptive, Hesserl
- Interpretive, Heidegger, for example, hermeneutics
- Existential—Merleau Ponty and others

Mixed Methods
Uses a combination of methods usually identified with qualitative and quantitative research within the same study.

Reviewers gave special attention to *propositional statements* as the "working backbone of science" (Walker & Avant, 2011. p. 59). Walker and Avant also noted that in the science of nursing practice many diagnoses, interventions, and outcomes are based on such scientific statements. *Proposition* is the term used to describe a statement of the relationship between variables or descriptors of variables asserted by theories and tested or discovered in research. Where possible the reviewers stated purposes or findings in propositional form. Later the authors of Part III would synthesize propositions as part of generating middle range theories.

PROCESS FOR EVALUATING STUDIES

The revised form for evaluating studies was aimed at the needs of this project so that each study would meet current standards of good research to generate further knowledge and evidence for practice. Assignment of reviewers to studies was done according to preference of qualitative or quantitative studies, using alphabetical order of the studies for specific assignments. The entire team participated in the screening and analyses that included descriptive and evaluation tables. Adjustments in assignments were made based on time commitments each team member could make. In the process of evaluating the studies, the team members conducted a process for establishing interrater reliability.

Form for Critique

The second set of forms included the criteria for analysis of the quality of the research, one for studies with quantitative designs and one for qualitative designs. The initial column named and described the criteria, two columns provided space to list strengths and weaknesses related to the criteria, and in the final column the reviewer provided an overall score for that criterion (scored from a high of 5 points to a low of 1 for how well the work met the criterion). Each study had the possibility of scores ranging from 20 to 4. In drafting the form the team members consulted a variety of current research textbooks and synthesized the criteria to use for evaluating the studies in this project.

The first criterion was called: *Design—Efforts to Control.* The two descriptive statements added were: (a) Threats to external validity: attempts to control the environment, representativeness of subjects, consistency of treatment, control of measurement, and control of extraneous variables; and (b) threats to internal validity, including: history, maturation, instrumentation, mortality, and sample. *Measurement* was the second criterion and included the descriptive statements: (a) Reliability of instruments addressed and (b) validity of instruments addressed. Next for the *Data Analysis* section the reviewer identified the extent to which the analysis was appropriate and accurate. Finally the criterion: *Interpretation of Results* listed for the reviewer the descriptor of consistency of findings with conclusions.

The team appropriately modified the criteria for qualitative studies and the rest of the form included the same spaces to list strengths and weaknesses related to the criteria, with a column for a summary score. The first criterion was *Method and Design*, which had descriptions in two categories, first, trustworthiness with the following descriptors: Credibility (prolonged engagement, member checking, search for disconfirming evidence); transferability (sufficient data to determine contextual similarity); dependability (consistency of data—peer debriefing and peer review); confirmability (neutrality of data). *Audit trail* was the second criterion and included the following descriptors for reviewers: raw data, data-reduction product, process notes, researcher intentions and dispositions, reflexive notes, instruments, and data reconstruction.

The last two criteria were the same as on the form for evaluation of quantitative studies, that is, *data analysis* and *interpretation of findings*, with their descriptors.

Interrater Reliability

The team handling the critical review of the studies was experienced working with each other and every effort was made to make the forms clear and straightforward to use. Consistency of use of the ratings was important to be able to rely on the results in generating new knowledge, meeting the goal of the project, and the focus of this book. The team conducted an interrater reliability check on a selection of studies. Studies were selected to represent the variety of methods used, that is, one qualitative study, one quantitative study, one mixed methods, and one intervention study. Three members of the team independently filled out the form evaluating the quality of the research. A conference call was held with the entire project team to discuss the ratings and to make final decisions on issues of the analysis and critique. Scores for all three raters were over 90% in agreement. The one area of difference was settled by discussion. In one of the studies used for this analysis the researcher had indicated in the article that the C-T-E structure for research had been used to link the model to the study. One member of the group was familiar with this approach taught by Fawcett (2010); it refers to relating theory and research by using Conceptual, Theoretical, and Empirical links. This is an appropriate way to cover the topic of links to the model and as it was explained, other members revised their judgments to have 100% agreement on scoring the forms proposed for the evaluation phase of the work. The team adopted the use of the evaluation forms and they were posted along with the form for describing the studies on the common real-time collaborative editing web site.

The team also agreed on the number of points required to judge a study strong enough on the criteria to be included in the next phase of the project, generating middle range theory and evidence for practice. For the *Evaluation*, the scores had to be mainly 4s and 5s, with no more than one score of 3. This meant that a study had to score between 16 and 20, that is, meet 80% to 100% of the expectations for good research. The team judgment of scores below which studies would be deleted for further knowledge development was posted on the shared work site.

RESULTS OF SELECTION AND EVALUATION

When the review team used the full text of studies to complete the critical analysis of description and evaluation, 28 additional studies were deleted as follows: 16 not research, 6 not authentic use of the RAM, and 7 were duplicates. At this stage of the project 172 studies remained and had description and evaluation forms filled out by the team for use in the writing phase of the project. Of these studies, 103 were referred journal publications and 69 were dissertations. Figure 2.1 shows the number of studies over time at 4 year intervals.

Among the studies retrieved were dissertations completed at 32 different universities in the United States and 1 in Finland. The schools with more than five dissertations each were: Widener University School of Nursing, PA–9, Wayne State University and University of Alabama at Birmingham–7 each, Medical College of Ohio–6, and Saint Louis University–5. The articles were published in 47 English-language journals. The six journals with the highest number of publications were: *Nursing Science Quarterly*–18, *Journal of Advanced Nursing*–6, *Oncology Nursing Forum*–6, *Nursing Research*–4, and *Issues in Comprehensive Pediatric Nursing and Pediatric Nursing* with 3 publications each. In addition the following journals have 2 publications each: *Advances in Nursing Science, AORN Journal, Issues in Mental Health Nursing, Journal of Clinical Nursing, Journal of Nursing Scholarship, The Journal of School Nursing,* and *Research in Nursing and Health.* Among the other research articles that used the RAM, 15 were in journals for specific clinical specialties such as *Cancer Nursing* and *Dimensions of Critical Care Nursing,* four were in other research journals such as *Clinical Nursing Research* and *Western Journal of Nursing Research,* and three were in practice journals such as *Clinical Excellence for Nurse Practitioners.* Finally, six other countries or regions published these research studies in English, that is, Korea, India, Scandinavia, Brazil, and Thailand, as well as the United Kingdom.

As noted on the evaluation forms each study was scored from 20 to 4 points on listed criteria for good-quality research. For a given study

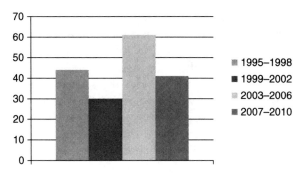

FIGURE 2.1   Number of Research Publications by 4-Year Intervals

to be considered adequate for use in further knowledge development or application to practice in this project, the research was scored between 20 and 16 points. When the evaluation forms for the 40 studies using various qualitative designs were reviewed the range of scores was from 20 to 16. A total of 17 qualitative studies received the highest score of 20; whereas 4 received the lowest score of 16. The lowest scores and all those in between were within the acceptable range. No studies of these 40 were eliminated from further consideration. More detail on the outcome of the numeric scoring is reported in Chapter 3 along with a summary of the strengths and weaknesses of the studies.

For the 126 studies using three types of quantitative designs the range was from 20 to 14 points. For the studies based on quantitative designs 27 were scored at the highest level of 20 points. The two lowest scores were 14 points and 15 points on two studies, which was the basis for removing these studies from further consideration in generating knowledge. Five studies with quantitative designs scored at the lowest level of being acceptable, each being evaluated at 16 points. All others were acceptable, being scored between 19 and 17. These studies are described and evaluated in Chapters 4, 5, and 6.

ORGANIZATION OF STUDIES

The aim of the project is to generate middle range theory-based knowledge for practice. The first step of synthesis of the studies for use in knowledge building was to find a way to organize the studies to present them and to make then useful in the knowledge-building phase. In particular the project required being able to provide evidence for the middle range theories created. Early in the project in June 2011, Sister Callista Roy, the principle investigator, reported to the team that 90% of the studies were not focused on one adaptive mode and the adaptive modes would not provide an organizing principle. The organization that emerged was to first divide the studies by research design, 40 of which were qualitative studies and 126 of which were quantitative. As noted in Table 2.1 there were subcategories of specific methods under each major method category. The 40 qualitative studies are described in Chapter 3 under the six subcategories for clarity in understanding the body of work and to provide the knowledge builders with levels of evidence to use. The subcategories included the qualitative designs of content analysis, grounded theory, ethnography, phenomenology, mixed methods, and analyses of cases.

Similarly the quantitative studies were divided into subcategories depending on the method used in the design of the study. As noted early

TABLE 2.1
Studies Organized By Method

Qualitative Studies ($n = 40$)
Content Analysis ($n = 7$)
Grounded Theory ($n = 4$)
Ethnography ($n = 3$)
Phenomenology ($n = 17$)
Mixed Methods ($n = 6$)
Case Study ($n = 3$)
Quantitative Studies ($n = 126$)
Descriptive ($n = 59$)
Explaining, Predicting and Prescribing ($n = 43$)
Interventions ($n = 25$)
Instrument Development ($n = 5$)

in the work, it was evident that investigators had gone beyond descriptive studies of associations and were using more multivariate analysis, which allows for explaining, predicting, and describing. In Table 2.1 there are 59 studies that fit the definition of descriptive designs and 43 that were considered designs that explain, predict, and describe. Further, this 15-year span yielded 25 studies based on the RAM classified as intervention designs. Each of these subcategories is covered separately in Chapters 4, 5, and 6.

The number of studies to be covered in each chapter on quantitative research warranted finding a way to organize the studies within the chapters. Given the importance of propositions in theory building and their potential for showing studies related in meaningful ways, the team chose to use clusters of RAM propositions for organization. The theorist had decided that the commonly used generic proposition list (BBARNS, 1999; Roy & Roberts, 1981) could be edited to put the related propositions together and could then be checked for completeness. The theorist completed the revision and sent it to the team. Table 2.2 shows the resulting update with clusters based on major concepts of the RAM: internal coping processes for the individual expanded to include the types of cognator processing; adaptive modes; stimuli; group adaptation; and nursing process that clarified two approaches to intervention according to the model, that is, managing stimuli and strengthening coping. This editing of the propositions was helpful for presenting studies within the clusters in each of the chapters on qualitative studies. This organization also grouped content areas in preparation for the knowledge-development process.

TABLE 2.2

Propositions From the Roy Adaptation Model—Clustered by Major Model Concepts

Cluster One: Internal coping processes—Individual
1. The adequacy of cognator and regulator processes affect adaptive responses
2. Specific cognator processes that affect adaptive responses are:
   a. perception
   b. information processing
   c. learning
   d. judgment
   e. emotion
3. Adaptation takes place over time as the regulator and cognator continue to process stimuli

Cluster Two: Observable behaviors in one or more adaptive modes
4. Adaptation in one mode is affected by adaptation in other modes
5. The adaptive modes change over time, both during development and throughout life
6. Behavior in adaptive modes is classified as effective and ineffective to determine adaptation levels of integrated, compensatory, and compromised

Cluster Three: Internal and external stimuli to the adaptive system
7. Internal and external stimuli influence cognator and regulator processes
8. Internal and external stimuli influence adaptive mode responses
9. The pooled effect of focal, contextual, and residual stimuli determines the adaptation level
10. Adaptation reflects the integration of the person with the environment

Cluster Four: Group Adaptation
11. At the group level, stabilizer and innovator processes affect adaptation
12. Adaptation of groups takes place over time as the stabilizer and innovator continue to process stimuli

Cluster Five: Nursing Process
13. Nursing assessment and interventions relate to identifying and managing input to adaptive systems
14. Supporting and enhancing coping processes are interventions to promote adaptation

CONCLUSION

With the analysis phase completed and the additional issue of organization addressed, the authors present the studies in Part II. The approach to middle range theory development was also developed and is described in the introduction to Part III "Middle Range Theories Derived From Research." The five selected middle range theories are the focus of that part.

REFERENCES

Boston-Based Adaptation Research in Nursing Society. (1999). *Roy adaptation model-based research: 25 years of contributions to nursing science.* Indianapolis, IN: Sigma Theta Tau International, Center Nursing Press.

Fawcett, J. (2010). Theory testing and theory evaluation. In J. Butts & K. Rich (Eds.), *Philosophies and theories for advanced nursing practice* (pp. 605–623). Sudbury, MA: Jones & Bartlett Learning.

Roy, C., & Roberts, S. (1981). *Theory construction in nursing: An adaptation model.* Englewood Cliffs, NJ: Prentice Hall.

Walker, L., & Avant, K. (2011). *Strategies for theory construction in nursing* (5th ed.). Upper Saddle River, NJ: Prentice Hall.

II

Data for Knowledge
Development

*I*n Part II the focus is on the preparation of the data to be used in knowledge development for both generating middle range theories and providing evidence for practice. As noted, the synthesis of the studies in knowledge building needed a way to organize the studies to present them and to make them useful in the knowledge-building phase. It is the task of this section to lay out for the project team and for the reader all of the studies in a way that makes them accessible for knowledge generation and for practice. The 172 studies based on the Roy adaptation model provided a rich reservoir of research based on related concepts. The studies provide the observations to be used in further cumulative knowledge. The remaining parts of this book draw on the advantage of having a body of research that uses similar concepts but multiple methods. Further, the studies have been meaningfully described and accurately evaluated.

The purpose of Part II is to use the processes described in Chapter 2 as devised by the research team for presenting and evaluating the studies as well as to provide examples of relating research to practice. The major applications of the cumulative research used to generate middle range theory and evidence-based practice will come in Parts III and IV. The work of those sections depends on the organization, description, and critique of the studies provided here.

The authors, Kathy Lauchner and Martha Whetsell, have organized Part II into four chapters based on the design of the studies. Each type of design contributes differently to knowledge for practice, as the authors describe at the beginning of each chapter. First studies were divided into qualitative and quantitative designs, and then the subcategories of each major design provided another level of organization. The 40 qualitative studies included those that used content analysis, grounded theory, ethnography, phenomenology, mixed methods, and case analysis. It might be noted that nearly half of the qualitative studies used one of the several types of phenomenology, providing the opportunity for findings based on meaning of the phenomenon. Organized in these five subcategories, the qualitative studies are described and evaluated in Chapter 3.

According to the processes designed by the project team, the 126 quantitative studies were divided into those that aim to be descriptive; to explain, predict, or describe; and to conduct interventions. The highest number of studies ($n = 59$) were descriptive and correlational (Chapter 4), which offers some insights into how key concepts and variables are related. The findings from these studies can be the basis for further research as well as offering some insights useful for practice. It is encouraging to see that 43 studies used multivariate statistical approaches to explain, predict, and prescribe (Chapter 5). These approaches provide greater insight into the phenomenon of study and can discern what level of effect an important variable will have on another within a set of interrelated variables. Finally, there were 25 intervention studies (Chapter 6) in the 15 years covered in this review. In the first research review project (Boston-Based Adaptation Research in Nursing Society [BBARNS], 1999), there were 27 intervention studies in the 25 years from 1970 to 1995. The quality of the studies seemed to improve over time as indicated by the fact that in the earlier review 6 of the 27 studies were omitted from further application because they did not meet the minimum criteria for empiric adequacy. In this review using essentially the same criteria but described more clearly and fully all 25 studies met the required level of adequacy and were available for further knowledge development and applications to practice.

The organization internal to each chapter in Part II followed the process designed by the project team. This was described earlier and is based on an understanding of grouping the main propositions of the Roy adaptation model into clusters of related concepts. In each chapter the authors described the organization within the chapter. The references are provided in two sections. The first is titled *References* and includes any works cited in the chapter. Second, for convenience of the project team and future scholars using the works for further applications to practice, the citations for all studies in that chapter are listed under the title *Bibliography*. Key definitions are provided. However, the reader is referred to texts on theory and research if more information is needed. This section serves the project by providing the research for the middle range theories to be generated and for evidence for practice to be derived.

REFERENCE

Boston-Based Adaptation Research in Nursing Society. (1999). *Roy adaptation model-based research: 25 years of contributions to nursing science.* Indianapolis, IN: Sigma Theta Tau International, Center Nursing Press.

3

Qualitative Studies

MARTHA V. WHETSELL AND KATHRYN LAUCHNER

The first set of studies based on the Roy adaptation model (RAM) to be reported on is those using qualitative research designs. Qualitative research in a broad sense has been described as "a form of systematic empirical inquiry into meaning" (Shank, 2002, p. 5). The author explained that the term *systematic* implies a specific methodology but that the empirical observations addressing the research questions are grounded in the world of experience. Denzin and Lincoln (2000) state that qualitative research involves an interpretive and naturalistic approach; this means that qualitative researchers study persons in their natural settings, thereby obtaining a complete picture of the person's health condition. This complete picture can lead the nurse to interpret phenomena in terms of the meanings of the experience of the person cared for and this leads to how to help the individual. The types of qualitative studies and a description of each type presented in this chapter are:

- *Content analysis*—a research tool used to determine the presence of certain concepts within a text. Researchers quantify and analyze the presence, meanings, and relationships of such concepts and make inferences about the messages within the concepts. The small set of concepts is chosen because of the theoretical importance of the concepts. An increasingly accepted approach to content analysis is directed content analysis (Hsieh & Shannon, 2005). Specifically, the concepts outlined in the RAM (Roy, 2009) can be used to provide direction for the content analysis.
- *Grounded theory*—part theoretical framework and part research methodology. It is based on symbolic interaction theory and uses inductive

thinking to combine theory and research. This approach grew from an effort to develop theories from an analysis of the sample, themes, and common categories discovered in observational research. The process involves formulation, testing, and redevelopment of propositions until theory is developed. The major assumption is that theories should be "grounded" in research and backed by authentic data.

- *Ethnography* is any qualitative research in which the intent is to investigate cultures by providing a detailed, in-depth description of everyday life and practice. The approach was developed in anthropology and is widely used in psychology and nursing as well as anthropology.
- *Phenomenological research* describes a "lived experience" of a phenomenon. Different phenomenological methods are derived from varying philosophical backgrounds. The method is an inductive qualitative analysis of narrative data. Appreciation of a given philosophical background directs the researcher to analyze data quite differently from other qualitative methods of analysis.
- *Mixed methods* draws from the strengths and minimizes the weaknesses of both qualitative and quantitative methods. There is a growing trend to have a planned integration of qualitative and quantitative data within a single study or a coordinated series of studies. Mixed-methods research offers great promise for practicing nurse researchers who would like to develop techniques that are closer to what nurses actually use in practice.
- *Case study analyses* guide the intensive exploration of any number of single units of study, such as a person, family, group, community, or organization with a given experience. This method explores particular aspects of phenomena under investigation in larger or mixed-methods studies. Nursing research is known for the high quality of its case study analysis.

The RAM provides a solid structure in which data from qualitative studies can be analyzed, either as planned in directed content analysis or as the best choice outcome for understanding concepts. In analysis of qualitative studies development of and refinement of nursing concepts can lead to an understanding of phenomena that provides a basis for designing nursing interventions (Morse, 2002). The purpose of this chapter is to review and analyze qualitative studies and to discover common concepts for data to generate middle range theories. The findings of the studies supporting the middle range theories will provide evidence for practice. The organization of the 40 qualitative research studies were divided into content analysis ($n = 8$), grounded theory ($n = 4$), ethnography ($n = 3$), phenomenology ($n = 17$), mixed methods ($n = 5$), and analysis of cases ($n = 3$).

OVERVIEW OF QUALITATIVE STUDIES

Using tables, the authors describe the 40 qualitative studies that met the criteria for review. The criteria for review included that the study used the RAM as the study's theoretical framework, that the study be published in the English language, and it had to be a research study. The descriptive tables that are included describe the purpose of each study, the sample for the study, the design of the study, and the major study findings. After these descriptive tables, the authors critique the studies and provide a summary of the strengths and weaknesses of the studies. Any study with major threats to quality was not included in further analysis, nor was the study used as a practice exemplar. Studies deleted based on quality were not used in Part III on generating middle range theory.

Thirty-two of the 40 studies (80% of the total) were conducted in the United States. Studies conducted in countries outside of the United States included Brazil ($n = 1$), Canada ($n = 1$), Sweden ($n = 1$), Kenya ($n = 1$), and Taiwan ($n = 4$). All studies were conducted in institutions or in the community. Institutional settings included hospitals, nursing homes, work settings, home hospice, and assisted-living facilities. Community settings encompassed outpatient hospital services and schools, as well as other agencies other than acute and chronic care facilities. Results showed that 72% of 40 studies were conducted in community settings, whereas the rest were conducted in an institutional setting. Of those studies conducted in an institutional setting 20% of the subjects were patients and 8% were nurses.

The populations of the studies included adults, elders (age 65 and over), children ages 5 to 14, adolescents, or a combination of age groups such as adults and elders or adolescents and adults, nurses, mothers, parents, home-hospice patients, and middle-age women. Additionally, studies included those adolescents, adults, or elders who had physical illnesses, including a diagnosis considered serious or terminal, pregnancy, victimization, bereavement, and women who had a stillborn baby of 18 weeks or more gestation. From the review of the studies the authors learned that 91% were of adults, 6% of the total studies were of adolescents, and 3% were of children. Overall, most of the 40 studies were conducted on convenience samples.

Description of Studies Using Content Analysis

Eight studies used content analysis as a method to answer research questions (see Table 3.1). All seven studies examined concepts related to coping and adaptation. Gagliardi, Frederickson, and Shanley (2002) examined the

TABLE 3.1
Description of Studies Using Content Analysis

Author and Date	Purpose	Sample	Design	Findings
1. Gagliardi, Frederickson, and Shanley (2002)	To examine the experience of living with multiple sclerosis (MS), as well as to identify the strengths and resources needed to adapt to MS	Adults with MS (n = 18)	Content analysis, conventional	Themes with corresponding adaptive modes: 1. Physiological changes (physiologic mode) 2. Future orientation (self-concept mode) 3. Feelings about illness (self-concept mode) 4. Work focused on (role function mode) 5. Relationships with others (interdependence mode)
2. Gandy (2003)	To explore the person's perception of living while dying	Adults diagnosed with a terminal illness (n = 2)	Content analysis, conventional	Themes 1. Strength 2. Living for today 3. Loss of independence 4. Loneliness 5. Being homebound Emphasis was placed on personal change, growth, and empowerment

3. Shyu (2000)	To develop a conceptual framework to explain the interaction between the caregiver and the care receiver during a discharge transition	Taiwanese elders being discharged from a hospital ($n = 12$) and their family caregivers ($n = 16$)	Content analysis, directed	Role tuning was the process used by caregivers and care receivers to adjust their behavior to the responses and expectations of each other. Three phases of role tuning were identified as role engaging, role negotiating, and role settling during the transition from hospital to home
4. Li and Shyu (2007)	To use the interdependence mode of the Roy adaptation model to explain the coping and adaptation processes of Taiwanese families	Taiwanese families providing care for an elderly family member after hospital discharge for a fractured hip ($n = 8$ families, 8 care receivers, and 12 family members)	Content analysis, directed	The core category of maintaining harmony between receiving and giving care emerged. Relationships were affected by external environmental factors, including the social network and cultural beliefs. Family coping styles used were instrumental, expressive, and distancing. Different family coping styles had different adaptation outcomes

(continued)

TABLE 3.1

Description of Studies Using Content Analysis (*continued*)

Author and Date	Purpose	Sample	Design	Findings
5. Lee and Ellenbecker (1998)	To compare the life stressors of Chinese elderly to American elderly	Elderly Chinese (*n* = 30)	Content analysis, conventional	Amount and sources of stress are different for Chinese elderly than for American elderly. The higher levels of family connection show lower stress
6. Gaines (1997)	To explore the levels of adaptation of adult males who were recovering from crack addiction	African American adult males who were recovering from crack addiction (*n* = 5)	Qualitative, descriptive	All participants experienced maladaptation in all four modes during addiction and all moved toward adaptation during recovery. A focal stimulus of low self-esteem and contextual stimuli of young age, effects of substances used, and factors within the family systems were contributors to addiction. A focal stimulus of death of a significant other and contextual stimuli of Narcotics Anonymous, prayer, tired of drug-abuse routine, and guilt were contributing factors to recovery

| 7. DeSanto-Madeya (2009) | To describe and compare spinal-cord–injured individuals' and family members' experiences of physical, emotional, functional, and social adaptation and their adjustment to spinal cord injury at 1 year and 3 years postinjury

To identify spinal-cord–injured individuals' and family members' perceptions of factors that help and factors that hinder their adaptation to spinal cord injury at 1 year and 3 years postinjury | n = 15 dyads, which were made up of a spinal-cord–injured person and an identified family member; eight spinal-cord–injured persons were quadriplegic, and seven were paraplegic | Qualitative, cross-sectional, descriptive | Spinal-cord–injured individuals and their family members, regardless of time since the initial injury, have a moderate level of adaptation and adjustment to spinal cord injury |

individual's adaptation to the experience of living with multiple sclerosis (MS). Shyu (2000), Li and Shyu (2007), and DeSanto-Madeya (2009) examined group adaptation, particularly individual and family adaptation to giving and receiving care. The study by Gandy (2003) explored the individual's perception of living while dying. Gaines (1997) explored adaptation while recovering from crack cocaine addiction. Adults were identified as the subjects for the studies by Gagliardi et al. (2002), Gandy (2003), and Gaines (1997). The subjects for the Shyu (2000) and Li and Shyu (2007) studies were elderly Taiwanese and their caregivers. DeSanto-Madeya (2009) looked at dyads of a person with spinal cord injury and an identified family member. The subjects for the Lee and Ellenbecker (1998) study were elderly Chinese immigrants.

The findings from two of the studies, Gagliardi et al. (2002) and Gandy (2003), identified themes reported by subjects describing their experiences. Gagliardi et al. (2002) further related the themes to the adaptive modes of the RAM. Lee and Ellenbecker (1998) reported that the amount and sources of stress are different for Chinese elderly immigrants than for American elderly and higher levels of family connection showed lower stress levels. Results from the Shyu (2000) study indicated that caregivers and care receivers adjust to each other in phases of role engaging, role negotiating, and role settling during the transition from hospital to home. Li and Shyu (2007) reported that caregiving and care receiving roles were affected by external environmental factors, such as social network and cultural beliefs. Additionally, family coping styles were identified and it was determined that different family coping styles had different adaptation outcomes. DeSanto-Madeya (2009) found that both persons with spinal cord injuries and their family members, regardless of time since injury, have a moderate level of adaptation to spinal cord injury. Gaines (1997) reported that all five African American males experienced ineffective adaptation in all four modes of adaptation during addiction and all moved toward adaptation during recovery. The focal stimuli of death of a significant other and contextual stimuli of Narcotics Anonymous, prayer, being tired of the drug-abuse routine, and guilt were contributing factors to recovery.

Description of Grounded Theory Studies

Four studies used the qualitative method of grounded theory (see Table 3.2). Both studies by Dobratz (2002, 2004) looked at aspects of coping of dying persons. In the Dobratz (2002) study, findings included the responses and reactions of the subjects, describing a pattern identified as becoming self

TABLE 3.2
Description of Studies Using Grounded Theory

Author and Date	Purpose	Sample	Design	Findings
1. Patterson (1995)	To develop a substantive theory to describe and explain human responses to urinary incontinence (UI) among older adults who reside in nursing homes	Older adults residing in nursing homes ($n = 10$)	Grounded theory	Two distinct responses to UI were discovered: making the best of it and suffering with it. Both are consequences of the core category, "Managing the Flow." Six strategies to manage the flow included limiting, improvising, learning, monitoring, speaking up, and letting it go
2. Dobratz (2002)	To describe basic sociopsychological processes of dying with support of caregiving in home-hospice patients	Dying home-hospice patients ($n = 15$) from a subset of 97 participants in a larger study	Grounded theory	The responses and reactions describe a pattern identified as becoming self that was shaped by self-integration, inner cognition, creation of personal meanings, and connection to others and a higher being
3. Dobratz (2004)	To describe perceptions of spirituality in home-hospice patients	Dying home-hospice patients ($n = 44$) from a subset of 97 participants in a larger study	Grounded theory	The responses supported the importance of spirituality and religious beliefs to end-of-life situations. Believing was linked to six other themes: comforting, releasing, connecting, giving, reframing, and requesting

(continued)

TABLE 3.2

Description of Studies Using Grounded Theory (*continued*)

Author and Date	Purpose	Sample	Design	Findings
4. Hamilton and Bowers (2007)	To explore the experience of adult genetic testing	Adults who had predictive genetic testing ($n = 24$) and five who did not ($n = 5$)	Grounded theory	The theory of genetic vulnerability was developed and was composed of five concepts: 1. Experiencing the family disease 2. Testing for a mutation 3. Foregrounding inherited disease risk 4. Responding to knowledge of genetic vulnerability 5. Altering or avoiding the family experience of inherited disease

that was shaped by self-integration, inner cognition, creation of personal meanings, and connection to others and a higher being. Dobratz (2004) looked at persons who were dying with the support of the caregiving of home hospice. Findings supported the importance of spirituality and religious beliefs to end-of-life situations.

Patterson (1995) used a sample of older adults residing in nursing homes to develop a substantive theory to describe and explain responses to urinary incontinence. Six strategies to manage the flow of urine included limiting, improvising, speaking up, and letting it go. The Hamilton and Bowers (2007) study explored the coping experience of genetic testing using 29 adults related to predictive genetic indicators for testing, 24 of whom decided to participate in testing and 5 who did not participate. A theory of genetic vulnerability was developed and was comprised of five concepts, experiencing the family disease, testing for a mutation, foregrounding inherited disease risk, responding to knowledge of genetic vulnerability, and altering or avoiding the family experience of inherited disease.

Description of Ethnographic Studies

Niska (1999a, 1999b, 2001) used ethnography to observe the adaptive behaviors of Mexican American families (see Table 3.3). In the 1999a study, the processes of nurturing, support, and socialization of the Mexican American family unit during early family formation were explored. Twenty-three couples were followed from the third trimester of pregnancy through the child's fourth year. Findings indicated that family socialization was kin-based, hierarchical in nature, and ritualistic with intergenerational repetition of traditional family events. In the 1999b study, 26 first-time parents were observed to assess whether the similarity to the culture of nursing interventions would enhance the processes of nurturing, support, and socialization in early family formation. Nursing interventions ranged from moderately high to highly similar to the ways the participants' own parents assisted their families. The third study aimed to identify how Mexican American families in early family formation establish basic patterns for family survival, continuity, and growth. These were the same 23 couples used in the initial study. Families linked their survival to factors such as being healthy, being a united couple, having supportive parents, and having a steady job. Continuity was derived from patterns such as routines of household tasks. Some key findings related to growth included shared communication and helping the child become part of the family.

TABLE 3.3
Description of Studies Using Ethnography

Author and Date	Purpose	Sample	Design	Findings
1. Niska (1999a)	To explore the distinctive nature of adaptive processes of nurturing, support, and socialization of the Mexican American family unit during early family formation	Couples followed from the third trimester of pregnancy through the child's fourth year (n = 23 couples)	Ethnographic	Family nurturing characterized by being kin based, intimate in nature (involving the reception of direct personal care in time of illness), and hierarchical, with trust invested in experienced elders. Material, emotional, and informational support were also kin based, and grounded in shared conversation, stories, problem solving, prayer, explanations, and practical guidance. Family socialization was kin based, hierarchical in nature, and ritualistic with intergenerational repetition of traditional family events
2. Niska (1999b)	To assess the similarity of nursing interventions that enhance the family processes of nurturing, support, and socialization in early family formation	Mexican American first time parents in Texas (n = 26)	Ethnographic	Nursing interventions ranged from moderately to highly similar to the ways their own parents assisted their families. Acceptability ranged from low to high for a nurse to intervene in the way specified by the nursing intervention

3. Niska (2001)	To identify how Mexican American families in early family formation establish basic patterns for family survival, continuity, and growth	Couples followed from the third trimester of pregnancy through the child's fourth year (*n* = 23 couples)	Ethnographic	Family survival was linked to being healthy, being a united couple, having supportive parents, and having a steady job with minimal dependence on the government for additional resources. Family continuity was derived from the continual pattern of performance of 25 to 34 household tasks grounding family life. Essential characteristics for family growth were shared communication, growing in togetherness, planning ahead, and helping the child become part of the family

Description of Studies Using Phenomenology

Seventeen studies used one of the several types of phenomenology (see Table 3.4). Aims included to examine: coping with grief, living with advanced breast cancer; coping with traumatic and violent events in emergency rooms; adapting to caring for children with cancer or children or adolescents adapting to cancer, cerebral palsy (CP), or attention deficit/hyperactive disorder (ADHD) or a newborn in the neonatal intensive care unit (NICU); termination of pregnancy for fetal anomaly (TOPFA); the essence of moral distress; and the effectiveness of adaptive modes for psychosexual concerns.

Six of the 17 studies explored the internal coping process of surviving the death or impending death of a significant other or termination of pregnancy. Martin (2003) explored the lived experience of five older surviving spouses in the second year of bereavement, whereas Smith (2001) explored spousal grief of five male employees who had been widowed. Although the themes identified in the studies differed, the studies indicated that grief was long lasting, pervasive, and intense. One difference in findings was that male survivors received social support by people bringing specifics such as food, whereas these survivors felt they also needed the social support of empathy. Short (2004) described the experience of mothers who were 18 or more weeks pregnant coping with the death of a stillborn infant, any time between 2 and 10 years previously. Findings indicated that there was an intense need to think that the stillborn was a real infant compounded by feelings that their experience was not understood by others. Additionally, subjects reported great discomfort when they see pregnant women. Watson (2006) examined the experience of survivors who have lost loved ones to sudden traumatic death. The emerged themes included the need to know that their loved one was okay, of perceiving certain events as being representative of their loved ones' presence, as well as a need to discuss the nature of their last encounters with their loved ones prior to death. The stressors of coping by parents following termination of pregnancy for fetal anomaly (TOPFA) was explored by Kruszewski (1999). Findings from this study indicated that several coping processes were used by these parents, including reconstructing meaning. The necessity of finding meaning in the death of a loved one was a pervasive finding in all five studies. Ryde, Strang, and Friedrichsen (2008) used interpretive phenomenology to explore the significance of family members crying in a palliative care setting. The findings discussed three categories that related to before crying, triggers for crying, or hiding crying to ease patient's burden.

How mothers cope with their child's cancer was the focus of a study by Clark (2001). Some of the themes that emerged were that the experience was hard and horrible with a life that was plagued with fears.

TABLE 3.4

Description of Studies Using Phenomenology

Author and Date	Purpose	Sample	Design	Findings
1. Martin (2003)	To describe the lived experience of older surviving spouses in the second year of bereavement	Older adult surviving spouses in the second year of bereavement (n = 5)	Phenomenological, descriptive	Analysis indicated that the second year of bereavement was one of intense emotion. The themes were: 1. Loneliness 2. Different life makeup 3. Making up your mind you are going to go on 4. Spiritual issues permeate life without the spouse 5. Feelings of gratitude and comfort for the past, present, presence of family, and memories 6. Health or abilities changed after the death of spouse
2. Smith (2001)	To explore the lived experience of spousal grief of working-age men	Male employees who work in a plant and who have been widowed at some point in life (n = 5)	Phenomenological, descriptive	Themes 1. Grief is profound and long lasting, challenges the coping abilities of the widower 2. Grieving can cause work to become of secondary importance 3. Role changes occur during the illness of the spouse and after the death 4. Men can adapt to the caregiver role 5. Men expect to be able to cope successfully with challenges presented by the death of their spouses 6. Attempts at support can generate positive or negative effect on the widower

(continued)

TABLE 3.4

Description of Studies Using Phenomenology (*continued*)

Author and Date	Purpose	Sample	Design	Findings
3. Short (2004)	To describe the experience of mothers coping with the birth of a stillborn infant	Women who were 18 or more weeks pregnant 2 to 10 years ago and who had a stillborn infant (*n* = 5)	Phenomenological, descriptive	Themes 1. Intense need to think that the stillborn was a real baby and the desire to celebrate the stillborn's life on their birth date 2. Profoundly difficult experience, compounded by feelings that they are not understood 3. Need to feel connected to the stillborn 4. Belief that coping with losing a stillborn is a complex phenomenon 5. Need for support from others; subjects reported great discomfort when they see pregnant women
4. Watson (2006)	To discover the lived experience of survivors who have lost loved ones to sudden, traumatic death	Adults, over 18 years of age, who have lost a loved one to sudden traumatic death (*n* = 5)	Phenomenological, descriptive	Themes 1. The traumatic nature of a loved one's death remains long term and becomes a contextual stimulus for survivors 2. There was a need to know that their loved one was okay and of perceiving certain events as being representative of their loved ones' presence 3. A need existed to have the significance of their loss acknowledged and acknowledging negative feelings when others minimized their loss

				4. There was a need to discuss the nature of their last encounters with their loved ones prior to death
				5. Participants sought closure after the sudden traumatic death of their loved one
5. Kruszewski (1999)	To describe stressors and coping of parents following termination of pregnancy for fetal anomaly (TOPFA) as the basis for midrange theory development regarding psychological adaptation to pregnancy termination for fetal anomaly	Parents who terminated a pregnancy for fetal anomaly (n = 18)	Phenomenological, descriptive	Before termination, stressors included dilemma of termination, mother's physical condition, including discomfort, and actual death of the fetus. After termination, stressors were ongoing loss, responsibility, regret, revealing the loss, and concerns about subsequent pregnancy; coping processes were decision making, transforming, avoiding awareness, constructing a cause, reconstructing meaning, backgrounding, displacing blame, and reconstructing one's personal moral code; five categories of contextual stimuli were identified: (1) societal controversy about abortion, (2) social attitudes about disability, (3) meaning of the baby, (4) parents' personal beliefs about abortion, and (5) social interactions that affected coping process

(continued)

TABLE 3.4
Description of Studies Using Phenomenology (*continued*)

Author and Date	Purpose	Sample	Design	Findings
6. Clark (2001)	To investigate the lived experience of mothers coping with their child's cancer	Mothers coping with their child's cancer ($n = 3$)	Phenomenological, descriptive	Themes 1. The experience was hard and horrible 2. Life was plagued with fears 3. A need to look for a bright side 4. A duty existed to be strong 5. A need to rely on others 6. A craving for normalcy
7. Ramini (2008)	To examine adaptive strategies of adolescents with cancer using the Roy adaptation model	Adolescents with cancer ($n = 4$)	Phenomenological, descriptive	Themes were evident in each of the four modes Physiological themes 1. Uncontrolled nausea and vomiting 2. Weakness and fatigue 3. Uncontrolled pain Self-concept themes 1. Increased confidence and psychosocial maturation 2. Embracing changes 3. Appreciation for life 4. Use of bandanas or wigs 5. Reliance on positive feedback from friends and family

				Role-function themes
				1. Desire to feel normal
				2. Resentful of sympathy and pity
				3. Increased freedom from teachers/parents
				4. Cancer camps are beneficial
				Interdependence themes
				1. Spiritual support and faith
				2. Support from family and friends
				3. Open family communication
				4. Sibling jealousy and appreciation from sibling(s)
				5. Respect for doctors, nurses, and teachers
				Unanticipated responses were the illegal behaviors of underage driving and the use of marijuana
8. Yeh (2001)	To understand how children adapt to cancer, changes in clinical status, and how these processes affect their lives	Taiwanese children with cancer at all stages (n = 34 in three age groups)	Phenomenological, descriptive	Participants changed their coping tasks and strategies as clinical events (e.g., diagnosis, side effects, or relapses) occurred. Included five interrelated aspects: sociological and psychological, cognitive (self-concept), interdependence, and future orientation (self concept and role). Children in different age groups expressed different ways of adapting

(continued)

61

TABLE 3.4

Description of Studies Using Phenomenology (*continued*)

Author and Date	Purpose	Sample	Design	Findings
9. Milbrath, et al. (2007)	To discover the adaptation process of women who gave birth to a child with cerebral palsy (CP)	Brazilian mothers of children with CP (*n* = 6)	Phenomenological, descriptive	Themes 1. Experience of being a woman with a child with CP 2. Support by the father and network are necessary to the mother with a child with special needs
10. Moore (2005)	To explore the lived experience of being a mother of a child with severe CP	Mothers of children from 4 to 11 years with CP (*n* = 5)	Phenomenological, descriptive	Themes 1. Mothers created unique ways of bonding and connecting with their child 2. Mothers describe positive aspects of their parenting experience 3. The child's diagnosis of CP was a lifelong journey of recurrent adversity, eliciting a series of individualized responses 4. The mothering experience necessitates dealing with many types of burden

11. Knipp (2006)	To describe teen's perceptions about attention deficit/ hyperactivity disorder (ADHD) and the use of medications	Adolescents with parent-reported ADHD (n = 15)	Phenomenological, descriptive	Themes with corresponding adaptive modes: 1. Use of medication helped (physiological mode) 2. Doing better in school with medications (role function mode) 3. Taking medication improved family relationships and friends do not see teen as being different (interdependence mode) 4. Feeling that with medication their teen was pretty much like other teens (self-concept and group identification)
12. Lazemby (2001)	To explore the stressors and adaptation of Mexican mothers who had infants in a neonatal intensive care units (NICU)	Mexican mothers (n = 5)	Phenomenological, descriptive	The NICU environment had a negative effect on maternal stress and adaptation. Mexican mothers experienced the same stressors as Caucasian mothers, but their inability to communicate with caregivers increased anxiety, emphasizing the importance of effective communication between parents and nurses

(continued)

TABLE 3.4

Description of Studies Using Phenomenology (*continued*)

Author and Date	Purpose	Sample	Design	Findings
13. Wright (2007)	To describe the experience of emergency nurses and to identify the most effective coping strategies used when faced with traumatic and violent events	Direct-care registered nurses who work in a level 1 trauma center (*n* = 5)	Phenomenological, descriptive	Themes 1. Behavior manifestations, such as sleep disturbances and having thoughts replay in one's mind 2. Communications 3. Empathy 4. Humor 5. Knowledge and skills 6. Distress of caring for critical pediatric patients 7. Support of peers and families 8. Teamwork 9. Uncertainty 10. Workload
14. Lemone (1995)	To evaluate the effectiveness of the adaptive modes for assessing psychosexual concerns of adults with diabetes mellitus	Hospitalized adult patients with insulin-dependent diabetes (*n* = 10)	Phenomenological, descriptive	Themes 1. Actual or potential discomfort or pain 2. Loss of control of body functions 3. Loss of love from others 4. Alterations in sensation of body parts

	Purpose	Sample	Design	Findings
15. Hanna (2005)	To discover the essence, properties, and full content domain of the concept of moral distress in order to develop a universal definition of the concept	Registered nurses (n = 10)	Phenomenological, descriptive	Themes (identified as properties of moral distress) 1. Perception 2. Pain 3. Valuing 4. Altered participation 5. Perspective Three types of moral distress identified were: shocked, muted, and persistent. Types of moral distress were related to situational conditions, recognition of moral ends, quality of common processes, and temporal breath
16. Pacsi (2010)	To illuminate the perceptions of Dominican women living with stage IV breast cancer (advanced breast cancer)	Second-generation U.S.-born women of Dominican immigrants, residing in the New York City (NYC) area (n = 6)	Phenomenological, descriptive	The four essences that unfolded were uncertainty, coping, loving, and believing. The overall meaning of the experience of stage IV breast cancer is described as one of uncertainty and unknowing; accepting the diagnosis so that thinking results in positive changes and healthy choices; enjoying life through meaningful participation in the lives of others and accepting support; and trusting in God through prayer, faith, and hope to create everlasting memories for their children

(continued)

TABLE 3.4
Description of Studies Using Phenomenology (*continued*)

Author and Date	Purpose	Sample	Design	Findings
17. Ryde, Strang, and Friedrichsen (2008)	To explore the significance of family members crying in a palliative care context with special reference to factors that influence crying	Family members of patients admitted to palliative care in two different advanced palliative hospital-based home-care units (HBHCs) in the southeast of Sweden (*n* = 14)	Phenomenological, interpretive	Three main categories emerged 1. Before the start of crying, some prerequisites for crying had to be fulfilled, such as an allowing attitude and courage, time, feeling secure, honesty, and trusting relationships. These prerequisites did not cause crying themselves; rather crying emerged when triggering factors occurred 2. Triggers for crying were circumstances that created uncertainty and turbulence (bad news), exhaustion due to lack of own time, and sympathy from others 3. Family members tried to do the best possible by adopting or hiding their crying to ease the patient's burden and to create a positive counterbalance to suffering and grief. As an interpretation of the whole, crying could be expressed as being shared with someone for support and consolation or escape to solitude for integrity and respite

The mothers reported the duty to be strong, a craving for normalcy, as well as a need to rely on others. Two other studies (Ramini, 2008; Yeh, 2001) examined internal coping with cancer for children and adolescents. Yeh (2001) explored how Taiwanese children and adolescents with the diagnosis of cancer adapted to the changes in clinical status and how these changes affected their lives. Yeh (2001) found that participants changed their coping tasks and strategies as clinical events occurred and that children in different age groups had different ways of adapting. Ramini (2008) reported that adolescents adapt to cancer using strategies in each mode of the RAM. Unanticipated strategies were the illegal behaviors of underage driving and the use of marijuana. For the Dominican immigrant women living with advanced breast cancer, Pacsi (2010) reported four essences of the experience: uncertainty, coping, loving, and believing.

Two studies (Milbrath, Cecagno, Soares, Amestoy & de Siqueira, 2008; Moore, 2005) explored the internal coping mechanisms of mothers of children with cerebral palsy (CP). Findings from the Milbrath et al. (2008) study indicated that the father's and network's support are necessary to the mother of a child with special needs. The Moore (2005) study found that mothers created unique ways of bonding and connecting with their children and that a child's diagnosis of CP was a lifelong journey of recurrent adversity eliciting a series of individual responses.

Adolescent internal coping as an outcome of perception was the subject of a study by Knipp (2006). The purpose of the study was to describe teens' perceptions about ADHD and the use of medications. The themes identified from the data corresponded with the modes of the RAM and included that medications improved relationships and schoolwork, helped the teens feel like other teens, and helped the participants control behaviors. Lazemby (2001) explored the stressors and internal coping of mothers from Mexico who had infants in a NICU. The NICU was very stressful and Mexican mothers experienced the same stressors as Caucasian mothers but their inability to communicate with caregivers increased anxiety.

A study by Wright (2007) examined the group adaptation and internal coping strategies used when emergency room nurses were constantly faced with traumatic and violent events. Themes that emerged were the behavioral manifestations such as sleep disturbances and having thoughts replay in one's mind as well as teamwork, humor, empathy, knowledge, and skills and the support of peers and families contributing to coping. The purpose of a study by Lemone (2005) was to evaluate the effectiveness of the RAM adaptive modes for assessing psychosexual concerns of adults with diabetes mellitus. The themes derived from the study included the actual or potential discomfort or pain, loss of control of body functions, loss of love from others, and alterations in sensations of body parts.

Hanna (2005) explored the concept of moral distress in order to develop a universal definition of the concept. Perception, pain, valuing, altered participation, and perspective were identified as properties of moral distress. These types of moral distress were related to situational conditions such as recognition of moral ends, quality of common processes, and time perspective.

Description of Mixed-Methods Studies

There were six studies that used a mixed-methods approach (see Table 3.5). These studies explored Taiwanese children's pain experiences (Cheng, 2002), children's perceptions of self-concept and associated emotional indicators of children living with HIV/AIDS in the United States and Kenya (Waweru, Reynolds, & Buckner, 2008), the relationship between self-concept and body image and the presence of spinal cord injury (Harding-Okimoto, 1997), maternal and infant stress and the perceptions of nurses in the NICU environment (Raeside, 1997), a research intervention using the RAM (Senesac, 2004), and hospice support for the decision to care for a family member at home.

Both Harding-Okimoto (1997) and Raeside (1997) explored how varying factors affected internal coping processes. Harding-Okimoto (1997) compared the body image of spinal-cord–injured patients with and without pressure ulcers and found that the presence of pressure ulcers affect adaptation in the self-concept mode and impacts body image. Raeside (1997) studied the maternal and infant stress in the NICU and perceptions of neonatal nurses in relation to these stressors. Findings indicated that maternal stress levels were lower than perceived by nurses and that the nurses' perceptions of the elements in the environment that caused the most maternal stress differed from those reported by mother.

Findings from Cheng's (2002) study of pain in children in Taiwan noted that the surgical pain intensity exceeded pain from medical conditions as reported by the children. Although pain did not vary by age, the expression varied with younger children using more affective words than older children. Another study looked at children's perceptions, but these were associated with living with HIV/AIDS (Waweru et al., 2008). The investigators compared children in the United States with children in Kenya. Children in the United States and in Kenya were both found to have an average self-concept. However, the associated emotional indicators differed in that one third of the children in the United States had indicators of an alteration in emotional well-being, whereas in Kenya half were found to have indicators of alteration in emotional well-being. Recurrent themes

TABLE 3.5
Description of Studies Using Mixed Methods

Author and Date	Purpose	Sample	Design	Findings
1. Cheng (2002)	To explore the pain experience of Taiwanese children and describe the relationship between pain and age, gender, and prior pain experience	Hospitalized Taiwanese children aged 5–14 years divided into three groups ($n = 90$)	Mixed methods	Most of the variance in overall pain explained the intensity of surgical pain better than medical pain, with surgical pain intensity exceeding medical pain. There was no significant difference in pain by age group, but a significant difference existed in pain description by age group with younger children using more affective words than older children
2. Harding-Okimoto (1997)	To describe the relationship between self-concept manifested by body image and the occurrence of pressure ulcers in spinal-cord–injured adults	Spinal-cord–injured adults with pressure ulcers ($n = 5$) and without pressure ulcers ($n = 5$)	Mixed methods	The presence of pressure ulcers affects adaptation in the self-concept mode and impacts body image

(continued)

TABLE 3.5
Description of Studies Using Mixed Methods (*continued*)

Author and Date	Purpose	Sample	Design	Findings
3. Waweru, Reynolds, and Buckner (2008)	To assess the perceptions of self-concept and associated emotional indicators of children living with HIV/AIDS	Children with HIV or AIDS living in the United States (*n* = 6) or living in Kenya (*n* = 42) between the ages of 7 and 12 years	Mixed methods	Children in the United States were found to have an average self-concept and one third demonstrated significant emotional indicators of an alteration in emotional well-being. In Kenya, 93% of the subjects had an average self-concept and half were found to have significant emotional indicators. Content analysis of interview questions revealed the recurrent themes of caring, healing, and companionship. Both groups had a large social network of friends, relatives, volunteers, and staff that, which also helped the children feel positive about themselves
4. Raeside (1997)	To explore maternal and infant stress within the neonatal intensive care unit (NICU) environment and to assess perceptions of neonatal nurses in relation to these stressors	Mothers and nurses in NICU (*n* = 12 of each)	Mixed methods	Maternal stress levels were lower than perceived by nurses; mothers of very low birth weight infants reported higher levels of stress than those of low birth weight infants; nurses' perceptions of the elements of the environment that caused most maternal stress differed from those reported by mothers

	Purpose	Sample	Design	Findings
5. Senesac (2004)	To conduct an action research intervention using a nusing conceptual framework	Nurses employed in a community hospital (*n* = 14)	Mixed methods	The intervention impacted planned organizational change in role, group identity, interdependence, and organizational structure. These changes were viewed as adaptive outcomes consistent with the American Nurses Association's Scope and Standards of Practice for Nurse Administrators
6. Raleigh, Robinson, Marold, and Jamison (2006)	The purpose of this study was to explore hospice support of family caregivers in their decision to provide care at home and to examine the relationships among hospice support, coping, and spiritual well-being	Recently bereaved family caregivers of hospice patients in the Detroit, Michigan, and Toledo, Ohio, metropolitan areas (*n* = 21)	Mixed methods	Study confirmed that families prefer to care for their dying family members at home, and cited three factors in this decision to be: patient request, desire to be with the patient, and desire to help the patient Caregivers noted the importance of hospice support in making the decision to keep the patient at home and in making that decision possible. The more contact the caregivers had with the hospice network, the fewer coping strategies were reported. Bereaved caregivers reported a low use of coping strategies, but rated those used as very effective There was no relationship between spiritual well-being and hospice support

from interviews of children in both countries included caring, healing, and companionship.

Senesac (2004) conducted an action research intervention using the RAM to examine the process of nurses carrying out a self-selected change project. The findings from this study indicated that the intervention changed organizational roles, group identity, interdependence, and organizational structure. These changes were viewed as adaptive organizational outcomes. Study confirmed that families prefer to care for their dying family members at home, and cited three factors in this decision to be: patient request, desire to be with the patient, and desire to help the patient.

In the mixed-methods study by Raleigh, Robinson, Marold, and Jamison (2006) the purpose was to explore hospice support of family caregivers in their decision to provide care at home and to examine the relationships between hospice support, coping, and spiritual well-being. Recently bereaved family caregivers of hospice patients were recruited (n = 21). Findings showed that caregivers noted the importance of hospice support in making the decision to keep the patient at home and found that the support made that decision possible. The authors further reported that the more contact the caregivers had with the hospice network, the fewer coping strategies were reported. Whereas the bereaved caregivers reported a low use of coping strategies, they rated those used as very effective. Finally, there was no relationship found between spiritual well-being and hospice support.

Description of Studies Using Analyses of Cases

Three studies used the method of analyses of cases (see Table 3.6). Gagliardi (2003) analyzed the experience of a small number of participants who had the same diagnoses. The author described the experience of sexuality for individuals living with multiple sclerosis. Three themes were derived from telephone interviews, including how the subject felt about his or her appearance and that both positive and negative emotions were associated with sexuality.

Cunningham (2002) used the RAM to implement the nursing process by managing stimuli to facilitate group member adaptation for Jamaican Canadian middle-aged women going through menopause. During the time of the study, first- and second-level assessments were conducted, and assessment data were analyzed to identify nursing diagnoses and goals. From the goals interventions were developed that focused on managing stimuli and promoting adaptation.

In another study (Weiss, Fawcett, & Aber, 2009), nursing students collected data on one patient each, so this is considered an analysis of

TABLE 3.6

Description of Studies Using Analyses of Cases

Author and Date	Purpose	Sample	Design	Findings
1. Gagliardi (2003)	To describe the experience of sexuality for individuals living with multiple sclerosis (MS)	Adults with MS (n = 8)	Naturalistic study of cases	Themes derived from three telephone interviews that each participant had: 1. How do I feel about my appearance 2. I have feelings about my sexuality 3. Sexuality has for me positive and negative emotions
2. Cunningham (2002)	To use the Roy adaptation model to manage stimuli to facilitate group member adaptation and develop nursing interventions based on group assessment data	Jamaican Canadian middle-aged menopausal women (n = 3)	Descriptive analysis of cases	First- and second-level assessments were conducted, and assessment data were analyzed to identify nursing diagnoses and goals. From the goals interventions were developed that focused on managing stimuli and promoting adaptation. All group members evaluated the group sessions as very satisfying

(continued)

TABLE 3.6

Description of Studies Using Analyses of Cases (*continued*)

Author and Date	Purpose	Sample	Design	Findings
3. Weiss, Fawcett, and Aber (2009)	To describe women's physical, emotional, functional, and social adaptation; postpartum concerns; and learning needs during the first 2 weeks following caesarean birth and identify relevant nursing interventions	Culturally diverse caesarean-delivered women in urban areas of the Midwestern and Northeastern USA between 2002 and 2004; nursing students collected data on one patient each (*n* = 233)	Descriptive analysis of multiple cases	Women with unplanned caesarean births and primiparous women reported less favorable adaptation than planned caesarean mothers and multiparas. Black women reported lower social adaptation, Hispanic women had more role-function concerns, and Black and Hispanic women had more learning needs than White women. Postdischarge nursing assessments revealed that actual problems accounted for 40% of identified actual or potential problems or needs. Health teaching was the intervention most commonly recommended

multiple cases. The focus was to study culturally diverse women who had infants born by caesarean section and to identify physical, emotional, functional, and social adaptation as well as concerns and learning needs during the first 2 weeks postpartum and to identify relevant nursing interventions. The findings of this study showed that women with unplanned caesarean births and primiparous women reported less favorable adaptation than mothers who had planned caesarean sections and multiparous women. Areas of adaptation varied to some extent by culture and health teaching was the common intervention recommended.

CRITIQUE OF STUDIES

The critique of the studies included in this chapter is presented in two ways. First we will summarize the results of the critical analysis done on a set of studies and then we will discuss the strengths and weaknesses of this work. Chapter 2 described the criteria used in the critique of qualitative studies. It was noted that each study could be scored with a maximum of 20 points, that is, 5 points for each category of the critique. To be considered adequate for a given study to be used in further knowledge development or application to practice in this project it is expected that the work scored between 16 and 20 points. This means that most areas were either 4 or 5 out of 5 points and not more than one could be scored at 3. Among the qualitative studies reported here the range of scores was 20 to 16. Only four studies scored one "three" and two of these were in the last category of method, that is, case analyses, the weakest of the methods. Based on the rules for deleting studies, no qualitative studies were dropped from further consideration in generating middle range theories and in evidence for practice.

In identifying strengths of the qualitative research, we noted that Dobratz (2002, 2004), Short (2004), Lemone (1995), Harding-Okimotto (1997), Clark (2001), Moore (2005), Ramini (2008), and Gandy (2003) completely described study populations and properly described the settings, as well as the circumstances under which the data were collected. Additionally, these researchers explained the ways in which data were analyzed to create the themes. In most of the studies the research questions were described adequately so the reader knew what was being asked and what type of methods were employed. Most of the studies did not have sufficient descriptive information given to allow the reader to conclude that the authors' interpretations were grounded in the data. A few of the researchers addressed internal validity through "triangulation," including Cheng (2002), Harding-Okimoto (1997), Waweru et al. (2008), Raeside (1997), and Senesac (2004).

In qualitative research the phenomena under study often is the coping abilities in handling a specific focal stimulus. According to Roy (2009), the focal stimulus is the internal or external stimulus most immediately confronting the individual. The focal stimulus and its effect on internal coping processes include both the cognator and regulator. This relationship is supported by most of the studies: Gandy (2003), Cheng (2002), and Lee and Ellenbecker (1998), Hamilton et al. (2007), Dobratz (2002, 2004), Short (2004), Smith (2001), Watson (2006), Clark (2001), Milbrath et al. (2008), Moore (2005), Kruszewski (1999), Ramini (2008), Yeh (2001), Wright (2007), Knipp (2006), Lazemby (2001), Raeside (1997), Gagliardi et al. (2002), Cheng (2002), and Harding-Okimoto (1997).

Several studies related the processes of adaptation to all four adaptive modes, which might be considered contextual stimuli. These are described by Roy as being "all other stimuli present in the situation that contribute to the effect of the focal stimulus" (Roy, 2009, p. 26). Niska (1999a, 1999b, 2001), Lemone (1995), Hanna (2005), and Gaines (1997) explored contextual stimuli. The concepts of family support and social support emerged as significant concepts in studies by Dobratz (2002, 2004), Martin (2003), Robinson (1995), Short (2004) and Watson (2006). Group adaptation was studied by Shyu (2000), Li and Shyu (2007), Senesac (2004), and Waweru et al. (2008). The impact of incoming stimuli was studied by Patterson (1995) and Martin (2003). Studies that were well conceived and constructed are those by Dobratz (2002, 2004). In the studies examining the loss of a loved one, the concept of social support emerges (Martin, 2003; Short, 2004). In the studies of certain groups and their adaptation, the passage of time that individuals required to adapt by way of the cognator subsystem is another recurrent theme that surfaced in these particular studies, Shyu (2000), Li and Shyu (2007), Senesac (2004), and Waweru et al. (2008).

IMPLICATIONS FOR PRACTICE

Two studies were selected as exemplars for practice. Both studies emphasized the need for changes in nursing practice. Dobratz (2002) explains human responses and family processes as well as her recognition that there is beginning evidence of an integrative metaparadigm, in which the human life processes at the end-of-life move in fluid and dynamic interaction with the total environment. This process is explicated in the philosophical assumptions of the RAM (Roy, 1988). Therefore, end-of-life care in hospitals and in hospice care will be based on a principle that explicates the human life processes of valuing, relating, feeling, and acting. Without a doubt, further study is needed to explore the bond that links life-closing spirituality to dying, to the philosophical principles of the RAM, and to the human life processes.

The work of Patterson (1995) on urinary incontinence demonstrated that misconceptions regarding the etiology and treatment of urinary tract infections (UTI) exist among nursing home residents. Thus efforts to educate residents and families about UTI and available treatment will be made. The notion of "continence programs" or "bowel and bladder programs" as operational in many nursing homes will be rethought. The singular goal of most programs is reduction of leakage, which is implemented through protocols developed without input from the patient. According to Patterson (1995) treatment will be an individualized approach considering the actual potential of the patient as well as appropriate management strategies already available. Teaching caregivers the proper physiological interventions also should be included to prevent harmful practices as limiting fluid intake.

CONCLUSION

This chapter reviewed the descriptions of the qualitative studies based on the RAM that were included in the database. Some rich insights were noted, particularly among the studies using phenomenological and mixed methods. Further, the formal critique of the studies was presented along with the strengths and weaknesses of the studies. It was noted that case analysis provided the weakest qualitative approach. However, no study was dropped from further consideration for knowledge development.

REFERENCES

Denzin, N., & Lincoln, Y. (Eds.). (2000). *Handbook of qualitative research*. London: Sage.

Morse, J. M. (2002). Where do interventions come from? *Qualitative Health Research, April*, 435–436.

Roy, C. (1988). An explication of the philosophical assumptions of the Roy adaptation model. *Nursing Science Quarterly, 1*(1), 26–34.

Roy, C. (2009). *The Roy adaptation model* (3rd ed.). Upper Saddle River, NJ: Prentice Hall Health.

Shank, G. (2002). *Qualitative research. A personal skills approach*. Upper Saddle River, NJ: Prentice Hall.

BIBLIOGRAPHY

Cheng, S. F. (2002). *A multi-method study of Taiwanese children's pain experiences* (Doctoral dissertation, University of Colorado Health Sciences Center). Retrieved from https://mail.bc.edu/Redirect/metaquest.bc.edu:4000/sfx_local ?sid=SP:NU&id=pmid:&id=&issn=&isbn=978-0

Clark, E. D. (2001). *The lived experience of mothers with their child's cancer.* Toledo, OH: Medical College of Ohio at Toledo. Retrieved from http://proquest.umi.com/pqdweb?index=60&did=729283541&SrchMode=1&sid=1&Fmt=2&Vinst=PROD&Vtype=PQD&RQT=309&Vname=PQD&TS=1224510743&clientId=7750

Cunningham, D. A. (2002). Application of Roy's adaptation model when caring for a group of women coping with menopause. *Journal of Community Health Nursing, 19*(1), 49–60.

DeSanto-Madeya, S. (2009). Adaptation to spinal cord injury for families post-injury. *Nursing Science Quarterly, 22*(1), 57–66.

Dobratz, M. C. (2002). The pattern of the becoming-self in death and dying. *Nursing Science Quarterly, 15*(2), 137–142.

Dobratz, M. C. (2004). Life-closing spirituality and the philosophic assumptions of the Roy Adaptation Model. *Nursing Science Quarterly, 17*(4), 335–338.

Lee, A. A., & Ellenbecker, C. H. (1998). The perceived life stressors among elderly Chinese immigrants: Are they different from those of other elderly Americans? *Clinical Excellence for Nurse Practitioners, 2*(2), 96–101.

Gagliardi, B. (2003). The experience of sexuality for individuals living with multiple sclerosis. *Journal of Clinical Nursing, 12*(4), 571–578.

Gagliardi, B. A., Frederickson, K., & Shanley, D. A. (2002). Living with multiple sclerosis: A Roy adaptation model-based study. *Nursing Science Quarterly, 15*(3), 230–236.

Gaines, G. (1997). A qualitative study of the levels of adaptation of African-American males who are recovering from crack addiction (drug abuse) (Master's thesis, D'Youville College). *Masters Abstracts International, 35*(6), 1774.

Gandy, L. L. (2003). *Through the voices of the dying.* Reno, NV: University of Nevada. Retrieved from http://proquest.umi.com/pqdweb? Index=47&did=766450981&SrchMode=1&sid=1&Fmt=2&Vinst=PROD&Vtype=PQD&RQT=309&Vname=PQD&TS=1224509768&clientId=7750

Hamilton, R. J., & Bowers, B. J. (2007, July). The theory of genetic vulnerability: A Roy model exemplar. *Nursing Science Quarterly, 20*(3), 254.

Hanna, D. R. (2005). The lived experience of moral distress: Nurses who assisted with elective abortions. *Research Theory Nursing Practice, 19*(1), 95–124.

Harding-Okimoto, M. B. (1997). Pressure ulcers, self-concept and body image in spinal cord injury patients. *SCI Nurse, 14*(4), 111–117.

Hsieh, H. F., & Shannon, S. E. (2005). Three approaches to qualitative content analysis. *Qualitative Health Research, 15*(9), 1277–1288.

Knipp, D. K. (2006). Teens' perceptions about attention deficit/hyperactivity disorder and medications. *Journal of School Nursing, 22*(2), 120–125. Retrieved from http://jsn.sagepub.com/cgi/reprint/22/2/120

Kruszewsk, A. (1999). Psychosocial adaptation to termination of pregnancy for fetal anomaly (Doctoral dissertation, Wayne State University). *Dissertation Abstracts International, 61*(01B), 194.

Lazemby, L. M. (2001). *The experiences of Mexican mothers in a neonatal intensive care nursery.* Reno, NV: University of Nevada. Retrieved from http://proquest.umi .com/pqdweb?index=59&did=727205361&SrchMode=1&sid=1&Fmt=2&Vinst= PROD&Vtype=PQD&RQT=309&Vname=PQD&TS=1224508512&clientId=7750

Lemone, P. (1995). Assessing psychosexual concerns in adults with diabetes: Pilot project using Roy's modes of Adaptation. *Issues in Mental Health Nursing, 16*(1), 67–78.

Li, H. J., & Shyu, Y. L. (2007). Coping processes of Taiwanese families during the postdischarge period for an elderly family member with hip fracture. *Nursing Science Quarterly, 20*(3), 273–279.

Martin, J. L. (2003). *Spousal grief in older adults: The lived experience of surviving spouses during the second year of bereavement.* Toledo, OH: Medical College of Ohio. Retrieved from http://proquest.umi.com/pqdweb?index=46&did=766679731& SrchMode=1&sid=1&Fmt=6&Vinst=PROD&Vtype=PQD&RQT=309&Vname= PQD&TS=1224509768&clientId=7750

Milbrath, V. M., Cecagno, D., Soares, C. D., Amestoy, S. C., & de Siqueira, H. (2008). Being a woman, mother to child with cerebral palsy. *Acta Paulista de Enfermagem, 21*(3), 427–431.

Moore, L. A. (2005). *The lived experience of being a mother of a child with severe cerebral palsy.* Toledo, OH: Medical College of Ohio. Retrieved from http://proquest.umi. com/pqdweb? Did=932417851&Fmt=6&clientId=7750&RQT=309&Vname=PQD

Niska, K. (1999a). Mexican American family processes: Nurturing, support, and socialization. *Nursing Science Quarterly, 12*(2), 138–142.

Niska, K. (1999b). Family nursing interventions: Mexican American early family formation. *Nursing Science Quarterly, 12*(4), 335–340.

Niska, K. J. (2001). Mexican American family survival, continuity, and growth: The parental perspective. *Nursing Science Quarterly, 14*(4), 322–329.

Pacsi, A. L. (2010). *The lived experiences of Dominican women with Stage IV breast cancer* (Doctoral dissertation, City University of New York).

Patterson, J. (1995). Responses of Institutionalized older adults to urinary incontinence: Managing the flow (Doctoral dissertation, University of Pennsylvania). *Dissertation Abstracts International, 56*(05B), 2563.

Raeside, L. (1997). Perceptions of environmental stressors in the neonatal unit. *British Journal of Nursing, 6*(16), 914–916, 918, 920–923.

Raleigh, E. D. H., Robinson, J. H., Marold, K., & Jamison, M. T. (2006). Family caregiver perception of hospice support. *Journal of Hospice and Palliative Nursing, 8*(1), 25–33.

Ramini, S. K. (2008). Embracing changes: Adaptation by adolescents with cancer. *Pediatric Nursing, 34*(1), 72.

Robinson, J. H. (1995). Grief responses, coping processes, and social support of widows: Research with Roy's model. *Nursing Science Quarterly, 8*(4), 158–164.

Rydé, K., Strang, P., & Friedrichsen, M. (2008). Crying in solitude or with someone for support and consolation: Experiences from family members in palliative home care. *Cancer Nursing, 31*(5), 345–353.

Senesac, P. M. (2004). *The Roy adaptation model: An action research approach to the implementation of a pain management organizational change project* (Doctoral dissertation, Boston College, William F. Connell Graduate School of Nursing).

Retrieved from https://mail.bc.edu/Redirect/metaquest.bc.edu:4000/sfx_local
?sid=SP:NU&id=pmid:&id=&issn=&isbn=&volume

Shank, G. (2002). *Qualitative research. A personal skills approach.* Upper Saddle River,
NJ: Prentice Hall.

Short, J. K. (2004). *The lived experience of mothers coping with the birth of a stillborn
infant.* Toledo, OH: Medical College of Ohio. Retrieved from http://proquest
.umi.com/pqdweb? Did=766854591&Fmt=6&clientId=7750&RQT=309&Vnam
e=PQD

Shyu, Y. (2000). Role tuning between caregiver and care receiver during discharge
transition: An illustration of role function mode in Roy's Adaptation Theory.
Nursing Science Quarterly, 13(4), 323–331.

Smith, W. C., III. (2001). *Spousal grief in working men: A qualitative study.* Toledo, OH:
Medical College of Ohio at Toledo. Retrieved from http://proquest.umi.com/
pqdweb?Index=58&did=727201391&SrchMode=1&sid=1&Fmt=6&Vinst=PROD
&Vtype=PQD&RQT=309&Vname=PQD&TS=1224508512&clientId=7750

Watson, S. A. (2006). *The lived experience of losing a loved one to a sudden traumatic
death.* Toledo, OH: Medical College of Ohio. Retrieved from http://proquest.
umi.com/pqdweb?Did=1428837291&Fmt=6&clientId=7750&RQT=309&Vname
=PQD

Waweru, S. M., Reynolds, A., & Buckner, E. B. (2008). Perceptions of children with
HIV/AIDS from the USA and Kenya: Self-concept and emotional indicators.
Pediatric-Nursing (PEDIATR-NURS), 34(2), 117–124. Retrieved from http://mail.
bc.edu/Redirect/www.cinahl.com/cgi-bin/refsvc?Jid=299&accno=2009910094;
http://mail.bc.edu/Redirect/metaquest.bc.edu:4000/sfx_local?sid=SP:NU&id=
pmid:18543836&id=&issn=0097

Weiss, M., Fawcett, J., & Aber, C. (2009). Adaptation, postpartum concerns, and
learning needs in the first two weeks after caesarean birth. *Journal of Clinical
Nursing, 18*(21), 2938–2948.

Wright, R. R. (2007). *Experiences of emergency room nurses: What has been learned
from traumatic and violent events?* New York, NY: Teachers College, Columbia
University. Retrieved from http://proquest.umi.com/pqdweb?did=1390306751&
Fmt=6&clientId=7750&RQT=309&VName=PQD

Yeh, C. (2001). Adaptation in children with cancer: Research with Roy's model.
Nursing Science Quarterly, 14(2), 141–148.

4

Quantitative Studies: Descriptive Designs

KATHRYN LAUCHNER AND MARTHA V. WHETSELL

Studies based on the Roy adaptation model (RAM) that use quantitative research designs are presented next. The quantitative designs were divided into three types for purposes of this project, that is, (1) descriptive; (2) those that aim to explain, predict, or prescribe; and (3) intervention studies. In general, quantitative research is a formal, objective, systematic process, which uses numerical data to obtain information, to test theory, and to verify whether explanations are true. The main value of research is the ability of research to contribute to knowledge development. Research is closely tied to theory in creating knowledge, especially knowledge for practice. This interrelationship has a sustained recognition in nursing and other fields (Fawcett, 1978, 1999; McGaghie, Bordage, & Shea, 2001). Quantitative research basically focuses on measuring social reality, viewing the world as reality that can be objectively determined. The quality of the processes of data collection and analysis become critical when research is used to determine the best evidence for practice. Nursing knowledge is developed using a range of strategies that include theory generation at all levels and multiple approaches to research, the findings of which are translated for use in nursing practice. An exemplar of this process is the focus of this book; here the authors begin looking at quantitative studies derived from a grand theory that cumulatively can be used to generate middle range theory and provide evidence for practice.

Quantitative research (Box 4.1) assumes some ability to represent reality. This research method is used: (1) to describe variables; (2) to examine relationships among variables; and (3) to determine cause-and-effect interactions between variables (Burns & Grove, 2009, p. 22). In this project we are defining descriptive studies as those that deal with the first two uses identified by these authors, that is, describing variables and examining relationships among them. Descriptive research aims to present an accurate conceptual account of given individuals, situations, or groups. Because the research reviewed used the RAM, the investigators often were using major concepts that were similarly defined and described. In an initial review of Roy-model–based studies, it was noted that a large number were describing relationships among the variables. Therefore studies such as those using correlational designs were included in the group called descriptive. The aim of such studies is to show that a relationship exists, but the approach does not determine cause and effect. Such designs can lead to findings that are useful in refining hypotheses to be tested in intervention research (Burns & Grove, 2009).

The purpose of this chapter is to analyze descriptive research using the RAM and articulate its relevance to developing knowledge for practice. Specific aims are to (1) describe the studies identified, (2) critique the research, and (3) provide an exemplar for change in practice based on research.

Given the large number of studies that used descriptive designs, a way to organize studies with similar concepts was needed. As described in Chapter 2, a useful approach was the propositions of the RAM. The generic propositions based on the model first published in 1981 (Roy & Roberts) were clustered by the major model concepts (see Table 2.2). The wording was clarified and extended into 14 propositions in five clusters of how the major model concepts were related. In this chapter the 56 studies are presented in four groups as listed in Box 4.2.

BOX 4.1
KEY DEFINITIONS OF RESEARCH

- Quantitative research—a formal, objective, systematic process that uses numerical data to obtain information, to test theory, and to verify whether explanations are true; basically focuses on measuring social reality and views the world as reality that can be objectively determined.
- Descriptive quantitative research—describing variables and examining relationships among them; aims to present an accurate account of given individuals, situations, or groups; the aim is to show that the concepts and relationships exist, but the approach does not determine cause and effect.

BOX 4.2
DESCRIPTIVE STUDIES BASED ON CATEGORIES OF
PROPOSITIONS (*n* = 56)

- Descriptive Studies Related to Internal Coping Processes-individual (*n* = 12)
- Descriptive Studies related to Adaptive Modes (*n* = 22)
- Descriptive Studies Related to Stimuli (*n* = 12)
- Descriptive Studies Related to Group Adaptation (*n* = 10)

OVERVIEW OF STUDIES USING DESCRIPTIVE DESIGN

A further understanding of the organization of studies for presentation is based on understanding the basic concepts of the RAM that are used in the proposition clusters. The RAM is generally considered a systems model. Persons or groups are viewed as adaptive systems with input, output, and internal processes. Basic to Roy's model are four concepts: the human being, environment, adaptation, and nursing. The human being is viewed as a holistic being that is continually interacting with the environment. The human being's goal through this interaction is adaptation. Nurses can promote adaptation by changing the environment or enhancing the person's ability to cope with it. The person as an individual adaptive system uses the cognator and regulator. The group uses the regulator and stabilizer. Environmental changes are viewed as stimuli to which the persons adapt with the help of nursing. The key concepts of the RAM used in the proposition cluster are defined in Box 4.3.

Roy (2009, p. 41) categorizes the "innate and acquired coping processes into two major subsystems, the regulator and the cognator." These subsystems respond to cope with changes in the internal and external environment. The regulator works primarily through neural, chemical, and endocrine systems. The cognator subsystem is a major coping process involving four cognitive–emotive processes: perceptual/information processing, learning, judgment, and emotion. The process of perception bridges the two subsystems (Roy & Roberts, 1981). It is the basic concept of persons using the cognator and regulator subsystem to respond to the changing environment that provided the structure for selecting studies reviewed in the section.

The next cluster of studies relates to the four adaptive modes described by Roy (2009): physiologic, self-concept, role function, and interdependence. The modes were originally conceptualized based on 500 samples of patient behavior to provide categories for assessing adaptive behavior. They have

---

BOX 4.3
DEFINITIONS OF KEY CONCEPTS OF THE RAM USED IN
PROPOSITION CLUSTERS

Internal coping processes of the person—Regulator subsystem that uses neural, chemical, and endocrine systems to maintain the system; cognator subsystem that uses four cognitive–emotive processes: perceptual/information processing, learning, judgment, and emotion to adapt and grow.

Adaptive modes—Four interrelated ways the person or group adapts: physiologic/physical, self-concept/group identity, role function, and interdependence.

Stimuli—A way of describing the environment; focal is the internal or external stimulus most immediately confronting the person or group; contextual are all other stimuli in the situation that contribute to the affect of the focal stimulus; residual are environmental factors, internal or external, that have an unclear affect.

Group adaptation—Groups of relating persons use internal coping processes of the stabilizer and the innovator to reach stability and to change; the stabilizer involves established structures, values, and daily activities to accomplish the primary purpose of the group and contribute to society; the innovator involves structures and processes for change and growth of human social systems.

---

proved useful in understanding people and the theoretical bases of the adaptive modes provide ways to describe research variables. The third set of studies relates to the stimuli, that is, the focal, contextual, and residual stimuli. Again these are abstract generalizations that help to classify the environment and also provide a basis for creating research variables. The last cluster of studies is about adapting groups. Possibly because this was a development of the model that occurred later in time, investigators have not used all the concepts of groups described by Roy. However, the team chose to report this set of studies as a group to clearly point out the different knowledge being created and to encourage investigators to further develop research with groups.

Description of Studies Related to Internal Coping Processes

Eleven of the twelve studies were conducted in the United States. The study that included data collection in other countries was one carried out in Sweden, Norway, and the United States, and was a part of a larger study (Kiehl & White, 2003). Studies were conducted in an institution or in the community. Institutional settings included hospitals, nursing homes, assisted-living facilities, and departments of health. Community settings encompassed outpatient hospital services and schools, as well as other agencies besides acute and chronic care facilities. Results showed that 58% of studies ($n = 7$) were conducted in community settings; mixed settings—institution and community—were used in 25% of the studies ($n = 3$); and for two studies (16%), the setting could not be identified from the information provided (see Table 4.1).

The populations of the studies included adults (ages 24 to 82), adolescents (ages 16 to 18), or a combination of age groups, such as adults and elders, women, mothers, parents of children with chronic conditions, spousal caregivers, primiparous women, postpartum women, postmenopausal women, marital partners with infertility, middle-age women, caregivers of elders with a terminal illness, end-stage renal disease patients, patients with cancer, and those with breast cancer. Results from the review of the studies indicated that over 90% were adults and of this percentage, 30% were chronically ill. One study involved adolescents, and a third involved all ages across the life span. Overall, most of the 12 studies were conducted on convenience samples (see Table 4.1).

The reviewers found the 12 studies contributed to nursing science and provided foundations to develop further research. From this knowledge generation the studies can contribute to meeting the challenges of a demanding and changing nursing practice. All of the 12 studies examined internal coping processes related to the individual.

Starner and Peters (2004) investigated the effect of the style of anger expression on blood pressure (BP) among adolescents. Using the RAM the authors hypothesized that adolescents' coping response to an anger-provoking stimuli would be through the behavior of anger expression. If the behavior was ineffective, the integrity of the person would be compromised as evidenced by increased BP. The study findings indicated that girls had an ineffective response of increased BP when scores were high on overall anger and anger suppression. The boys in the study may have adaptive behavioral responses, as high scores on anger in and anger out did not result in elevated BPs. The study also found that there is a relationship between the impostor phenomenon (cognator system) and perceptions of competency, which provided support for the RAM proposition that "the adequacy of cognator and regulator processes affect adaptive responses." This study also raises questions about gender differences in the effectiveness of anger coping responses.

TABLE 4.1

Descriptive Studies Related to Internal Coping Processes—Individual

Author(s) and Date	Purpose	Sample	Design	Findings
1. Starner and Peters (2004)	To investigate the effect of the style of anger expression on blood pressure (BP) among adolescents	Urban public high school seniors between 16 and 18 years of age ($n = 66$)	Descriptive, correlational	Hypertension was noted in 43% of the sample. Increased B/P was significantly related to increased body mass index
2. Dell, Weaver, Kozempel, and Barsevick (2007)	To compare pain and activity after two types of transverse rectus abdominis myocutaneous (TRAM) flap breast reconstruction	Women who had TRAM flap breast reconstruction ($n = 16$)	Descriptive, comparative cohort study	No differences in pain scores at baseline or 8 weeks or in activity limitation scores at baseline, 4 weeks, and 8 weeks. Abdominal pain scores were higher for the free TRAM flap group at 4 weeks. Educational information about managing pain and resuming usual activities was rated as very helpful
3. Domico (1997)	To determine the impact of social support, the meaning and purpose in life on the quality of life of spousal caregivers	Spousal caregivers to persons with dementia ($n = 104$)	Descriptive, correlational	Caregivers reported a moderately high perception of social support related to quality of life with an undifferentiated purpose and meaning-of-life impact on quality of life

| 4. Kiehl and White (2003) | Investigate the relationship between maternal adaptation during pregnancy and postpartum | Healthy primiparous women in Sweden, Norway, and the United States ($n = 147$) | Descriptive, survey | Prenatal identification with the motherhood role affected formation of maternal identity and confidence in ability to cope with motherhood and affected satisfaction with motherhood. Greater adaptation during pregnancy indicated greater adaptation postpartum |
| 5. Martin (1995) | To identify common postpartum problems and coping strategies | Postpartum women 2 to 8 weeks following delivery of a full-term healthy newborn ($n = 300$) | Descriptive, survey | The common postpartum problems identified in frequency of descending order were loss of sleep, being tired, feeling tense, increased household chores, feeling tied down, loss of income, concerns for personal appearance, inability to concentrate, feeling lonely, trouble coping with the mothering role, and changes in sexual feelings. The subjects reported being able to find adaptive coping strategies |

(continued)

TABLE 4.1

Descriptive Studies Related to Internal Coping Processes—Individual (*continued*)

Author(s) and Date	Purpose	Sample	Design	Findings
6. Burns (2004)	To identify the psychosocial and physiological problems and coping strategies of hemodialysis patients	Black adults with a diagnosis of end-stage renal disease (ESRD) requiring hemodialysis (*n* = 102)	Descriptive correlational	The number of perceived problems was associated with coping ability. Putting trust in God was the most frequently used coping strategy. Clients who reported fewer perceived problems reported higher self-esteem and better psychosocial adaptation
7. Morgan, Gaston-Johansson, and Mock (2006)	To explore the relationships of spiritual well-being, religious coping, and quality of life among women in the acute stages of coping with breast cancer	African American women receiving treatment for breast cancer (*n* = 11)	Descriptive, correlational	Positive religious coping was used more than negative coping. Increased spiritual well-being was associated with increased physical, emotional, and functional well-being. No significant correlations existed between medical characteristics and spiritual well-being
8. Taylor (1997)	To determine the relationships among coping, attitude toward menopause,	Women who are postmenopausal in southwest Arkansas (*n* = 194)	Descriptive correlational	A positive relationship existed among attitude toward menopause, coping style use; coping style effectiveness and

			attitude toward menopause. The more positive the attitude toward menopause, the higher the self-esteem
	self-esteem and demographic variables		
9. Ciambelli (1996)	To test the usefulness of midrange nursing theory of adaptation	Marital partners with infertility ($n = 104$)	Descriptive, correlational	Coping strategies and effectiveness were related to levels of physical demands, self-esteem, home and work functioning and social support. Gender differences existed in coping strategies, self-esteem, interpersonal support, reciprocity and subjective well-being
10. Tanyi and Werner (2003)	To examine the relationship between spirituality and self-perception with adjustment to end-stage renal disease (ESRD)	Women aged 24 to 82 receiving hemodialysis in a large metropolitan area ($n = 65$)	Descriptive, correlational	Increased spiritual well-being moderately correlated with a better adjustment to ESRD. As the self-perceived health variables (general health, symptoms, and feeling ill) improved, adjustment to ESRD improved as well

(continued)

TABLE 4.1
Descriptive Studies Related to Internal Coping Processes—Individual (continued)

Author(s) and Date	Purpose	Sample	Design	Findings
11. Hovey (2005)	To identify concerns and coping strategies of fathers parenting chronically ill children, and to compare them with father's perceptions of their wives concerns and coping strategies	Fathers of children with chronic conditions, from immunology, oncology, and pulmonary clinics of a large children's hospital in the Midwest ($n = 48$)	A descriptive design	Fathers saw themselves and their wives as concerned about their children's health, extra demands on their time, and not enough time alone with spouse. 98% perceived their wives as worn out compared to 73% who were concerned about that for themselves. 87% of fathers were concerned about the sexual relationship with their spouse; 72% perceived this to be of concern to their wives. Fathers reported they and their wives commonly used five coping strategies: trying to figure out what to do, looking at options, reading about the problem, getting information, and weighing choices. Reading about the problem was used more extensively by wives. Health care providers have a window of opportunity to intervene and facilitate positive adaptation at the time of diagnosis, when fathers are usually present.

90

| 12. Al-Atiyyat (2009) | To examine the relationships among cancer pain, coping strategies, and quality of life among Arab American adults with cancer, and to test the Adaptation to Cancer Pain (ACP) model | Arab American ($n = 170$) oncology outpatients with cancer pain recruited at a community site in a mid town metropolitan area, and five community sites in a Midwest metropolitan area | Descriptive, Cross-sectional, correlational | Reported pain scores of Arab Americans varied when compared to those of White Americans, African Americans, and Hispanic Americans. Statistically significant relationships were found between worst cancer pain and coping process. Worst cancer pain and coping strategies explained 27% variance in quality of life. Behavioral coping (analgesics use) correlated significantly and negatively with self-control |

A study by Dell, Weaver, Kozempel, and Barsevick (2007) used a descriptive comparative cohort design that compared pain and activity after two types of transverse rectus abdominis myocutaneous (TRAM) flap breast reconstruction. They found no differences in pain scores at baseline or 8 weeks or in activity limitation scores at baseline, 4 weeks, or 8 weeks. Abdominal pain scores were higher for the free TRAM flap group at 4 weeks. What emerged was the presence of pain as the patients attempted to adapt to activity and educational information about managing pain and resuming usual activities. Further, the findings showed that postoperative pain and activity limitations influence recovery. Findings from the study supported the RAM proposition that "Adaptation takes place over time as the regulator and cognator continue to process stimuli."

The impact of social support and of the meaning and purpose in life on the quality of life (QOL) of spousal caregivers was examined by Domico (1997). The researcher reported a moderately high perception of social support and QOL with an undifferentiated purpose and meaning of life. She further noted that the RAM was most helpful in choosing the appropriate variables and the methods of measurements used to assess the adaptive levels of the spousal caregivers. Findings included that the QOL was influenced by the focal stimulus of the caregiving role. High levels of social support increased caregiver adaptation. An increase in caregiver's age was correlated with an increase in perceived QOL, and a decrease in caregiver's health correlates with a decrease in QOL. The study is an example of support of the general RAM proposition that cognator information processing affects adaptive responses. This study is important because it encourages nurses' participation in support groups, the use of advanced assessments based on the RAM, and administration of the Quality of Life Index (QLI) as an indicator of the effectiveness of intervention for caregivers of dementia patients.

A study by Kiehl and White (2003) conducted in Norway, Sweden, and the United States investigated the relationship between the maternal adaptation during pregnancy and postpartum. Prenatal identification with the motherhood role affected formation of maternal identity and confidence in ability to cope with motherhood and affected satisfaction with motherhood. The author asserts that when individuals find stressors, by either volume or intensity, falling outside their "zone of adaptation," they do whatever is necessary to cope with the stressor until they bring about adaptation. These findings support the Roy adaptation proposition that "The characteristics of the internal and external stimuli influence the adequacy of cognator and emotional processes." An additional finding is that greater adaptation during pregnancy indicated greater adaptation postpartum.

The findings of Martin (1995) identified common postpartum problems and coping strategies. The common postpartum problems identified in frequency of descending order were loss of sleep, being tired, feeling tense, increased household chores, feeling tied down, loss of income, concerns for personal appearance, inability to concentrate, feeling lonely, trouble coping with the mothering role, and changes in sexual feelings. The subjects reported finding adaptive coping strategies as another example of support for the RAM proposition that "The adequacy of cognator and regulator processes will affect adaptive responses."

Burns (2004), using a descriptive correlational design, identified the psychosocial and physiological problems and coping strategies of hemodialysis patients. The findings of the study included that the number of perceived problems was associated with coping ability. Age, perceived problems, and socioeconomic status are directly related to coping ability. The level of trust in God was the most frequently used coping strategy with clients who reported fewer perceived problems, reported higher self-esteem, and better psychosocial adaptation. These findings support the RAM proposition that "cognator processes of perception and learning affect adaptive responses."

The relationships of spiritual well-being, religious coping, and QOL among African American women in the acute stages of coping with breast cancer were explored by Morgan et al. (2006). The researchers focused on the cognator coping subsystem exploring the involvement of religious coping and spiritual well-being in promoting adaptation to breast cancer. Positive religious coping was used more frequently than negative coping by this population. Increased spiritual well-being was associated with increased physical, emotional, and functional well-being, supporting the RAM proposition that specific cognator processes such as perception, information processing, and emotion affect adaptive responses.

No significant correlations existed between medical characteristics and spiritual well-being. The researchers state that nurses should recognize cultural differences among populations in order to promote coping strategies used by women from diverse ethnic backgrounds undergoing breast cancer treatments.

Taylor (1997) addressed the relationships among coping, attitude toward menopause, self-esteem, and demographic variables. Findings included a positive relationship among attitude toward menopause and coping style use; coping-style effectiveness and attitude toward menopause, that is, the more positive the attitude toward menopause, the higher the self-esteem. This finding supports the RAM proposition that adequacy of cognator processing affects adaptive responses.

In a study that tested the usefulness of midrange nursing theory of adaptation by Ciambelli (1996), coping strategies and effectiveness were related to levels of physical demands, self-esteem, home and work functioning, and social support. Using a cross-sectional design the study tested nine hypotheses developed from a midrange theory derived from the RAM and previous research with marital partners with fertility problems. The variables included were coping strategies, physical demands, self-esteem, home and work functioning, social support and conflict, subjective well-being, and marital satisfaction. Findings included that the nature of fertility problems influences adaptation. The researcher also reports that she found that infertile partners with more stress from physical demands, social conflict, and lower self-esteem tend to use avoidance, pessimism, and emotional expression as coping strategies. Her results also show that gender affects coping strategies in infertile partners; women in infertile partnerships report lower self-esteem. She also found that there are gender differences in adaptation to fertility problems by fertile partners. The findings may add to understanding of how the cognator activity of information processing varies with gender in given situations. The model tested is important for practice. Further directions for model-based research were identified, and further testing is indicated to identify implications for clinical research and practice.

Tanyi and Warner (2003) examined the relationship between spirituality and self-perception with adjustment to end-stage renal disease. She reported that spiritual well-being correlated moderately with a better adjustment to ESRD. As the self-perceived health variables, that is, general health, symptoms, and feeling ill, improved, adjustment to ESRD improved as well. This supports the general role of perception in adaptation.

Hovey (2005) studied 48 fathers of children with chronic conditions to compare their concerns and coping strategies with their perceptions of their wives' concerns and coping strategies. Fathers saw themselves and their wives as concerned about their children's health, with extra demands on their time and not enough time alone with spouse. There were some differences in the fathers' perceptions of their concerns and of their wives' concerns. For example, 98% perceived their wives as worn out compared to 73% who were concerned about that for themselves. Also reading about the problem was a coping strategy perceived to be used more often by wives. The researcher noted that health care providers have a window of opportunity to intervene and facilitate positive adaptation at the time of diagnosis, when fathers are usually present.

In a study that examined the relationships among cancer pain, coping strategies, and QOL, Al-Atiyyat (2009) included 170 Arab American patients recruited at oncology outpatient sites. The findings of this cross-sectional, correlational descriptive study noted that the reported pain scores varied when compared to those of White Americans, African Americans, and Hispanic Americans. Significant relationships were found between worst cancer pain and coping processes.

Description of Studies Concerning Adaptive Modes

According to Roy, viewing the person as an adaptive system is to see an individual who is constantly influenced by his or her environment; people have the opportunity to respond to their environment and adapt, or fail at adapting. As noted previously, the four modes of adaptation according to Roy (2009) are:

1. Physiologic adaptation involves physical and chemical processes in the function and activities of living organisms; the underlying need is physiologic integrity as seen in the degree of wholeness achieved through adaptation to change in basic needs such as oxygenation, nutrition, elimination, activity and rest, and protection as well as complex processes of the senses; fluid, electrolyte, and acid–base balance; neurologic function; and endocrine function.
2. Self-concept adaptation focuses on psychic and spiritual integrity and on the sense of unity, meaning, and purposefulness of people in the universe; the composite of beliefs and feelings that the person holds about the self at a given time, which is formed from internal perceptions and perceptions of others.
3. Role-function adaptation begins with positions that individuals occupy in society, fulfilling the need for social integrity; it is to know self in relation to others; role-function adaptation is defined by a set of expectations and how the individual behaves toward others in related positions.
4. Interdependence adaptation includes the close relationships of people; focusing on interactions related to giving and receiving love, value, and respect; need for relational integrity, the feeling of security in nurturing relationships.

Of the 22 studies described under adaptive modes (95%), 21 were conducted in the United States and 1 was conducted in Taiwan. Studies were carried out in an institution or in the community. Institutional settings included hospitals, nursing homes, and assisted-living facilities. Community settings encompassed homes, outpatient hospital services, and schools, as well as other agencies besides acute and chronic care facilities.

Results showed that 64% of studies ($n = 14$) were conducted in community settings. Mixed settings, institution, and community were used in 23% of the studies ($n = 5$), and for three studies (14%), the setting could not be identified from the information provided in the study (see Table 4.2).

The populations of the studies included community-dwelling women with urinary incontinence; adult women with a diagnosis of HIV; residents of senior housing; service members with war injuries; adults who sustained extremity amputation; parents whose adult children died a traumatic death; women in the 6 weeks following coronary artery bypass graft (CABG) surgery; primiparous and postpartum women; adolescents; individuals with ostomies; and individuals with heart failure (HF), diabetes, and cancer. Most of the studies were conducted on convenience samples. The reviewers found that the 22 studies are empirical and related to the RAM. Meeting the screening criteria, they provided a basis for further analysis in this project to meet the new challenges of nursing practice (see Table 4.2).

Gallagher (1998) posed four research questions to investigate the existence of a relationship between urogenital distress and psychosocial impact of urinary incontinence (UI) in community-living women over 60 years of age ($n = 17$). The researcher founded a strong positive relationship between urogenital distress and the psychosocial impact of UI. Physical activity, travel, social relationships, and emotional health are negatively affected by the distress caused by UI. Loneliness relates to satisfaction with living arrangements. The relationship between adaptation to the stimulus of UI and behaviors in physiological, role function, interdependence, and self-concept modes was also supported.

The immunologic and nutritional responses of women with human immune virus (HIV) were examined by Orsi et al. (1997). The researchers reported that the RAM was a useful guide for this study because the model provided for the continual holistic assessment of the HIV-positive women to help maintain their health. They also reported that the use of the RAM helped them to discover coping strategies that contribute to adaptation in the four modes. The small cohort pilot study supports the proposition of the RAM that "Adaptation in one mode is affected by adaptation in other modes through cognator and regulator connectives." The findings report coping strategies that can be used in clinical practice.

Modrcin-Talbott, Pullen, Ehrenberge, Zandstra, and Muenchen (1998a), using a descriptive correlational study, examined the relationship of levels of self-esteem and selected variables in adolescents in an outpatient psychiatric treatment program ($n = 140$). The research question of whether the level of self-esteem differs by age group, gender, exercise participation, and smoking was addressed using analysis of variance (ANOVA). The results show that self-esteem in this clinical adolescent sample was higher

TABLE 4.2
Descriptive Studies Related to Adaptive Modes

Author(s) and Date	Purpose	Sample	Design	Findings
1. Gallagher (1998)	To discern the existence of a relationship between urogenital distress and psychosocial impact of urinary incontinence (UI)	Community-living women over age 60 experiencing UI at least once a week (*n* = 17)	Descriptive, correlational	A strong positive relationship exists between urogenital distress and the psychosocial impact of UI. The relationship between adaptation to the stimulus of UI and behaviors in physiological, role function, interdependence, and self-concept modes was supported
2. Orsi, Grandy, Tax, and McCorkle (1997)	To examine the immunologic and nutritional responses of women with human immune virus (HIV)	Adult women with diagnoses of HIV (*n* = 13)	Descriptive, survey	The women's nutritional and protection responses were judged to be relatively adapted
3. Modrcin-Talbott, Pullen, Zandstra, Ehrenberger, and Muenchen (1998b)	To evaluate adolescent's self-esteem and how smoking, exercise, depression, anger, and parent use of alcohol affected self-esteem	Male and female adolescents (*n* = 77)	Descriptive, correlational	Lower self-esteem was seen in older adolescents who were more depressed and did not exercise

(continued)

TABLE 4.2
Descriptive Studies Related to Adaptive Modes (*continued*)

Author(s) and Date	Purpose	Sample	Design	Findings
4. Modrcin-Talbott, Pullen, Ehrenberger, Zandstra, and Muenchen (1998a).	To examine adolescent's self-esteem and identify factors that correlate with self-esteem	Male and female adolescents receiving outpatient mental health services ($n = 140$)	Descriptive, correlational	Exercise was significantly and positively related to self-esteem. Self-esteem was related to age. Older adolescents had lower scores. There was no relationship between self-esteem and gender
5. Salisbury (2005)	To explore the sexual awareness, body image, and self-esteem of individuals with ostomies	Individuals with ostomies from two different support groups ($n = 18$)	Descriptive, correlational (pilot)	Disturbances existed among sexual awareness, body image, and self-esteem. Males had higher scores on some subscales related to body image, self-esteem, and sexual awareness
6. Thomas (2007)	To gain an understanding of the influence of self-concept on adherence to prescribed regimens in individuals with heart failure	Adults diagnosed with HF ($n = 97$)	Descriptive, correlational	Subjects were more challenged than threatened by health regimens and had high adherence to medications and diet. Inverse relationships were found between adherence and threat to the self-concept mode

				Positive relationships were found between adherence and challenge to the self-concept mode
7. DiMattio and Tulman (2003)	To describe the influence of comorbidity, household composition, fatigue, and surgical pain on functional status following coronary artery bypass graft surgery	Women in the 6 weeks following CABG surgery ($n = 42$)	Descriptive, correlational	Significant increases in overall functional status over 6 weeks, with significant increases between each time period. At 6 weeks functional status had not returned to presurgery levels and fatigue and pain were still present
8. Samarel et al. (1998)	To test the clinical impression that cancer patients benefit from contact with other cancer patients	Women who had previously participated in a study of social support and educational groups ($n = 70$)	Descriptive, correlational	Positive attitudes toward breast cancer and study participation emerged. Breast cancer and group participation affected adaptation in each of the four modes of the RAM
9. Chiang (1998)	To examine the direct and interactive relationships of stimuli and adaptive modes to help-seeking behaviors and quality of life	Married-cohabiting women with breast cancer ($n = 102$)	Descriptive, correlational	The need for social support, the number and interaction among individuals in the social network, and the number of symptoms contribute to help-seeking behaviors and satisfaction with social support

(continued)

TABLE 4.2
Descriptive Studies Related to Adaptive Modes (*continued*)

Author(s) and Date	Purpose	Sample	Design	Findings
10. Arcamone (2005)	To describe and compare postpartum adaptation to motherhood as assessed by the RAM modes, 2 weeks after childbirth	Three groups of primiparous women who gave vaginal birth to healthy infants; two groups attended childbirth classes with or without baby care, and one group without classes (*n* = 158)	Descriptive, comparative cohort	There were no differences among the three groups in overall adaptation. Significant differences existed among the groups on the pain scores and on age, race, education, and type of insurance
11. Black (2004)	To investigate the relationships of psychological responses, well-being, availability of social support, and stress to the progression of pregnancy-induced hypertension (PIH)	Postpartum women diagnosed with PIH during pregnancy (*n* = 100)	Descriptive, correlational, comparative cohort	On the day of birth, physiological symptoms, self-monitoring, well-being, stress, and perceived social support did not accurately predict worsening PIH. Women with worsening PIH did not report significantly lower perceived social support, sense of well-being, or self-efficacy for self-monitoring than women with mild PIH

12. Black (2007)	To investigate the relationships of psychological stress, preeclampsia/gestational hypertension symptoms, confidence in self-monitoring, well-being, and perceived social support with preeclampsia/gestational hypertension disease progression in outpatient women	$n = 100$ postpartum women with preeclampsia/gestational hypertension	Descriptive, correlational	Women with worsening/severe preeclampsia/gestational hypertension reported a significantly higher number of symptoms than women with mild preeclampsia/gestational hypertension. Psychological stress was significantly higher in women with worsening/severe preeclampsia/gestational hypertension. There were no differences in well-being, self-confidence in self-monitoring, or perceived social support between women with mild preeclampsia/gestational hypertension and those with worsening preeclampsia/gestational hypertension
13. Ryan (1996)	To determine the relationships among loneliness, social support, depression and cognitive status	Residents of senior housing over age 60 ($n = 74$)	Descriptive, correlational	No significant relationships were found among the variables of loneliness, social support, depression, and cognitive status

(continued)

TABLE 4.2

Descriptive Studies Related to Adaptive Modes (*continued*)

Author(s) and Date	Purpose	Sample	Design	Findings
14. Willoughby (1995)	To examine the extent to which social support, personal resources, coping, and psychosocial adjustment to illness influenced metabolic control	Adult women with diabetes (*n* = 115)	Descriptive, correlational	Social support was positively related to personal resources, coping was associated with fewer problems in psychosocial and illness adjustment. Better adjustment was associated with better metabolic control
15. Grimes (1997)	To examine the relationship of daily hassles, life-change events, and pain to hopelessness	Adult men (*n* = 37 and women (*n* = 40) patients with cancer ages 21 to 89 (*n* = 77)	Descriptive, correlational	Pain was the only predictor of hopelessness. Daily hassles, or life-change events did not predict hopelessness
16. Huang (2002)	To describe the characteristics of postpartum sleep and daytime sleepiness and examine the interrelationships among these characteristics in	First-time mothers at 2 to 3 weeks postpartum (*n* = 189)	Descriptive, correlational	Only the variable of co-sleep practices had statistically significant contributions to both sleep quality and perceived sleep debt, after controlling other predictors. Sleep quality was not a prominent contributor to any of the four types

Author (year)	Purpose	Sample	Design	Findings
	first-time mothers early postpartum in Taiwan			of daytime sleepiness. Mothers' perceptions of sleep debt were a significant contributor to the type of daytime sleepiness related to interdependence mode
17. Sabatini (2003)	To determine the relationship among exercise and adaptation to aging in older women	Community-dwelling women (n = 107)	Descriptive, correlational	Exercise was positively related to health status, functional status, and self-esteem, but not to satisfaction with interpersonal relationships
18. Kowalski (2007)	To identify differences found in self-reports of pain intensity, information-seeking behavior, and adjustment between Japanese American and European American men treated for prostate cancer	Japanese American and European American men (N = 89) living in Hawaii or North America who had received or are currently receiving treatment for prostate cancer	Descriptive, correlational	No significant differences in self-reported pain or adjustment when comparing Japanese American and European American men treated for prostate cancer. Differences in information-seeking with European American tending toward more open communication
19. Aktan (2010)	To explore relationships between functional	Pregnant and postpartum women, ages	Descriptive, correlational	This group had relatively low levels of anxiety and high levels of social support

(continued)

TABLE 4.2

Descriptive Studies Related to Adaptive Modes (*continued*)

Author(s) and Date	Purpose	Sample	Design	Findings
	status after childbirth and related concepts	19 to 40 years, with no complications ($n = 177$)		and functional status after childbirth. The State–Trait Anxiety Inventory (STAI) demonstrated coefficient as from .90 to .93, the Pre-Review Questionnaire (PRQ) 85-Part 2 as .87 to .93, and the Inventory of Functional Status after Childbirth (IFSAC) .90. The relationship between state anxiety in the postpartum period and IFSAC ($r = -.204$, $p = .008$) was significant. Additional significant findings among social support, anxiety, and subscales of the IFSAC were found
20. Bingham et al. (2009)	To assess sleep disturbance and posttraumatic stress disorder (PTSD) symptoms in injured service members with extremity	Service members, all but one were males; age range 19 to 47; most were active combat injuries in Iraq;	Comparative descriptive	Sleep disturbance for 3 or more nights/week was reported by 66%; the most frequent sleep disturbance characteristics were decreased quality of sleep ((95%) and awakenings

in mid sleep (95%). Other characteristics included trouble initiating sleep (89%), early awakenings (86%), and decreased quantity of sleep (71%). Significant PTSD symptoms were found in 22 of the injured service members. As compared to service members without PTSD symptoms, those service members with symptoms reported significantly poorer sleep quality, more difficulty initiating sleep, and daytime sleepiness

trauma sustained during service in Operation Enduring Freedom (OEF) or Operation Iraqi Freedom (OIF)

45 had primarily orthopedic injuries (including 30 who had undergone one or multiple amputations), 36 had primarily burn injuries, and 4 had a combination of both orthopedic and burn injuries (n = 85)

21. Santarlasci (2009)

To explore the extent to which pain, functional ability, depression, and social support predicted the ability to cope and return

Convenience sample of male and female patients, 18 years or older who had sustained a lower extremity amputation as a

Quantitative, descriptive, correlational

Pain, functional ability, depression, and social support demonstrated no relationship with coping. More than half of the study sample had at least one co-morbidity; therefore,

(continued)

TABLE 4.2
Descriptive Studies Related to Adaptive Modes (*continued*)

Author(s) and Date	Purpose	Sample	Design	Findings
	to work for persons with lower extremity amputation	result of an injury or illness (amputation could have occurred at any time in patient's life) (*n* = 101)		the most evident need is for education of the public as a whole to understand the significance and risk of hypertension, diabetes, and renal disease
22. Baden (2004)	To describe the grief experience of parents of adult children who died a traumatic death using the RAM and the Grief Experience Inventory in the second year of bereavement	33 parents (13 men and 20 women); mean age 52.9 years	Descriptive, correlational	Strong positive correlation between physiological mode scores and self-concept scores; between physiological and interdependence; and self-concept and interdependence; though not statistically significant, indicated the men and women grieve differently

than the researchers expected for a population receiving outpatient mental health treatment. Exercise was significantly and positively related to self-esteem. Self-esteem was related to age and it was the older adolescents who had lower scores. There was no relationship between self-esteem and gender.

In another study with a broader focus, Modrcin-Talbott, Pullen, Zandstra, Ehrenberge, and Muenchen (1998b) evaluated adolescent's self-esteem and how smoking, exercise, depression, anger, and parent use of alcohol affected self-esteem ($n = 77$). The researchers reported a lack of a significant relationship among parental alcohol use, anger, and self-esteem. The relationships among the variables remain inconclusive. They state that a larger sample size may be needed to discover these relationships. The authors noted that anger may be an adaptive response depending on the situation.

The sexual awareness, body image, and self-esteem of individuals with ostomies were explored by Salisbury (2004). Using the RAM the ostomy was viewed as the focal stimulus, which may potentiate ineffective adaptive responses or behaviors resulting in disruptions of role function, self-concept, or physical aspects of the individual's life. The author reported that males had higher scores on some subscales of body image, self-esteem, and sexual awareness than females. Despite some weaknesses such as sample size, this study showed that pre- or postoperative nursing assessment based on theory helps to identify the individual's adaptive responses and the nurse can plan for enhancing better adaptation. Salisbury asserts that studies addressing how sexual awareness, body image, and self-esteem are affected by an ostomy need to be conducted with larger and different populations.

A study by Thomas (2007) examined the influence of self-concept on adherence to prescribed regimens in individuals with HF. The RAM was used to examine the relationships among the identified components of the self-concept and to what extent aspects of self-concept could predict adherence to health regimens. The researcher reported that subjects were more challenged than threatened by health regimens and had high adherence to medications and diet. Inverse relationships were found between adherence and threat to body sensation, self-ideal, and self-consistency. Positive relationships were found among adherence and challenge to body sensation, body image, self-consistency, self-ideal, and moral–ethical–spiritual self. Challenge to self-concept accounted for 13% of the variance in adherence.

DiMattio and Tulman (2003) described the changes in functional status and the influence of co-morbidity, household composition, fatigue, and surgical pain in women during the first 6 weeks at home following coronary artery bypass surgery. The researchers reported that women experienced increase in functional status over 6 weeks. The most significant changes for many role activities occur between 2 and 4 weeks with improvement in the role activity of work occurring between 4 and 6 weeks. Most women perceived an improvement in their functioning and most experienced less fatigue and pain during the first 6 weeks. By 6 weeks after discharge, women were able to perform many activities that they performed prior to CABG surgery. However, an important finding was that they did not return to their previous level of performance. Women experienced the most role conflict when resuming household activities because of the desire to resume these activities earlier than they were physically able; others experienced dissatisfaction with the help they received.

Samarel et al. (1998) reported the findings from a quantitative analysis of responses to structured interviews with a sub sample of the women who participated in an experimental study. The aim was to test the clinical impression that cancer patients benefit from contact with other cancer patients. Positive attitudes toward breast cancer and study participation emerged. In particular, breast cancer and group participation affected adaptation in each of the four modes of the RAM. The authors conclude that participation in groups can contribute to adaptive physiological, self-concept, role function, and interdependence-mode responses.

Using a secondary analysis, Chiang (1998) examined the direct and interactive relationships of stimuli and adaptive modes to help-seeking behaviors and QOL. Stimuli were external (social network characteristics and social support) and internal (age, severity of symptoms, and satisfaction with social support). Stepwise multiple regressions were used to test the research hypotheses. Need for social support had a direct effect on help seeking. The number and interaction among individuals in the social network, and the number of symptoms contributed to help-seeking behaviors and satisfaction with social support. Self-care had a direct effect on QOL. This study demonstrated that nurses need to be aware of women's levels of social need and help them to increase the number of persons in their social network, and that they need to be aware of women with less education who may not seek help.

A study by Arcamone (2005) described postpartum adaptation to motherhood by assessing the four modes of the RAM 2 weeks after childbirth and compared the adaptation with prenatal preparation. The variables measures were perineal pain, confidence in the ability to cope with the tasks of motherhood, satisfaction with motherhood and infant care, and quality of relationship with husband. She used three groups of primiparous women who gave birth vaginally to healthy infants. Two groups attended childbirth classes with or without baby care, and one group was without classes ($n = 158$). There were no differences among the three groups in overall adaptation. Significant differences existed among the groups on the pain scores and on age, race, education, and type of insurance.

Black (2004, 2007) conducted a dissertation study and then published her work in a journal. The description of this work is combined here although the studies are listed as two published works in Table 4.2. The author investigated the relationships of physiological responses, sense of well-being, self-efficacy for self-monitoring, perceived availability of social support, and perceived stress to the progression of pregnancy-induced hypertension (PIH), and compared women whose disorder is mild with those whose PIH worsened or became severe. Study findings included that women with worsening or severe preeclampsia/gestational hypertension had a higher number of physical symptoms and psychological stress than women with mild preeclampsia/gestational hypertension. No differences were found in well-being, self-confidence in self-monitoring, or perceived social support.

The relationships among and between loneliness, social support, depression, and cognitive status on adults over 60 living in senior housing in a metropolitan area were examined by Ryan (1996). Life satisfaction and ability to perform activities of daily living were also measured to determine their relationships with the main variables. No significant relationships were found among the variables of loneliness, and only social support seems to help depression in some of the participants.

A study by Willoughby (1995) examined the extent to which social support, personal resources, coping styles, metabolic control, and psychosocial adjustment to illness differ among women with diabetes living in different types of household structures. A second purpose was to explore the influence of social support, personal resources, coping styles, and household structure on the psychosocial adjustment and metabolic control of women with diabetes. Multiple analyses of variance showed that women living in varying household structures differ in both personal resources and coping skills. Further, those women with divergent levels of metabolic control differed in both personal resources and psychosocial adjustment to illness. The results affirm the importance of contextual variables on adjustment and control for women with diabetes.

Grimes (1997) recruited adults with cancer ($n = 77$) to examine the relationship of daily hassles, life-change events, and pain to hopelessness. Pain was the only predictor of hopelessness in ambulatory cancer subjects. The researcher examined and identified the relationships of three stimuli to hopelessness. Using multiple regression a positive relationship was found between pain and hopelessness. The author reported that daily hassles, or life-change events, did not predict hopelessness. Grimes reported that although results supported the contention that pain and hopelessness were related, this study demonstrated that examination of stressors in isolation does not contribute to the knowledge of the impact of stressors in combination with many others. The researcher asserted that to successfully influence a stressor, the nurse must identify the influence of other stressors.

In a study of first-time mothers in early postpartum in Taiwan ($n = 189$), Huang (2002) aimed to describe the characteristics of sleep and daytime sleepiness in this sample and to examine the interrelationships among sleep characteristics. Only the variable of co-sleep practices had statistically significant contributions to both sleep quality and perceived sleep debt, after controlling other predictors. Sleep quality was not a prominent contributor to any of the four types of daytime sleepiness. Mothers' perceptions of sleep debt were a significant contributor to one type of daytime sleepiness in the interdependence mode.

A study by Sabatini (2003) investigated whether a relationship exists between exercise and adaptation to aging in older women who live in the community. Gathering a convenience sample ($n = 107$), the author used Pearson's correlation to test the relationships of exercise with four variables. In her findings the researcher reports that exercise was positively related to health status, functional status, and self-esteem, but not to satisfaction with interpersonal relationships.

The purpose of the study by Kowalski (2007) was to identify differences in self-reported pain intensity, information-seeking behavior, and adjustment between Japanese American and European American men treated for prostate cancer. The sample of this descriptive correlational study included Japanese American and European American men ($n = 89$) living in Hawaii or North America. There were no significant differences in self-reported pain or adjustment between the two groups. In information seeking European American men tended toward more open communication.

Aktan (2010) explored the relationships between functional status, related to the role function adaptive mode, after childbirth with pregnant and postpartum women without complications ($n = 177$). The findings of this descriptive correlational study showed that this group had relatively low levels of anxiety and high levels of social support and functional status after childbirth. The relationship between state anxiety in the postpartum period and functional status was significant. Additional significant findings were found among social support, anxiety, and subscales of the functional status scale.

A study by Bingham, Young-McCaughan, and Miaskowski (2009) assessed sleep disturbance and posttraumatic stress disorder symptoms in injured service members with extremity trauma sustained in Operation Enduring Freedom or Operation Iraqi Freedom. The 45 members of the Army or Marines had primarily orthopedic injuries. The injuries included

30 service members who had undergone one or multiple amputations; 36 had primarily burn injuries; and 4 had a combination of both orthopedic and burn injuries. Sleep disturbance for 3 or more nights each week were reported by 66% of the participants. The most frequent sleep-disturbance characteristics were decreased quality of sleep ((95%) and awakenings in mid sleep (95%)). Other characteristics included trouble initiating sleep (89%), early awakenings (86%), and decreased quantity of sleep (71%). Significant PTSD symptoms were found in 22 of the injured service members. As compared to service members without PTSD symptoms, those service members with symptoms reported significantly poorer sleep quality, more difficulty initiating sleep, and daytime sleepiness.

Santarlasci (2009) explored the extent to which pain, functional ability, depression, and social support predicted the ability to cope and return to work for persons with lower extremity amputation. In this study the adults had the amputation as a result of injury or illness that occurred at any time in their lives. Findings showed that pain, functional ability, depression, and social support demonstrated no relationship with coping. More than half of the study sample had at least one co-morbidity, showing the need for education of the public to understand the risks of hypertension, diabetes, and renal disease.

To describe the grief experience of parents of adult children who died a traumatic death, Baden (2004) used 33 parents (13 men and 20 women) to fill out a Grief Experience Inventory in the second year of bereavement. The author found strong positive correlations between physiological mode scores and self-concept scores, between physiological and interdependence, and between self-concept and interdependence. They summarize that though not statistically significant, the findings provided some indication that men and women grieve differently.

Description of Studies Related to Stimuli

A stimulus is input that produces a reaction. According to the RAM, the environment can be looked at as stimuli that are constantly changing and to which people adapt. At times it is a health condition that the person had to handle to reach higher levels of adaptation. Sometimes it is events or people surrounding the health situation that requires responses and adapting. Any of these factors can be considered stimuli. The three classes of the stimuli were described previously. The 12 studies described here mainly looked at focal and contextual stimuli.

Eight studies (67%) were conducted in the United States, whereas studies also were conducted in Zimbabwe, Thailand, and two in Canada.

One study was a part of a larger study, one study was a secondary analysis of archival data, and one study was a retrospective chart review. Studies were conducted in institutions or in the community. Institutional settings included hospitals, nursing homes, and assisted-living facilities. Community settings encompassed homes, outpatient hospital services and schools, as well as other agencies besides acute and chronic care facilities. Results showed that 50% of studies (n = 5) were conducted in community settings. Mixed settings—institution and community—were used in 30% of the studies (n = 3). The hospital was the setting for 30% of the studies (n = 3) and for one study the setting could not be identified from the information included.

The populations of the studies included adults with epilepsy, women who had hysterectomy, children (ages 7–12) and adults diagnosed with multiple sclerosis (MS), cancer patients, community-dwelling women, adult women with diagnosis of type 2 diabetes, teen parents, patients on medical units, caregivers of children in body casts, archived medical records of spinal-cord-injured patients, and medical records of patients with spontaneous labor. Three of the 12 studies obtained their data from existing medical records. Overall convenience samples were used (see Table 4.3).

Saburi et al. (2006) as a part of a larger study in Harare, Zimbabwe, examined the effects of epilepsy on the QOL of adults who have taken medication for their condition for at least 3 years (n = 66). The sample was a convenience sample. The instrument used to test QOL in epilepsy was composed of 12 open-ended questions using the four adaptive modes of the RAM. Findings indicated epilepsy adversely affected QOL only in the role-function mode and that the physiologic, self-concept, and interdependence modes were not affected. The researchers also report that achieving control of seizures enhances QOL. The RAM helped to identify family reactions as positively correlated to the QOL of adults with epilepsy.

Using a descriptive exploratory design, Sheppard and Cunnie (1996) investigated whether diuresis was greater following hysterectomy for conditions that could cause obstruction of the urinary tract than for other conditions that necessitate hysterectomy. A retrospective chart review of 140 posthysterectomy patients was conducted. The sample records were divided into one nonobstructive and three potentially obstructive conditions for surgery. A ratio of total intake divided by total output was devised for each patient and contrasted between the groups. Statistically significant differences were reported between two of the obstructive groups and the nonobstructive group. Results of this research indicated that certain obstructive conditions such as uterine prolapse and endometrial cancer increased the risk of hypovolemia. The researcher stated that

TABLE 4.3

Descriptive Studies Related to Stimuli

Author(s) and Date	Purpose	Sample	Design	Findings
1. Saburi, Mapanga, and Mapanga (2006)	To examine the effects of epilepsy on quality of life	Adults with epilepsy for at least 3 years taking medications (*n* = 66)	Descriptive, correlational	Epilepsy adversely affected QOL only in the role-function mode; the physiologic, self-concept, and interdependence modes were not affected
2. Sheppard and Cunnie (1996)	To investigate whether or not diuresis is greater following a hysterectomy for conditions that cause enlargement of the uterus such as leiomyoma, endometrial cancer, and uterine prolapse than for conditions without uterine enlargement	Women who had a hysterectomy for conditions that cause enlargement of the uterus such as leiomyoma, endometrial cancer, and uterine prolapse and women who had a hysterectomy for conditions without uterine enlargement (*n* = 140 charts)	Descriptive, correlational, retrospective chart review	Women who had hysterectomies for the identified conditions that cause uterine enlargement had significantly higher postoperative urine outputs than women who had hysterectomies for other conditions
3. LeBlanc and Morin (2004)	To compare depressive symptoms in children with attention deficit hyperactivity	Children ages 7 to 12 years with and without ADHD (*n* = 68)	Descriptive, comparative	Depressive symptoms were higher in children with ADHD. There were no significant

(continued)

TABLE 4.3
Descriptive Studies Related to Stimuli (*continued*)

Author(s) and Date	Purpose	Sample	Design	Findings
	disorder (ADHD) to those in healthy children and to explore the influence of individual and family factors on level of depression			effects of individual or family factors on severity of depression
4. Fawcett, Sidney, Riley, Lawless, and Hanson (1996)	To explore the relationship of alternative health therapies and symptom severity to functional status in adults with multiple sclerosis	Adults diagnosed with MS (*n* = 16)	Descriptive, correlational	All respondents reported seeking traditional medical treatment and at least one alternative therapy. The greater the number of therapies used, the lower the functional status. MS symptoms were less severe following use of alternative therapies
5. Poirier (2007)	To determine the factors affecting the performance of usual activities during radiation treatment	Cancer patients (*n* = 77)	Descriptive, survey	The ability to perform activities decreased over time with fatigue being the main factor

Study	Purpose	Sample	Design	Findings
6. Newman (2005)	To examine the relationship between health and self-esteem to functional status and to develop nursing interventions to attain optimal functional status while caring for children in body casts	Caregivers of children in a body cast; children were divided into two groups by age ($n = 30$)	Descriptive, correlational (pilot)	Parents of children aged 3 to 12 years of age experienced more changes than parents of younger children. Caregiver comments included lack of information provided by some nurses after the cast was applied
7. Sander (2004)	To explore the functional status of people with spinal cord injuries	Archived records of spinal-cord-injured people ($n = 782$)	Descriptive, secondary analysis of archival data, instrument development	People with tetraplegia were significantly less functional than people with paraplegia. The use of the Modified Functional Independence Measure (FIM) indicated the need for continued revision
8. Platner (2004)	To determine whether moon phase affects the rate of spontaneous labor	Medical records of patients with spontaneous labor ($n = 100$)	Descriptive, retrospective review	There was no difference in the rate of spontaneous labor for the different moon phases
9. John (1997)	To determine whether perceptions of QOL change over time in patients with	Cancer patients with stages IIIa or IIIb NSCLC receiving XRT ($n = 23$)	Descriptive, comparative cohort study	Although QOL declined significantly during XRT, it improved following XRT to a higher level than prior to

(continued)

TABLE 4.3
Descriptive Studies Related to Stimuli (*continued*)

Author(s) and Date	Purpose	Sample	Design	Findings
	non-small cell lung cancer (NSCLC) receiving curative radiation therapy (XRT) alone or in combination with other treatment modalities			treatment, and then returned to a pretreatment level
10. Harner (2001)	Compare outcomes of teenage pregnancy fathered by adult men to those fathered by peer-age boys; prenatal and obstetric outcomes were explored	Teenagers under 18 at time of conception who presented to the antepartum/ postpartum floor at University of Pennsylvania Medical Center (*n* = 86)	Descriptive, comparative	Study yielded few statistically significant results, i.e., age of father not a factor in prenatal and obstetric outcomes. Also found no significant difference between adult men vs. peer-age boys and outcomes such as violence, abuse, prenatal care or gestational age at birth. One difference was breastfeeding was significantly more common among those with peer-age fathers vs. adult fathers

Study	Purpose	Sample	Design	Findings
11. Siripitayakunkit et al. (2008)	To examine the causal relationships among personal, psychological, and health care system factors that contribute to integrating lifestyle in Thai women with type 2 diabetes	Women with type 2 diabetes from 3 hospitals in Bangkok, Thailand ($n = 490$)	Descriptive, correlational	Personal (education income), psychological (family and friend social support), and health system factors (quality of patient–provider relationships) supported the relationships proposed by Roy's conceptual model of nursing. Education had a nonsignificant negative and direct effect on perceived integrating lifestyle and had a slightly moderate positive direct effect on perceived demands of diabetes
12. Lynch (2007)	To explore and describe the visitation preferences of patients on acute medical units	Adults hospitalized on three general medical units in a large tertiary care hospital in Manitoba, Canada ($n = 128$)	Descriptive, correlational	Visiting hours do matter to a patient in a hospitalized environment. Age is a significant factor in influencing visiting preferences. Younger patients prefer more frequent visiting. Women are more likely to experience greater perceived stress than men in hospital. Married couples were less likely to perceive social situations of low social support, and older patients were more likely to perceive experiences of low social support

early recognition of a patient's volume status is essential to ensure timely nursing intervention and maintain physiological homeostasis.

In a study by LeBlanc and Morin (2004), depressive symptoms in children with attention deficit hyperactivity disorder (ADHD) were compared to those in healthy children and the influence of individual and family factors on level of depression were explored. The participants included children ages 7 to 12 years with and without ADHD ($n = 68$). Family factors were viewed as focal and contextual stimuli. There were no significant effects of the contextual stimuli of education and working status of parents on levels of depression. Results indicated that depressive symptoms were higher in children with ADHD.

The Fawcett et al. (1996) study was a pilot study that explored the relationship of alternative health therapies and symptom severity to functional status in adults with multiple sclerosis and was used to plan a larger study. The authors reported the effects of the focal stimulus of alternative therapies and their resulting responses in each of the four modes. The role-function response was self-reported functional status, whereas the physiological-mode response was the self-rated severity of MS symptoms. The researchers reported moderate correlation among alternative therapies, functional status, and the improvement of severity of symptoms on adaptation to MS. There was a relatively high correlation between severity of symptoms and functional status, showing that adaptive-mode responses are interrelated as proposed by the RAM.

Poirier (2007) examined the factors that might affect the performance of activities of daily living during radiation treatment; more specifically, the role function adaptive mode of the RAM guided the selection of variables for the research. Contextual stimuli in this study included age, gender, employment patterns, and living conditions. Confirmatory regression analysis was conducted using the simultaneous regression procedure, entering all independent variables supported by the literature review into the regression model at the same time. Data were collected at baseline prior to starting radiation treatment, weekly during treatment, and 1 month after completion of treatment. The analysis included cross-sectional and longitudinal regression, which allowed for identification of changes over time. Overall, the findings of this study reported that subjects maintained fairly high role performance through the course of radiation treatment. However, performance ability decreased significantly from baseline to the end of the treatment. Ability to perform correlated negatively with fatigue and side effects. The author concluded that fatigue and side effects negatively affected patient's ability to perform usual activities.

The relationship of personal health and self-esteem to the functional status of caregivers of children in a body casts was explored by Newman

(2005). For this study functional status of roles was defined as performance of household activities, social and community activities, care of the child in the body cast, care of other children, personal care activities, and occupational activities. The author reported the finding that the relationship between personal health and self-esteem is weak. However, she also noted that both have a stronger relationship to role function, which supports the RAM proposition that the RAM adaptive modes of physiologic, self-concept, and role function are interrelated.

Sander (2004) examined the psychometric characteristics of the Modified Functional Independence Measure and explored the functional status of people with spinal cord injury. The main hypothesis was that an individual has the capability to adapt to the trauma of spinal cord injury. In this study the author performed a secondary analysis of archival data to explore functional adaptations in physical activity and neurological function related to feeding, locomotion, and expression. The measurement tool reflected the theoretical elements of the RAM and quantified the patient's level of physical functional status related to severity of disability using observed behavior. As expected, people with tetraplegia were significantly less functional than people with paraplegia. The modified Functional Independence Measure tool is a reliable and valid instrument, yet the author noted the need for continued revision.

Platner (2004) investigated whether or not moon phase affects the rate of spontaneous labor. The results reported that there was no difference in the rate of spontaneous labor for the different moon phases. This study used power analysis to ensure an adequate sample for meaningful results. Still the author concluded that no absolute conclusion can be made regarding the effect of the full or new moon on spontaneous labor. Rather, it can be concluded that if there is a difference, it is probably weak.

John (1997) explored the perceptions of QOL changing over time for patients with non-small cell lung cancer receiving curative radiation therapy alone or in combination with other treatment modalities. The author reported that although QOL declined significantly during XRT, it improved following XRT to a higher level than prior to treatment, and then returned to a pretreatment level. Sampling over time provided important insights. The author used a pilot study to determine feasibility and a useful measurement tool, Functional Assessment of Cancer Therapy-Lung (FACT-L).

In a study of pregnancy outcomes, Harner (2001) examined teenagers who were under 18 at the time of conception and compared the pregnancies of those fathered by adult men to those fathered by peer-age boys. Prenatal and obstetric outcomes were explored. The study yielded few statistically significant results, that is, the age of father was not a factor in prenatal and obstetric outcomes. The author also found no significant difference between adult men compared to peer-age boys and outcomes such as violence, abuse, prenatal care, or gestational age at birth. One difference was that breastfeeding was significantly more common among teens whose partner was a peer-age boy than with adult fathers.

Siripitayakunkit et al. (2008) examined the relationships among personal, psychological, and health care system factors that contribute to integrating lifestyle in Thai women with type 2 diabetes ($n = 490$). Personal factors such as education and income, psychological factors of family and friend social support, and health system factors of quality of patient–provider relationships supported the interrelationships affecting the outcome as proposed by the RAM. The contextual stimuli of education level had a nonsignificant negative and direct effect on perceived integrating lifestyle and had a slightly moderate positive direct effect on perceived demands of diabetes.

The stimulus of visiting hours in hospitals was explored by Lynch (2007), who described the visitation preferences of patients on acute medical units. A large tertiary care hospital in Manitoba, Canada, was used with adult hospitalized patients as participants ($n = 128$). The author reported that visiting hours do matter to a patient in a hospitalized environment and that age is a significant factor influencing visiting preferences. Younger patients prefer more frequent visiting. Women are more likely to experience greater perceived stress than men in the hospital. Married couples were less likely to perceive situations of low social support, and older patients were more likely to perceive experiences of low social support.

Descriptive Studies Concerning Relationships in Adapting Groups

According to Roy (2009), adaptation is the process and outcome whereby thinking and feeling people, as individuals or in groups, use conscious awareness and choice to create human and environmental integration. Adaptation leads to optimal health and well-being, to QOL, and to death with dignity. The processes of coping as well as the processes for sustaining the system and allowing it to grow differ for individuals and groups. The RAM identifies central coping processes at the individual level as the regulator and the cognator processes, and at the group level they are stabilizer and innovator. The studies described in this section included looking at groups such as nurses, yet the nurses were individuals adapting rather than nurses such as a work group functioning as a system. This category of studies is included to encourage researchers to look at groups and to use as is helpful the more recent published theoretical work on groups as adaptive systems (Roy, 2009).

Out of the 10 studies, eight studies (80% of the total) were conducted in the United States, one was done in eastern Ontario, Canada, and one in Hong Kong. The studies were carried out in institutions or in the community. Data for two studies were obtained from the medical charts, that is, one of intensive care unit (ICU) patients and one of perioperative nurses. For one study data were collected from six hospitals in Canada. The populations of the studies included ICU patients admitted from the emergency department, nursing organizations, nurses with families, members of Association of Rehabilitation Nurses and American Association of Spinal Cord nurses, perioperative nurses, pediatric nurses, generic senior nursing students, faculty and junior-level students, and licensed practical nurses (see Table 4.4).

A study by Powell (2005) examined the relationship of time spent in the emergency department (ED), overall length of stay (LOS), and medical ICU outcomes. Study findings included that the longer the time spent by critically ill medical patients in the ED, the higher the mortality rate and the greater the LOS in medical ICU. A formula for a Mortality Probability Model developed by Lemeshow et al. (1993) was adopted to determine the probability that a patient would die while in the hospital based on data from 15 physiological variables present at the time of admission to the ED. Reliability of the formula was not addressed.

The preoxygenation practice of nurses who perform tracheal suctioning for spinal-cord-injury patients and the identified decision-making factors when altering the frequency or method of preoxygenation was described by Stevens (2005). The author reported that 50% of nurses preoxygenate. Clinical improvement in oxygenation and ventilatory function were related to the decision to do less suctioning. Abnormal pulse oximetry readings were related to the decision to suction more frequently. Hyperoxygenation was used most frequently, whereas hyperinflation was used less frequently. This study had a national representative sample. The author had a frame set for data collection; however, it was developed by the researcher and there with no mention of reliability.

Using a descriptive survey, Cook, Green, and Topp (2001), explored the incidence and impact of physician verbal abuse on perioperative nurses. The authors reported that 91% of the nurses experienced some type of verbal abuse from a physician at least once over the past year. Adaptive behaviors included problem-focused behaviors by nurses in response to the verbal abuse, which were rated as effective to very effective. The incidence and types of verbal abuse influenced the interpretation, severity of stress, interpretation of the abuse, and coping methods used by nurses.

TABLE 4.4
Descriptive Studies Related to Group Adaptation

Author(s) & Date	Purpose	Sample	Design	Findings
1. Powell (2005)	To examine the relationship of emergency department length of stay and medical ICU outcomes	Consecutive charts of ED patients sent to the medical ICU (n = 50)	Descriptive, retrospective chart review	The longer the time spent by critically ill medical patients in the ED, the higher the mortality rate and the greater the LOS in medical ICU
2. Stevens (2005)	To describe preoxygenation practice of nurses who perform tracheal suctioning with individuals with spinal cord injury and to identify decision-making factors when altering frequency or method of preoxygenation	Members of Association of Rehabilitation Nurses & American Association of Spinal Cord Nurses (n = 232)	Descriptive survey, correlational	Fifty percent of nurses preoxygenate. Clinical improvement in oxygenation and ventilatory function were related to the decision to do less suctioning, whereas abnormal pulse oximetry readings were related to the decision to suction more frequently. Hyper-oxygenation was used most frequently, whereas hyperinflation was used less frequently
3. Cook, Green, and Topp (2001)	To explore the incidence and impact of physician	Perioperative nurses (n = 78)	Descriptive, survey	Ninety-one percent reported experiencing some type of verbal abuse from a physician

Study	Purpose	Sample	Design	Findings
	verbal abuse on perioperative nurses			at least once over the past year. Nurses reported adaptive, problem-focused behaviors in response to verbal abuse, and rated these behaviors as effective to very effective
4. Pejic (2005)	Determine the incidence, characteristics, and personal and professional reactions to verbal abuse.	Registered pediatric nurses working in six hospitals in eastern Ontario, Canada (n = 35)	Descriptive, survey	Ninety-four percent reported being the victim of at least one episode of verbal abuse in the 3-month study period. Common types of abuse were condescension, abusive anger, being ignored, and humiliation. Patients, parents, visitors, and physicians were equally ranked as common perpetrators. Increased stress and decreased job satisfaction were the most frequent reactions to verbal abuse
5. Klein (2000)	To explore relationships among anxiety, self-concept, the impostor	Generic senior baccalaureate	Descriptive, correlational	Positive relationships existed between anxiety and the imposter phenomenon and perceptions of competency

(continued)

TABLE 4.4
Descriptive Studies Related to Group Adaptation (*continued*)

Author(s) & Date	Purpose	Sample	Design	Findings
	phenomena and adaptation to the professional nurse role	nursing students (*n* = 181)		The influence of contextual stimuli alone or when combined with the focal stimuli of role function were not confirmed
6. Jenkins (2006)	To study the relationships among emotional intelligence (EI) of nursing faculty, the climate of learning environment, and empowerment of generic junior-level baccalaureate nursing students	Faculty and junior-level nursing students in public and private colleges and universities in Maryland (faculty *n* = 17) (students *n* = 317)	Descriptive, correlational	Significant positive relationships existed between facilitating thoughts and student empowerment, learning environment and student empowerment, task orientation with perceiving emotions and understanding emotions, task orientation with the total EI score
7. Evans (2008)	To examine the feasibility of family presence in the operating room during breast biopsy by ascertaining perioperative nurses' attitudes toward the concept	Perioperative registered nurses who were members of a local chapter of Association of Periopertive of Registered Nurses (AORN; *n* = 338)	Descriptive, correlational	Eighty-six percent believe that providing psychosocial and emotional support to patients and family members is part of their practice. Four percent had experience with family-member presence during breast biopsy with 35% feeling hampered by family presence

8. Williams (2003)	To explore the relationships among job stress, job satisfaction, and intent to leave employment	Registered nurses and licensed practical nurses working full time in obstetrics (*n* = 30)	Descriptive, correlational	A moderate inverse relationship was demonstrated between job satisfaction and intent to leave employment
9. Chung (2007)	To examine the relationship of nurses' spirituality to their understanding and practice of spiritual care	Nurses from a part-time Bachelor of Science program in nursing in Hong Kong (*n* = 61)	Descriptive, correlational	A positive significant correlation existed between self and dimension beyond self, understanding of spiritual care, and practice of spiritual care. A negative statistically significant correlation was found between religious affiliations and the dimension beyond self
10. Gipson-Jones (2005)	To determine the levels of and examine the relation of work–family conflict and job satisfaction to psychological well-being among nurses	African American nurses with families (*n* = 79)	Descriptive, correlational	Psychological well-being was influenced by negative or positive work to family spillover, school to family spillover, work–family balance, spirituality, single parenting, racism/discrimination, autonomy/role modeling

A study by Pejic (2005) examined the incidence, characteristics, and personal and professional reactions to verbal abuse by nurses working in six hospitals in Canada. Study findings included 94% reported being the victim of at least one episode of verbal abuse in the 3-month study period. Common types of abuse were condescension, abusive anger, being ignored, and humiliation. Ineffective behaviors were reported from patients, parents, visitors, and physicians. Ineffective adaptation, such as stress and decreased job satisfaction, were the most frequent reactions to verbal abuse. This study was a retrospective design and used a convenience sample; the research questionnaire did not have internal validity or reliability reported.

Klein (2000) explored the relationships among anxiety, self-concept, the impostor phenomenon, and adaptation to the role of the professional nurse by generic baccalaureate nursing students. Adaptation to the role was measured by perceptions of clinical competency. The author found positive relationships between anxiety and the imposter phenomenon and role-function behaviors and the students' perceptions of competency. A statistically significant inverse relationship was identified between the focal stimulus of self-concept and the role-function behavior of students' perceptions of competency. The author reported that when the focal stimuli of anxiety, self-concept and the impostor phenomenon were entered into a step wise multiple regression on the role-function behavior, self-concept accounted for 19% ($p < .001$) of the variance in perceptions of competency. This study revealed that the focal stimuli of anxiety and the imposter phenomenon both had a positive statistically significant and moderate correlation with role-function behavior.

Jenkins (2006) described the relationships among emotional intelligence of nursing faculty, the climate-of-learning environment, and empowerment as effective behaviors of generic junior-level baccalaureate nursing students. Seven public and private colleges and universities met the criteria for inclusion in the study and 17 faculty and 317 students were included. The College and University Classroom Environmental Inventory (CUCEI) was used and had good psychometric properties. Empowerment was viewed as adaptation in the self-concept mode that was influenced by faculty emotional intelligence and the learning environment. The data were analyzed with multiple regressions and showed positive relationships between the following:

- facilitating thoughts and student empowerment
- learning environment and student empowerment
- task orientation with perceiving emotions and understanding emotions
- task orientation with the total EI score

A study by Evans (2008) questioned the feasibility of family presence in the operating room during breast biopsy by examining perioperative nurses' attitudes toward the concept of having close family present during the biopsy. The study sought to identify psychosocial factors that influenced the nurses' decisions ($n = 338$). The author reported that 86% believe that providing psychosocial and emotional support to patients and family members is part of their practice. Four percent had experience with family member presence during breast biopsy with 35% of those feeling hampered by family presence. Findings suggested that although nurses believe that providing emotional support is part of their job or practice, not all feel comfortable providing this support in this situation. The author addressed validity and reliability of the instrument and there was a survey response rate of 53%, which was representative of the population of perioperative nurses.

Williams (2003) studied the relationships among job stress, job satisfaction, and intent to leave employment of registered nurses and licensed practical nurses in obstetrics ($n = 30$). A moderate inverse relationship was demonstrated between job satisfaction and intent to leave employment. The study used a convenience sample from one hospital and a good return of instruments (100%) and reported psychometrics on original scale. Because the researcher used only eight items of the instrument and her subjects were both RNs and LPNs, the generalizability is limited.

The relationship of nurses' spirituality to their understanding and practice of spiritual care was examined by Chung (2007). The participants were nurses from a part-time bachelor of science program in nursing in Hong Kong ($n = 61$). The author reported that a positive significant correlation existed between self and the dimension beyond self, understanding of spiritual care, and practice of spiritual care. A significant negative correlation was found between religious affiliation and the dimension beyond self. The researcher addressed well the validity and reliability of the new instrument that she used in this study. She also performed test–retest reliability, established internal consistency, and did factor analysis.

Gipson-Jones (2005) aimed to determine the levels of and to examine the relation of work–family conflict and job satisfaction to psychological well-being among African American nurses with families ($n = 79$). The author used the RAM concepts of adaptive system, stimuli, and the self-concept and role-function modes. Psychological well-being was influenced by negative or positive work to family spillover, school to family spillover, work–family balance, spirituality, single parenting, racism/discrimination, autonomy/role modeling. Qualitative data showed that work–family conflict and job satisfaction were found to be independent constructs that tested different aspects of the role-function mode. The author reported that

African American nurses used spirituality to cope with work and family conflict and to increase psychological well-being.

CRITIQUE OF STUDIES

To present the critique of studies the research team devised two approaches. The first approach is a summary of the results of the evaluation done on the studies included in the chapter and the second is to discuss the strengths and weaknesses of the studies. These approaches are discussed in Chapter 2 along with a description of the criteria for critiquing the quantitative studies. There are four basic categories of evaluation: (1) efforts to control for threats to validity, (2) measurement, (3) data analysis, and (4) interpretation of results. A 5-point scale was used for each category with 5 being the highest score. Each study had a possible maximum of 20 points, that is, 5 points for each of four categories. The method and results of inter-rater reliability among the reviewers was also described. As noted, to be considered adequate for a given study to be used in further knowledge development or application to practice in this project, the research was scored between 16 and 20 points. This means that most categories for evaluation were either 4 or 5 out of 5 points and not more than one could be scored at 3. In this way 80% to 100% of the expectations for quality were met.

The range of scores for the 56 descriptive quantitative studies included in this chapter was 14 to 20. Two studies received the highest score of 20, whereas 12 studies received at least one score of 3. The two studies dropped from further use in this project based on the rules for determining quality of research were the one with the lowest score of 14, which included two 3s (Sheppard & Cunnie, 1996) and one that had a score of 15 with one 3 and three 4s (Tanyi & Warner). Thus they were not used for creating middle range theories or evidence for practice.

In looking at the strengths and weaknesses identified by reviewers, the two studies with the highest scores demonstrate common strengths found in this selection of studies based on the RAM. Morgan and colleagues (2006) and Jenkins (2006) clearly identified their samples and use of eligibility criteria; for example, Jenkins used all seven public and private colleges and universities that met the stated criteria for inclusion in the study so that the sample included 17 faculty and 317 students. Also for both studies the investigators carefully selected the tools to measure the concepts and reported on the psychometric properties of these. Morgan used the Brief Religious Coping Scale (RCOPE) subscales measuring positive and negative religious coping and clarified these concepts. Specifically the investigators of this study used the Functional Assessment and Cancer therapy scale (Fact-B) with nine questions (treatment, side effects, hair loss, sexuality, attractiveness, and stress illness), specific to patients with breast cancer. The methods of data analyses for both studies were appropriate and clearly described. Finally, the interpretation of their results matched the findings and provided new insights. Morgan and colleagues stated that nurses will recognize cultural differences among populations in order to promote coping strategies utilized by women from diverse ethnic backgrounds undergoing breast cancer treatments. Jenkins provided a good example of the RAM proposition that perception influences adaptation in her linking of emotional intelligence of nursing faculty, the climate-of-learning environment, and empowerment as effective behaviors of generic junior-level baccalaureate nursing students.

Other strengths noted were seen in Kiehl and White's (2003) study of 147 healthy primiparous women in Sweden, Norway, and the United States that aimed to explore the relationship between the maternal adaptation during pregnancy and postpartum. The findings showed that prenatal identification with the motherhood role affected formation of maternal identity and confidence in ability to cope with motherhood and affected satisfaction with motherhood. As is needed in a multisite study, there was a consistency of method in that the researcher used two questionnaires, back translated in Swedish and Norwegian, and all the instruments had reliability and validity reported. The author's discussion shows the advantages of the using the RAM concepts for practice. Kiehl and White asserted that when individuals find stressors, by either volume or intensity, falling outside their "zone of adaptation," they do whatever is necessary to cope with the stressor until they bring about adaptation. The nursing role in helping to deal with stressors is emphasized.

Mostly the studies shared the weakness of using convenience samples and sometimes the size was too small for the aims of the study or the instruments used, for example, Gallagher, 1998, Dell et al. (2007), and Tanyi and Warner (2003). In one example, Starner and Peters (2004) asked all the students in class to participate in the study; however, the sample was self-selected by the students and more girls than boys responded to the questionnaires. In this study as in most there was an underrepresentation of people of color. Studies of immigrants were the exception, for example, Al-Altiyyat (2009) studied Arab American oncology patients and Kowalski (2007) compared Japanese American and European American men receiving treatment for prostate cancer. Three studies specifically choose African American subjects, those who had breast cancer, ESRD, and nurses with families. There is increasing global representation although the studies were limited to English publications. These 56 studies included the countries of Sweden, Norway, Taiwan, Zimbabwe, Thailand, Hong Kong, and three studies from Canada.

Overall, the studies on descriptive quantitative research reviewed in this chapter address the holistic nature of the individual. Reliability and validity were not addressed for all instruments used in the reviewed research. Therefore, threats to internal and external validity remain an issue for some studies. As noted, most samples are convenience samples, which limits their generalizability. Generalizability also was compromised by the lack of ability to control the environment and extraneous variables or the localized nature of the data collection. In some reports demographic data did not include socioeconomic status or gender. This lack of information had implications for the interpretation of findings and the comparison of findings of some studies with previous ones.

IMPLICATIONS FOR PRACTICE

Descriptive studies can provide implications for practice, particularly when linked with the RAM. The types of description reflected in these studies included individual coping processes, the adaptive modes, stimuli, and group adaptation. We can identify both needs in these areas and possibilities for helping people to cope. Selecting two studies describing coping processes, we can identify knowledge that had an impact on practice. Domico (1997) studied spousal caregivers to persons with dementia. The caregivers reported moderately high perceptions of social support related to QOL. Having supportive others who can pay attention to the caregivers' needs is helpful to their adaptation. Knowledge in these areas has developed over time and likely has improved the experience of spousal caregivers. The second finding, however, indicates the need for further developments to help spouses in this demanding role. The researcher noted that meaning and purpose in life had an undifferentiated impact on QOL. This impact can be made explicit with nursing intervention that helps individual caregivers to focus on what is meaningful to them and leads them to see purpose in the role they have taken on. The philosophical assumptions of the RAM point to the significance of purpose in life and the shared purposefulness of human life. As nurses help caregivers cope with the demands of caring for a spouse with dementia, in addition to social supports, they can also help them turn inward to their own sense of meaning and purpose.

The study by Kiehl and White (2003) provides specific guidance in helping new mothers adapt during pregnancy and the postpartum period. Nurses can focus on the finding of a relationship between prenatal identification with the motherhood role and maternal identity, confidence in ability to cope, and satisfaction with motherhood postpartum. In the care of maternity patients the nurse can help the pregnant woman begin to develop an identification with the motherhood role. Efforts in this direction can be reinforced and new opportunities provided. Role cues that show the mother where to focus attention, what is expected in the role, and specific information on how to carry out what is expected can enhance identification with the role. According to Kiehl and White's research, this can lead to maternal identity, confidence in ability to cope, and greater satisfaction with the maternal role. Each study can be examined for evidence that may be ready for use in practice.

CONCLUSION

In this chapter we reviewed the rich set of quantitative descriptive studies based on the RAM from the database of this project. The studies were described in the categories of individual coping processes, the adaptive modes often as outcomes, stimuli as that with which persons need to cope, and group adaptation. A summary of the evaluation of the research was provided along with general strengths and weaknesses and specific examples of these. The implications for practice were illustrated, particularly in understanding the individual coping processes.

REFERENCES

Burns, N., & Grove, S. (2009). *The practice of nursing research: Appraisal, synthesis and generation of evidence* (6th ed.). St. Louis, MO: Saunders Elsevier.

Fawcett, J. (1978). The relationship between theory and research: A double helix. *Advances in Nursing Science. 1*(1), 49–62.

Fawcett, J. (1999). *The relationship of theory and research* (3rd ed.). Philadelphia, PA: F. A. Davis.

McGaghie, W. C., Bordage, G., & Shea, J. (2001). Problem statement, conceptual framework, and research question. *Academic Medicine, 76*(9), 923–924.

Roy, C. (2009). *The Roy adaptation model* (3rd ed.). Upper Saddle River, NJ: Prentice Hall Health.

Roy, C., & Roberts, S. (1981). *Theory construction in nursing: An adaptation model.* Englewood Cliffs, NJ: Prentice-Hall.

BIBLIOGRAPHY

Aktan, N. M. (2010). Functional status after childbirth and related concepts. *Clinical Nursing Research, 19*(2), 165–180.

Al-Atiyyat, N. M. H. (2009). *Pain, coping strategies, and quality of life in Arab American cancer patients* (Doctoral dissertation, Wayne State University).

Arcamone, A. A. (2005). *The effect of prenatal education on adaptation to motherhood after vaginal childbirth in primiparous women as assessed by Roy's four adaptive modes* (Doctoral dissertation, Widener University).

Baden, T. M. (2004). *Roy's adaptation model and parental grief of adult children who died a traumatic death* (Doctoral dissertation, Medical College of Ohio).

Bingham, M., Young-McCaughan, S., & Miaskowski, C. (2009). Sleep disturbance and PTSD symptoms in injured service members. *Communicating Nursing Research, 42,* 200.

Black, K. D. (2004). *Physiologic responses, sense of well-being, self-efficacy for self-monitoring role, perceived availability of social support, and perceived stress in women with pregnancy-induced hypertension* (Doctoral dissertation, Widener University).

Black, K. D. (2007). Stress, symptoms, self-monitoring confidence, well-being, and social support in the progression of preeclampsia/gestational hypertension. *Journal of Obstetric Gynecologic and Neonatal Nursing, 36*(5), 419–429.

Burns, D. (2004). Physical and psychosocial adaptation of blacks on hemodialysis. *Applied Nursing Research, 17*(2), 116–124.

Chiang, H. (1998). Help-seeking and quality of life in women with breast cancer (Doctoral dissertation, University of Arizona). *Dissertation Abstracts International,* 59(04B), 1582.

Chung, L. Y. F. (2007). Relationship of nurses' spirituality to their understanding and practice of spiritual care. *Journal of Advanced Nursing, 58*(2), 158.

Ciambelli, M. (1996). Adaptation in marital partners with fertility problems: Testing a midrange theory derived from Roy's Adaptation Model (Doctoral dissertation, Wayne State University). *Dissertation Abstracts International,* 57(12B), 7448.

Cook, J. K., Green, M., & Topp, R. V. (2001). Exploring the impact of physician verbal abuse on perioperative nurses. *AORN-Journal, 74*(3), 317–318, 320, 322–327.

Dell, D., Weaver, C., Kozempel, J., & Barsevick, A. (2007). Assessment of recovery post TRAM (transverse rectus abdominis myocutaneous) flap breast surgery. *Oncology Nursing Forum, 34*(2), 477.

DiMattio, M. J. K., & Tulman, L. (2003). A longitudinal study of functional status and correlates following coronary artery bypass graft surgery in women. *Nursing Research, 52*(2), 98–107.

Domico, V. (1997). The impact of social support and meaning and purpose in life on quality of life of spousal caregivers of persons with dementia (Doctoral dissertation, University of Alabama at Birmingham). *Dissertation Abstracts International,* 58(12B), 6485.

Evans, L. (2008). Feasibility of family member presence in the OR during breast biopsy procedures. *AORN Journal, 88*(4), 568–570, 573–578.

Fawcett, J., Sidney, J. S., Riley-Lawless, K., & Hanson, M. J. S. (1996). An exploratory study of the relationship between alternative therapies, functional status, and symptom severity among people with multiple sclerosis. *Journal of Holistic Nursing, 4*(2), 115–129.

Gallagher, M. (1998). Urogenital distress and the psychosocial impact of urinary incontinence on elderly women. *Rehabilitation Nursing, 23*(4), 192–197.

Gipson-Jones, T. L. (2005). *The relationship between work–family conflict, job satisfaction and psychological well-being among African American nurses* (Doctoral dissertation, Hampton University, Hampton, VA).

Grimes, C. (1997). The relationship of daily hassles, life change events, and pain to hopelessness in the ambulatory cancer patient (Doctoral dissertation, The Catholic University of America). *Dissertation Abstracts International, 58*(02B): 0632.

Harner, H. M. (2001). *Obstetrical outcomes of teenagers with adult and peer age partners* (Doctoral dissertation, University of Pennsylvania).

Hovey, J. K. (2005). Fathers parenting chronically ill children: Concerns and coping strategies. *Issues in Comprehensive Pediatric Nursing, 28*(2), 83.

Huang, C. (2002). *Sleep and daytime sleepiness in first-time mothers during early postpartum in Taiwan* (Doctoral dissertation, University of Texas at Austin).

Jenkins, B. E. (2006). *Emotional intelligence of faculty members, the learning environment, and empowerment of baccalaureate nursing students.* New York, NY: Teachers College, Columbia University.

John, L. D. (1997). *Quality of life in patients receiving curative radiation therapy for non-small cell lung cancer* (Doctoral dissertation, Texas Woman's University, Denton, TX).

Kiehl, E. M., & White, M. A. (2003). Maternal adaptation during childbearing in Norway, Sweden and the United States. *Scandinavian Journal of Caring Sciences, 17*(2), 96–103.

Klein, G. (2000). The relationships among anxiety, self-concept, the imposter phenomenon, and generic senior baccalaureate nursing students' perceptions of clinical competency (Doctoral dissertation, Widener University School of Nursing). *Dissertation Abstracts International, 61*(10B), 5236.

Kowalski, M. O. (2007). *A comparative study of pain intensity, information seeking and adjustment to prostate cancer in Japanese American and European American men* (Doctoral dissertation, New York University).

LeBlanc, N., & Morin, D. (2004). Depressive symptoms and associated factors in children with attention deficit hyperactivity disorder. *Journal of Child and Adolescent Psychiatric Nursing, 17*(2), 49.

Lynch, M. A. (2007). *Hospital visitation preferences and perceived stress in adults on medical units* (Doctoral dissertation, University of Manitoba).

Martin, B. (1995). An analysis of common post partum problems and adaptation strategies used by women during the first two to eight weeks following delivery of a full term health newborn (Doctoral dissertation, University of Mississippi). *Dissertation Abstracts International, 56*(06B), 3128.

McGaghie, W. C., Bordage, G., & Shea, J. (2001). Problem statement, conceptual framework, and research question. *Academic Medicine, 76*(9), 923–924.

Modrcin-Talbott, M. A., Pullen, L., Ehrenberger, H., Zandstra, K., & Muenchen, B. (1998a). Self-esteem in adolescents treated in an outpatient mental health setting. *Issues in Comprehensive Pediatric Nursing, 21*(3), 159–171.

Modrcin-Talbott, M. A., Pullen, L., Zandstra, K., Ehrenberger, H., & Muenchen, B. (1998b). A study of self-esteem among well adolescents: Seeking a new direction. *Comprehensive Pediatric Nursing, 21*(4), 229–241.

Morgan, P. D., Gaston-Johansson, F., & Mock, V. (2006). Spiritual well-being, religious coping, and the quality of life of African American breast cancer treatment: A pilot study. *ABNF Journal, 73*(7), 73–77.

Newman, D. M. L. (1997). The inventory of functional status-caregiver of a child in a body cast. *Journal of Pediatric Nursing: Nursing Care of Children and Families, 12*(3), 142–147.

Newman, D. M. L. (2005). Functional status, personal health, and self-esteem of caregivers of children in a body cast: A pilot study. *Orthopaedic Nursing, 24*(6), 416–423.

Orsi, A. J., Grandy, C., Tax, A., & McCorkle, R. (1997). Nutritional adaptation of women living with HIV: A pilot study. *Holistic Nursing Practice, 12*(1), 71–79.

Pejic, A. R. (2005). Verbal abuse: A problem for pediatric nurses. *Pediatric-Nursing, 31*(4), 271–281.

Platner, E. A. (2004). *How does the full and new moon affect the spontaneous labor rate.* Lubbock, TX : Texas Tech University Press.

Poirier, P. (2007). Factors affecting performance of usual activities during radiation therapy. *Oncology Nursing Forum, 34*(4) 827–834.

Powell, J. R. W. (2005). *The relationship between time spent in the emergency department and patient outcomes in the medical intensive care unit* (Master of Science thesis, D'Youville College).

Ryan, M. C. (1996). Loneliness, social support, and depression as interactive variables with cognitive status: Testing Roy's model. *Nursing Science Quarterly, 9*(3), 107–114.

Sabatini, M. (2003). *Exercise and adaptation in older women* (Doctoral dissertation, Widener University).

Saburi, G. L., Mapanga, K. G., & Mapanga, M. B. (2006). Perceived family reactions and quality of life of adults with epilepsy. *Journal of Neuroscience Nursing, 38*(3), 156.

Salisbury, M. (2004). *Sexual awareness, body image, and self-esteem of individuals who have ostomies* (Doctoral dissertation, Medical College of Ohio).

Samarel, N., Fawcett, J., Krippendorf, K., Piacentino, J. C., Eliasof, B., Hughes, P., … Ziegler, E. (1998). Women's perceptions of group support and adaptation to breast cancer. *Journal of Advanced Nursing, 28*(6), 1259–1268.

Sander, R. A. (2004). *Measurement of functional status in the spinal cord injured patient* (Doctoral dissertation, Saint Louis University, St. Louis, MO).

Santarlasci, P. R. (2009). *The relationships among pain, functional ability, depression, and social support with coping and return to work for persons who have sustained a lower extremity amputation* (Doctoral dissertation, Widener University).

Sheppard, V. A., & Cunnie, K. L. (1996). Incidence of diuresis following hysterectomy. *Journal of Post Anesthesia Nursing, 11*(1), 20–28.

Siripitayakunkit, A., Hanucharurnkul, S., Melkus, G. D. E., Vorapongsathorn, T., Rattarasarn, C., & Arpanantikul, M. (2008). Factors contributing to integrating lifestyle in Thai women with type 2 diabetes. *Thai Journal of Nursing Research, 12*(3), 166–177.

Starner, T. M., & Peters, R. M. (2004). Anger expression and blood pressure in adolescents. *Journal of School Nursing, 20*(6), 335–342.

Stevens, K. A. (2005). *Preoxygenation practices prior to tracheal suctioning by nurses caring for individuals with spinal cord injury* (Doctoral dissertation, Loyola University, Chicago, IL).

Tanyi, R. A., & Werner, J. S. (2003). Adjustment, spirituality, and health in women on hemodialysis. *Clinical Nursing Research, 12*(3), 229.

Taylor, H. (1997). Self-esteem, coping and attitude toward menopause among older rural Southern women (Doctoral dissertation, University of Alabama at Birmingham). *Dissertation Abstracts International,* 58(05B), 2359.

Thomas, C. M. (2007). The influence of self-concept on adherence to recommended health regimens in adults with heart failure. *Journal of Cardiovascular Nursing, 22*(5), 405–416.

Williams, A. (2003). *Job stress, job satisfaction, and intent to leave employment among maternal-child health nurses.* Huntington, WV: The Graduate College of Marshall University.

Willoughby, D. (1995). The influence of psychosocial factors on women's adjustment to diabetes (Doctoral dissertation, Georgia State University). *Dissertation Abstracts International,* 56(08B), 4247.

5

Quantitative Studies: Explaining, Predicting, and Prescribing Designs

MARTHA V. WHETSELL AND KATHRYN LAUCHNER

In presenting the research that has been conducted based on the Roy adaptation model (RAM), the quantitative studies are presented by types of design. We have grouped the second set of quantitative studies as those that explain, predict, or prescribe. By the nature of these designs the studies go beyond identifying concepts and their relationships. To explain, predict and prescribe are all purposes of research. These types of studies are tied to theories that provide the rationale for the relationships to be tested. To explain is to identify systematic relationships underpinning a natural phenomenon (Polit & Beck, 2012). Explaining is dependent on looking for the pathways of relationships whereby the phenomenon exists or works. For example, we can explain becoming a mother by using a given role theory and outlining the interconnected relationships among concepts. Predicting and prescribing depend on identifying established relationships whether or not they explain the phenomenon. This kind of knowledge is crucial in making clinical decisions.

We can predict a lunar eclipse by knowing the predictable pathways of the sun, moon, and Earth. The example shows that some phenomenon that we can predict we cannot control or prescribe to change. We can predict anxiety in a given patient awaiting surgery or predict the probability of a genetic defect. Still not all the pathways for anxiety have been confirmed. Nor do we know the protein sequence changes whereby the genetic defect occurs. It takes understanding the individual underpinnings of anxiety for a given patient to prescribe interventions to decrease anxiety. Likewise, it is necessary to know the specific genetic sequence changes needed to be able to prescribe interventions to prevent the defect. Still, in nursing knowledge, each of these types of research—explaining, predicting and prescribing—is important to practice.

Researchers refer to this type of research as determining cause and effect. However, in the role that nursing takes in health care many clinical situations defy the principles of causality, that is, identifying the cause of a given effect. Rather, nurses think in terms of contemporary empiricism (Weiss, 1995), which considers the many factors influencing the situation and the context in which it occurs. The explanations and predictions discovered in nursing research generally relate to probabilities of occurrence of a given pattern in given situations. In this chapter most of the quantitative studies to explain, predict, and proscribe use multivariate analyses to identify pathways with probabilities of influence on the phenomenon being studied. Box 5.1 summarizes some key definitions of research useful in clarifying the approaches used in the studies being reported in this chapter.

The purpose of this chapter is to describe and analyze the studies identified as explaining, predicting, and prescribing and to show how these studies relate to developing knowledge for practice. Specifically the aims

---

BOX 5.1
KEY DEFINITIONS OF RESEARCH

Contemporary empiricism—to look for the probabilities that given factors will influence given outcomes; considers the context in which the effect occurs, that is, provides a full description of the conditions under which the phenomenon occurs.

Explain—to identify systematic relationships underpinning a natural phenomenon; looks for the pathways of relationships whereby the phenomenon exists or works.

Predict—to identify an established relationship that makes it possible to see one phenomenon and know the other will follow.

Prescribe—to understand pathways of occurrence in such a way that one can create an intervention to change the pathway.

Multivariate analysis—to use statistical procedures that analyze relationships among three or more variables, such as, multiple regression.

are to (1) describe each study in text and table, (2) report the critique of the studies, and (3) provide exemplars for change in practice based on the research.

OVERVIEW OF STUDIES THAT EXPLAIN, PREDICT, OR PRESCRIBE

There are 45 studies judged to fit the category of explaining, predicting or prescribing. Given the bases in the RAM, the main clusters of concepts for the model provided the outline for the order used to present the studies, as described in Chapter 2. The categories for related studies in this chapter include internal coping processes of individuals, adaptive modes, and stimuli as noted in Box 5.2. The next section describes the studies related to internal coping processes.

Description of Studies Related to Internal Coping Processes

Of the 15 studies related to internal coping processes, 12 studies (80% of the total) were conducted in the United States and 3 were carried out in Taiwan. Studies were executed in rural communities, institutions, or in the community. Institutional settings included hospitals ($n = 8$). Other studies were done in mixed settings, community residences, hemodialysis clinics, and universities. The populations for the studies included elderly women, children ages (8–12 years), Taiwanese mothers, patients in intensive care units (ICUs), Judeo-Christian individuals in the community, informal caregivers, African American women, women with infertility, patients with end-stage renal disease (ESRD) and those on hemodialysis, patients having first time coronary artery bypass graft (CABG) surgery, mothers of children with cancer, and university students. The reviewers found that the studies contributed to nursing science and provided foundations to develop further research and, therefore, met the challenges of a demanding and changing nursing practice. All of the 16 studies described here either

---

BOX 5.2
DESCRIPTIVE STUDIES BASED ON CATEGORIES OF RAM
PROPOSITIONS ($n = 45$)

- Descriptive studies related to internal coping processes—individual ($n = 15$)
- Descriptive studies related to adaptive modes ($n = 18$)
- Descriptive studies related to stimuli ($n = 12$)

explain, predict, or prescribe related to internal coping processes of an individual (see Table 5.1).

Kessenich (1996) described the effects of sociodemographic characteristics, bone density, bone fractures, perceived health, medications, and exercise on the quality of life of elderly women with spinal fractures secondary to osteoporosis. The study used a causal nonexperimental model, and a conceptual framework based on the RAM and quality of life. The assumptions from the RAM are derived from the principles of humanism and veritivity (Roy, 1988). The two specific assumptions were that the person "possesses intrinsic holism, and strives to maintain integrity" (Roy, 1988, p. 32). Veritivity is the principle that sees the individual as "viewed in the context of value and meaning of life" (Roy, 1988, p. 32). Descriptive statistics and regression path analysis were used to analyze the data. Findings showed that transportation by a friend, spinal fracture, and health perceptions had a direct effect on quality of life, providing empirical support for the cognator subsystem.

Bournaki (1997) examined the relationship of children's age, gender, painful experiences, temperament, fears, and child-rearing practices to venipuncture pain responses. In this study the sensory dimension was represented by children's behavioral and heart rate responses. The perceptual dimension of pain, which is processed by both the regulator and cognator subsystems, was portrayed by children's subjective responses about the location, intensity, and quality of pain. Empirical support was found for the contextual stimuli of age, medical fears, the temperamental dimensions of distractibility, and threshold. The contextual stimuli that affect developmental stage (age), self-concept (medical fears), and interdependence between parent and child (temperamental dimensions of distractibility and sensory threshold) were supported. Most important, findings from the correlational and canonical analyses support the multidimensionality of pain as conceptualized by the RAM. This empirical evidence is consistent with the need for clinicians and researchers to use a comprehensive approach to assess pain by integrating valid and reliable subjective, behavioral, and physiological measures. Such a global approach to understanding pain is in accordance with the RAM.

A study by Huang (2002) described the characteristics of postpartum sleep and daytime sleepiness. The purpose of the study was to assess factors contributing to the loss of sleep during the early postpartum period in first-time Taiwanese mothers'. The RAM was employed as the theoretical framework to explain the relationships among the variables. Postpartum sleep was defined as the focal stimuli that caused the responses of daytime sleepiness observed in each of the four adaptive modes. Contextual stimuli, including maternal and psychological influencing

TABLE 5.1
Studies That Explain, Predict, or Prescribe Related to Internal Coping Processes—Individual

Author(s) and Date	Purpose	Sample	Design	Findings
1. Kessenich (1996)	To describe effects of bone density, bone fractures, perceived health, drugs and exercise on quality of life	Elderly women in a rural New England community with spinal fractures due to osteoporosis ($n = 105$)	Explain–predict–prescribe, regression based on path analysis	Transportation by a friend, spinal fracture, and health perception had a direct effect on quality of life. No effect on quality of life was found by bone density, hip fracture, drugs, and exercise
2. Bournaki (1997)	To examine the relationship of children's age, gender, painful experiences, temperament, fears, and child-rearing practices to venipuncture pain responses	Children, aged 8–12, and their female caregivers ($n = 94$)	Explain–predict–prescribe, canonical correlations	Age and threshold correlated with pain quality, behavioral responses, and heart rate response, explaining 12% of the variance. Additionally, age, distractibility, and medical fears explained 5.7% of the variance in pain quality and heart rate. Significant correlations between pain intensity, quality, behavioral responses, and heart rate responses support the multidimensionality of pain

(continued)

TABLE 5.1

Studies That Explain, Predict, or Prescribe Related to Internal Coping Processes—Individual (*continued*)

Author(s) and Date	Purpose	Sample	Design	Findings
3. Huang (2002)	To describe the characteristics of postpartum and sleep and daytime sleepiness and to examine the interrelationships among these characteristics	First-time Taiwanese mothers 2 to 3 weeks postpartum (*n* = 189)	Explain–predict–prescribe, hierarchical multiple regression and path analysis	Only the variable of sleep practices significantly contributed to both sleep quality and perceived sleep debt. Sleep quality was not a prominent contributor to any of the four types of daytime sleepiness. Mothers' perception of sleep debt was a significant contributor to one type of daytime sleepiness
4. Robinson (1995)	To explore the grief response and the variables impacting grief using a nursing perspective	Women whose husbands had died within the past 13–24 months (*n* = 65)	Explain–predict–prescribe	Social support had moderate positive direct effect on total combined coping and was inversely and weakly related to total grief response. Stimuli and coping response explained 18% of variance in grief response
5. Hamner (1996)	To test a Roy adaptation model (RAM) proposition	General medical surgical ICU patients (*n* = 60)	Explain–predict–prescribe	Severity of illness, perceived control over visitation (PCV), hardiness, and state anxiety explained 18% of the variance in length of stay (LOS) in ICU

				The perceived control over visitation, hardiness, state anxiety, and length of stay in an intensive care unit	The path between hardiness and PCV was the only path supported by data
6. Dunn (2001)	To test the relationships among chronic pain; the use of religious and nonreligious coping; and the health outcomes of functional ability, depression, and spiritual well-being	Judeo-Christian community-dwelling older adults with chronic pain of at least 3 months duration ($n = 200$)	Explain– predict– prescribe, structural equation modeling	The level of self-reported pain intensity was not related to cultural or racial background, age or gender. Women and non-White participants reported using religious coping strategies significantly more often than did men and White participants
7. Dunn (2005)	To test the relationships among total chronic pain intensity, compensatory life processes, and adaptive responses	Judeo-Christian community-dwelling older adults with chronic pain of at least 3-months duration ($n = 200$)	Explain– predict– prescribe, structural equation modeling	The level of self-reported pain intensity was not related to cultural or racial background, age or gender. Women and non-White participants reported using religious coping strategies significantly more often than did men and White participants

(continued)

TABLE 5.1

Studies That Explain, Predict, or Prescribe Related to Internal Coping Processes—Individual (*continued*)

Author(s) and Date	Purpose	Sample	Design	Findings
8. Ducharme, Ricard, Duquette, Levesque, and Lachance (1998)	To pool empirical data from studies exploring the same variables but involving different populations, and then to verify the pattern of relationships among these variables	Informal caregivers of the psychiatrically ill (*n* = 161) and of demented relatives (*n* = 111), professional caregivers of elderly patients (*n* = 498), elderly spouses (*n* = 98)	Explain–predict–prescribe, structural equation modeling	Reciprocal effects were noted between psychological distress and level of conflict, between psychological distress and passive/avoidance coping strategies, and between active coping strategies and perceived stress
9. Henderson, Fogel, and Edwards (2003)	To determine coping strategies used by African American women with breast cancer and explore the effects of sociodemographic variables on coping strategies	African American women with a diagnosis of breast cancer in United States (*n* = 86)	Explain–predict–prescribe, regression analysis	No significant relationships found among sociodemographic variables and coping strategies. The most frequently used coping strategies were positive reappraisal and social support, followed by problem solving. Accepting responsibility was the least frequently used coping strategy

10. Yeh (2003)	To test the hypothesis that coping style mediates social support, parenting stress, psychological stress, and psychological distress for both parents	Parents (*n* = 246 mothers and 195 fathers) of children (*n* = 270) diagnosed with cancer and receiving treatment at either an outpatient department and/ or hospital ward in Taiwan	Explain–predict–prescribe, structural equation modeling	The relationship of social support and parenting stress to psychological distress was mediated through coping style. Parents who had less social support had higher parenting stress and higher psychological distress. Social support had a direct and lowering effect on parental stress
11. Zbegner (2003)	To explore the variables of physical energy level, self-esteem, marital satisfaction, and parenthood motivation as predictors of coping behaviors	Women with primary infertility who discontinued treatment comprised the three resolution groups of adoption, childbirth, or living without children (*n* = 140)	Explain–predict–prescribe, structural equation modeling	Physical energy level, self-esteem, marital satisfaction, and parenthood motivation did not predict coping behavior better than any single variable. Data suggested that predictive variables were best for classifying the in-treatment and adoption groups and least effective for predicting women who choose to live childfree
12. Chiou (1997)	To examine the relationship of physical symptoms, cultural variables, and developmental	ESRD patients on hemodialysis in Taiwan (*n* = 160)	Explain–predict–prescribe, structural equation modeling	Diabetic subjects who are older, have religious beliefs, have no spouse, and do have higher physical symptom distress have lower

(continued)

145

TABLE 5.1
Studies That Explain, Predict, or Prescribe Related to Internal Coping Processes—Individual (*continued*)

Author(s) and Date	Purpose	Sample	Design	Findings
	variables in patients with end-stage renal disease			functional status. Symptom distress contributed most to functional status
13. Burns (1997)	To describe the relationships among socioeconomic status (SES), social support, perceived problems, coping, physiological status, and psychosocial status	Hemodialysis patients (*n* = 127)	Explain–predict–prescribe, path analysis	The coping method used most often was prayer and trust in God. Perceived problems were positively related to coping. The use of fatalistic, emotive, and supportive coping methods was related to low self-esteem, whereas evasive coping methods were related to poorer adjustment. Optimistic coping was related to higher systolic blood pressure
14. Polichnowski (2008)	To explore adaptation to dating violence through spiritual well-being	Catholic undergraduate university students (*n* = 444)	Explain–predict–prescribe, regression analysis	Students who experienced dating violence were more likely to be positive for symptoms of depression. Both religious well-being and existential well-being facilitate adaptation by moderating and mediating the effects of dating violence

15. Zhang (2004)	To identify the variables that influence the decision-making responses related to advance directives (ADs)	Public data study of aging 1984–2000 (*n* = 938)	Explain–predict–prescribe, causal modeling with path analysis	• Age and gender significantly contributed to the number of hospital and nursing home admissions • Number of hospital and nursing home admissions was significantly associated with physical impairment • Physical impairment had greatest effect on decision-making responses • The degree of physical impairment also had indirect effects on AD completion through its influence on self-perception about health and role-function mode • Less likely to work or do volunteer work also less likely to complete ADs

factors, were hypothesized to have direct and indirect influences on the responses of daytime sleepiness. The author reports that the relationships between the focal stimuli (postpartum sleep quality and quantity) and the responses of four types of daytime sleepiness were partially supported by the study's findings. Higher levels of depression were found in mothers who experienced more sleep disturbances, short sleep duration, and more daytime dysfunctions. The highest correlation coefficient was 0.29 ($p < .001$), found between postpartum sleep and daytime sleepiness.

Robinson (1995) explored the grief response and the variables impacting grief. Using the RAM, she identified that the contextual stimuli of social support, social network, income/education and spiritual beliefs were related to the cognator coping processes and to adaptation viewed as the grief response. Significant relationships were found between coping processes and grief and moderate relationships existed between social networks and coping. The postulated relationships were deduced from three of Roy and Robert's (1981) cognator subsystem propositions: "The optimum amount and clarity of input of internal and external stimuli positively influences problem solving and decision making"; "the optimum amount and clarity of input of internal and external stimuli positively influences the adequacy of defenses to seek relief"; and "the higher the level of adequacy of the cognator processes the more effective the response" (Roy & Roberts, 1981, p. 65). It is important to remember that in this study compensatory processes affected adaptation level of the surviving spouse. This study supports the proposition of the RAM that "At the individual level the regulators and the cognator processes affect innate and acquired ways of adapting." This study has many implications for practice in hospitals as nurses assess the factors that influence coping processes in order to promote coping effectiveness and increase adaptive grief response. Additionally, in the community, because of the multivariate nature of grief response, interpersonal and personal resources are warranted.

A study by Hamner (1996) used a descriptive co-relational methodology to test the relationships of severity of illness, perceived control over visitation, hardiness, state anxiety, and length of stay in an ICU. Severity of illness, PCV, hardiness, and state anxiety explained 18% of the variance in LOS in ICU. The path between hardiness and PCV was the only path supported by data. The author used severity of illness as the focal stimulus. The contextual stimuli was the PVC. State anxiety and hardiness were viewed as residual stimuli. The researcher investigated whether freedom of communication patterns would positively influence the adequacy of seeking and receiving affection by using a series of regression analyses with blocks of independent variables. The focal stimulus of severity of illness was first entered into the equation, the contextual stimuli were entered next, and the residual were entered last. The hypothesis that LOS could be predicted by the severity of illness, state anxiety, hardiness, and PVC was supported; 18% of the variance in LOS was explained by the variables in the model at a significance level of 0.5. The proposed model demonstrated inadequate support; as noted only the path between hardiness and PVC was supported at the significance level of 0.1. The author states that many reasons contribute to the inadequacy of the model: restriction of the range in the Acute Physiological and Chronic Health Evaluation (APACHE) scores, a new PVC scale, small sample size, and limited number of variables and underidentification of the model.

Dunn (2001; 2005) reported her research in her dissertation, then in a journal article. The purpose of a study, using a cross-sectional, co-relational survey design, was to explore the use of religious and nonreligious coping strategies to manage chronic pain among Judeo-Christian elderly adults. Specifically, this study examined the relationship among the contextual variables of age, gender, and race, self-reported pain intensity, the use of religious and nonreligious coping as mediating factors, functional ability, depression, and spiritual well-being (SWB). The hypothesized relational statement was based on findings of empirical research and a proposed middle range theory derived from the RAM. Findings suggest that elders used pharmacological and nonpharmacological interventions to manage their pain. Elders who were more disabled reported using more pain medications. Elders who reported using religious coping more often were less depressed and had greater SWB. The RAM theoretical framework provided adequate fit for the data and supported the majority of the hypothesized relationships and findings from prior research.

A study by Ducharme et al. (1998) reports the steps and results of the empirical testing of a theoretical longitudinal model. The model was developed and empirically supported the results of four longitudinal studies related to mental health problems, exploring the same variables but using subjects from different populations. The purpose of this study was to report the results of the empirical testing of the theoretical model derived from the RAM. The results showed that the model was stable over time. This study proposed a systematic procedure for the support of a theoretical model. The procedure described by the authors allows data from different studies to be combined for the development of knowledge, and middle range theories to support nursing interventions. This study supports a theoretical model of reciprocal effects between psychological distress and level of conflict, between psychological distress and passive/ avoidance coping strategies, and between active coping strategies and perceived stress, which can be used in research and in practice.

Henderson, Edwards, and Fogel (2003) examined coping strategies that are used by African American women with breast cancer. The authors examined the relationships between sociodemographic variables, such as age, income, education, marital status, length of time since diagnosis, and the coping strategies used by the subjects. No significant relationships were found among sociodemographic variables and coping strategies. The most frequently used coping strategies were positive reappraisal and social support, followed by problem solving. Accepting responsibility was the least frequently used coping strategy. Findings indicate that coping strategies are related to how women adapt to breast cancer, yet it remains unclear how demographic variables predict coping strategies. This study uses multiple regression analysis, which was appropriate and adequate, and also compared raw scores obtained from each coping subscale to those from a previous study. The researchers caution that this study has a number of limitations, one of which was recruitment. No direct cultural comparisons were made with women from other ethnic or racial backgrounds.

A study by Yeh (2003) was designed to examine the relationships among social support, parenting stress, coping style, and psychological distress in parents caring for children with cancer. Mothers ($n = 246$) and fathers ($n = 195$) of children ($n = 270$) diagnosed with cancer and receiving treatment at either an outpatient department and/or hospital ward in Taiwan were recruited. Structural equation modeling (SEM) was used to test the hypothesis. The theoretical framework for this study was based on selected concepts of the RAM. Findings from this study should be reviewed in the context of the study limitations, including that the study tested mothers and fathers separately. One hundred and seventy-one pairs of parents had cared for their child and were not independent from each other. The relationship of social support and parenting stress to psychological distress was mediated through coping style. Psychological distress measured the self-concept mode. In the RAM, the self-concept mode specifically focuses on psychological and spiritual aspects of the human system. Support of this study suggests that adaptation to focal stimuli is connected to the contextual and focal stimuli. Parents who had less social support had higher parenting stress and higher psychological distress. Social support had a direct and lowering effect on parental stress. This study supports that in children with cancer, environmental stimuli influence biobehavioral responses. Communication with others, severity of illness, and age are a good explanation for biobehavioral responses and are considered focal stimuli.

Zbegner (2003) conducted a retrospective exploratory study using as subjects women diagnosed with primary infertility who were in treatment for 6 months or longer. The variables included energy level, self-esteem, marital satisfaction, and parenthood motivation. The variables were studied as predictors of coping behaviors identified as infertility resolution or non resolution. Relationships among the variables of age, education, income, and total time in treatment were also examined. Even though the data analysis included multiple regression and correlation, none of the hypotheses were supported. The adaptive-mode variables did not collectively discriminate group membership of the resolution and nonresolution groups. Inspection of Eigen values, canonical correlation, and Wilk's lambda results revealed that the overall ability of the linear functions to discriminate among the four outcome groups was poor. The regression of each adaptive mode on the contextual variables accounted for only 5% to 8% of the variance, and none of the variables explained motivation. The contextual variables were not strongly related to the adaptive-mode variables. Data suggested that predictive variables were best for classifying the in-treatment and adoption groups and least effective for predicting women who choose to live childfree.

Chiou (1997) used the RAM to examine the relationship of the focal stimulus of physical-symptom distress; the contextual stimuli of cultural variables; and environmental variables to physiological, self-concept, role function and interdependence modes of the RAM. SEM was used to analyze data collected from a sample of 160 patients with ESRD. The model developed by the author for this study explained 66% of the variance in functional status. People who are older, have diabetes, have religious beliefs, do not have a spouse, and have higher physical-symptom distress experience lower functional status. Study findings can guide nurses in practice to refine assessment and design nursing interventions for this population. Also, study findings shed light on how important it is to assess focal and contextual stimuli.

A study by Burns (1997) examined a middle range theory deduced from the RAM on coping with hemodialysis, to describe the relationships among the concepts of age, time on hemodialysis, socioeconomic status, social support network, perceived problems, coping, and the physiological and psychological status of hemodialysis patients. Correlation, multiple regression, and path analysis were used to examine relationships. Although the population had a multitude of problems, the highest ranked problem for this sample was fatigue. The coping methods used most often were prayer and trust in God. Perceived problems were positively related to coping. The use of fatalistic, emotive, and supportive coping methods was related to low self-esteem, whereas evasive coping methods were related to poorer adjustment. Optimistic coping was related to higher systolic blood pressures.

Polichnowski's (2008) cross-sectional, predictive, correlational study tested the relationship of depression and the influence of SWB among a sample of university students who had been dating within the last year and may have experienced dating-violence victimization. Analysis shows that 32.2% of the sample recalled experiencing dating violence in the previous year with a significantly higher percentage of women compared to men. From the total sample, 2.02% of students were identified as positive for symptoms of posttraumatic stress disorder (PTSD). Measurements of

SWB revealed that women reported significantly higher mean scores of religious well-being (RWB), existential well-being (EWB), and SWB than men. The author concludes that both RWB and EWB facilitate adaptation by moderating and mediating the effects of dating-violence victimization controlling for gender, childhood exposure to family violence, and problem drinking. Their symptoms of depression were also lower. These findings empirically support an association between spirituality and mental health.

In a 2004 study, Zhang identified the variables that influence the decision-making responses related to advance directives by using a public data study of aging persons from 1984 to 2000 ($n = 938$). Using causal modeling with path analysis, the researcher found that age and gender significantly contributed to the number of hospital and nursing home admissions; that the number of hospital and nursing home admissions was significantly associated with physical impairment and that physical impairment had greatest effect on decision-making responses. Further, the findings showed that the degree of physical impairment also had indirect effects on AD completion through its influence on self-perception about health and role-function mode and that those who were less likely to work or do volunteer work also were less likely to complete ADs.

Description of Studies Related to Adaptive Modes

The RAM recognizes the person as an adaptive system; this system is open and constantly influenced by internal and external changes within the environment. This process of adaptation results in the system being and becoming an integrated and whole person (Roy, 2009). The four adaptive modes—physiologic, self-concept, role function, and interdependence—were derived from 500 samples of patient behavior to create categories for describing the adaptive behavior. Nursing interventions can be designed to manage stimuli and promote adaptation in each adaptive mode. In promoting adaptation the nurse contributes to improving health, quality of life, and dying with dignity.

The samples of the 18 studies included in this section on adaptive modes are patients with myasthenia gravis (MG), pregnant women, postpartum mothers in Thailand, adult men, adult women, Korean mothers, Taiwanese men with chronic obstructive pulmonary disease (COPD), Thai men who had experienced mild traumatic brain injury (MBTI), Judeo-Christian community-dwelling elders, women with urinary incontinence, caregivers, first-time percutaneous transluminal coronary angioplasty (PTCA) patients, students, mothers, and children ages 8 to 12 years (see Table 5.2).

TABLE 5.2

Studies That Explain, Predict, or Prescribe Related to Adaptive Modes

Author(s) and Date	Purpose	Sample	Design	Findings
1. Kittiwatanapaisan (2002)	To determine the level of fatigue compared to illness severity, depression, and to develop the Myasthenia Gravis Fatigue Scale	Patients with myasthenia gravis ($n = 67$)	Explain, predict, or prescribe; regression analysis	Significant correlations existed between fatigue scores and depression. The best predictor of fatigue severity was activity restriction followed by number of years since diagnosis
2. Corbett (1995)	To examine the relationships of iron and zinc, pica, social support, and birth weight	Socioeconomically disadvantaged pregnant women ($n = 128$)	Explain, predict, or prescribe; step-wise multiple regression	Predictors of increased infant birth weight were increased dietary vitamin iron levels and decreased plasma iron and plasma zinc levels
3. Jarczewski (1995)	To determine whether there are relationships among social support, self-esteem, symptom distress, and anxiety among adults with AIDS	Adult men ($n = 49$) and women ($n = 11$) with AIDS (total $n = 60$)	Explain, predict, or prescribe; multiple regression	A positive relationship existed between social support and self-esteem and a negative relationship existed between social support and anxiety. No relationship was found between social support and symptom distress. Self-esteem and symptom distress predicted anxiety

(continued)

TABLE 5.2

Studies That Explain, Predict, or Prescribe Related to Adaptive Modes (*continued*)

Author(s) and Date	Purpose	Sample	Design	Findings
4. Shin, Park, and Kim (2006)	To search for predictors of maternal sensitivity	Korean mothers 6 weeks postpartum (*n* = 196)	Explain, predict, or prescribe; hierarchical regression analysis	Maternal–fetal attachment was the strongest predictor of maternal sensitivity
5. Chen (2005)	To examine the relationships among physiologic and psychosocial factors and hospital readmission to predict chronic obstructive pulmonary disease hospital readmission	Taiwanese patients with COPD (*n* = 145)	Explain–predict–prescribe, linear multivariate model testing	Daily functioning was the only significant variable to predict COPD readmission at 90 days. Age was significantly correlated with 14 days readmission
6. Chen and Narsavage (2006)	To develop a model predicting COPD readmission following hospital discharge at 14 days and 90 days	Taiwanese patients with COPD living in rural areas (*n* = 145)	Explain–predict–prescribe, predictive, multivariate model testing	Daily functioning was the only significant variable to predict COPD readmission at 90 days. Age was significantly correlated with 14 days readmission
7. Narsavage and Chen (2008)	To identify predictors of depressed mood, which in turn could identify individuals at risk for the development of depression	Participants who were discharged from five community hospitals after treatment of their COPD exacerbation (*n* = 65 women, *n* = 59 men Total = 124)	Predict	After the use of control for physiologic status (forced expiratory volume in 1 second percent predicted), the factors of anxiety, perceived health competence, daily functioning, and family emotional coping predicted depressed mood

Study	Purpose	Sample	Approach	Findings
8. Wunderlich (2003)	To develop and test the Psychological Observation Weaning Evaluation Rating Scale (POWERS)	Adults weaning from mechanical ventilation ($n = 66$)	Explain–predict–prescribe, instrument development and structural equation modeling	Higher POWERS scores were associated with failure to wean. The model was effective at predicting successful weaning but was problematic in identifying possible failures to wean
9. Chen et al. (2005)	To test the goodness-of-fit exhibited by the Roy adaptation model for studying nutritional health of community-dwelling elders	Elders dwelling in a public housing complex ($n = 243$)	Explain–predict–prescribe, structural equation modeling	Functional status, oral health, depressive symptoms, and satisfaction with social support affect nutritional health directly
10. Toughill (2001)	To describe the impact of age, severity of urinary incontinence, and adaption on quality of life (QOL)	Women with self-reported urinary incontinence aged 23–85 years ($n = 141$)	Explain–predict–prescribe, regression analysis	Adaptation had the largest impact on QOL and had a mediating effect between urinary incontinence and QOL
11. Levesque, Ricard, Ducharme, Duquette, and Bonin (1998)	To derive a model of psychological adaptation from the RAM and to empirically verify the model from five studies	Formal and informal caregivers and community-dwelling elders from five different studies ($n = 2,187$)	Explain–predict–prescribe, structural equation modeling	The percentage of variance of psychological distress explained by the models varied from 17% for professional caregivers to 56% for informal caregivers of psychiatric patients in crisis

(continued)

TABLE 5.2

Studies That Explain, Predict, or Prescribe Related to Adaptive Modes (*continued*)

Author(s) and Date	Purpose	Sample	Design	Findings
12. Rees (1995)	To determine the relationships among coronary artery disease (CAD) knowledge, anxiety, social support, self-efficacy, and adaptive health behaviors for percutaneous transluminal coronary angioplasty patients	First-time PTCA patients ($n = 82$)	Explain–predict–prescribe, regression analysis	Knowledge, anxiety, social support, and self-efficacy influenced one or more of the adaptive health behaviors of diet modification, exercise, and smoking. Self-efficacy was the single most predictive variable that was consistently related to adaptive behavior
13. Lin (2005)	To assess role adaptation within maternal and student roles in RNs who returned to school for BS degrees and to explore relationships among demographics, physical, psychosocial factors, and multiple role adaptation	Female students who had at least one child younger than 18 and were students in Taiwanese nursing programs ($n = 118$)	Explain–predict–prescribe, regression analysis	The highest correlations were found between activity and role accumulation. Forty-three percent of the variance was explained by activity, sleep quality, and maternal role expectation
14. Kan (2007, 2009)	To describe the perspectives of recovery of patients with coronary artery bypass graft during postoperative period in their home environment	First-time CABG surgery patients ($n = 41$)	Predictive	High level of recovery at 6 weeks. Perceptions of recovery related to role function. Role function and social support predicted perceptions of recovery better than one variable

15. Lu (2001)	To explore the relationship among caregiving stress, functional capability, and self-care behavior and to determine whether there is a mediating effect of functional capability on the relationship between care giving stress and self-care behavior for elderly caregivers of persons with Alzheimer disease	Caregivers over 50 years of age recruited from registry of caregiving core of the University Alzheimer's Center in Cleveland, OH ($n = 99$)	Explaining	Depression and anxiety are strong mediator variables that accounted for most of the effect of caregiving stress on actual self-care behavior
16. Pecthprapai (2007)	To explore adaptation, determine factors associated with adaptation, and identify the predictors of adaptation among Thai adults who experienced mild traumatic brain injury in the previous 3 to 12 months	Thai middle-age men, half of whom are married, who experienced mild traumatic brain injury ($n = 130$)	Predicting	QOL was positively associated with social support but did not significantly correlate with other stimuli. The mediator effect of coping and depression symptoms was not supported. All stimuli together with coping and depressive symptoms significantly explained 15.8% of the variation of QOL, with social support as the most powerful variable in the equation. However, all stimuli, coping, and depressive symptoms were not able to explain successfully the GOSE

(continued)

TABLE 5.2

Studies That Explain, Predict, or Prescribe Related to Adaptive Modes (*continued*)

Author(s) and Date	Purpose	Sample	Design	Findings
				Despite the fact that coping and depressive symptoms were not supported as mediators in the original conceptual model, the interactions among coping, social support, and depressive symptoms could explain QOL. This finding suggested that coping and depressive symptoms are the moderators of QOL
17. Phahuwatanakorn (2004)	To examine the relationships among social support, maternal employment, postpartum anxiety, and maternal role competencies in Thai primiparous mothers	Thai primiparous postpartum mothers at a well-baby clinic and a postpartum clinic in a public hospital in Thailand (*n* = 124)	Predicting	Social support and employment had an effect of postpartum anxiety, but only social support had an effect on maternal competencies. Support from families and significant persons affected maternal competencies as evidenced by caring for the babies. Only social support could predict the level of postpartum anxiety

Kittiwatanapaisan (2002) performed the initial psychometric testing of the Myasthenia Gravis Fatigue Scale (MGFS). The researcher examined the relationships among fatigue in MG patients and disease severity, depression, and selected demographic and clinical characteristics. The research subjects were given four questionnaires, the MGFS, the Chalder Fatigue Scale, the Center for Epidemiologic Studies Depression Scale, and a demographic severity assessment. The MGFS demonstrated high internal consistency both for total scale and each subscale, with high alpha coefficients. Test–retest reliability was high. In the presence of five demographic and clinical characteristics, the fatigue score did not correlate with the disease severity score but positively correlated with depression. The results from the regression analyses revealed that there was a relationship between the fatigue scores and two of nine selected demographic and clinical characteristics. In conclusion the MGFS can be used to investigate the relationship between fatigue and demographic and clinical variables. In this study the author used the conceptual theoretical–empirical structure (Fawcett, 2010).

A study by Corbett (1995) examined the relationships of iron and zinc, pica, social support, and birth weight among socioeconomically disadvantaged pregnant women. In the context of the RAM, pregnancy was the focal stimulus; contextual stimuli included ethnicity, marital status, and inadequate preconceptual nutritional environment, which were comprised of the nutritional needs of pregnancy. For this study the women at risk for lower birth weight were African America single women. The author stated that the RAM was applicable in guiding the study and in investigating the relationships among trace elements, pica, social support, and infant birth weight in rural socioeconomically disadvantaged pregnant women. This study also has implications for practice in rural areas where multiple measurements of iron and zinc ought to be in considered in pregnant women during pregnancy and in infants after birth.

A study to determine whether there are relationships among social support, self-esteem, symptom distress, and anxiety among adults with AIDS was conducted by Jarczewski (1995). Findings indicated that 50% of the subjects perceived their general health as fair, whereas four subjects (6.7%) perceived their health as good or excellent. Ninety-five percent identified one or more sources of support. A positive relationship existed between social support and self-esteem and a negative relationship existed between social support and anxiety. No relationship was found between social support and symptom distress. Self-esteem and symptom distress predicted anxiety. Further analysis revealed that those subjects with higher self-esteem had lower symptom distress. Self-esteem was, therefore, the single best predictor of anxiety followed by symptom distress. The researcher stated that the results of this study cannot be generalized, but of importance is that adults with AIDS who have higher self-esteem may have lower anxiety, which can help nurses to promote self-esteem in patients with AIDS.

Shin, Park, and Kim (2006) aimed to explore the levels of maternal–fetal attachment, maternal identity, and to identify significant predictors of maternal sensitivity, among the characteristics of mother and infant. The conceptualization of this study views maternal sensitivity as a combination of the four RAM modes. Findings indicated that the levels of maternal sensitivity postpartum were somewhat high. The mother's employment status and infant's gestational age at birth were the statistically significant predictors of maternal sensitivity among characteristics of mother and infant. The strongest predictor of maternal sensitivity was maternal–fetal attachment, accounting for about a half (31%) of the total variance (60%) explained in maternal sensitivity. Mothers who had more maternal–fetal attachment during pregnancy were more likely to report better maternal sensitivity postpartum. The researcher stated that the results show that nursing interventions to help develop maternal sensitivity ought to be started during pregnancy and be directed at enhancing maternal–fetal attachment.

In 2005 Chen conducted her dissertation and later published two related papers with Narsavage. The original study was designed to predict hospital readmission for patients with COPD by examining relationships among physiologic and psychosocial factors. The sample was Taiwanese patients with COPD (n = 145) contacted at home or in the hospital. Data analyses included linear multivariate model testing. Main findings noted that daily functioning was the only significant variable to predict COPD readmission at 90 days. Age was significantly correlated with 14 days readmission.

When the study was published in a research journal by Chen and Narsavage (2006), the authors reported on the development of a model predicting hospital readmission for people with COPD living in rural Taiwanese communities and reported on the relationships among physiological, psychological factors, family support, and hospital readmission. The influence of the variables predicting COPD readmission was specific to 14 and 90 days following discharge. Within the framework of the RAM, COPD hospital readmission was viewed as an ineffective adaptive response that occurs with the failure to handle repeated symptoms. The focal stimulus was the stress of the exacerbations with contextual stimuli, including age, gender, and education. Three of Roy's adaptive modes, physiological, self-concept, and interdependence, were examined as adaptation to the disease. The physiological mode included physiological factors, such as daily functioning, comorbidity, and severity of illness. The self-concept mode was seen as the psychological factors of self-efficacy and depressive symptoms. The interdependence mode was comprised of perceived informal support. The study findings did not confirm the hypotheses regarding readmission with COPD following hospital discharge. Daily functioning was the only variable that was found to have significance and was an influential factor on readmission at 90 days. This study pioneers the exploration of readmission among patients with COPD and the results are an important first step in understanding COPD readmission.

In another publication (Narsavage & Chen, 2008) the investigators identified predictors of depressed mood, which in turn could identify individuals at risk for the development of depression. The sample was participants who were discharged from five community hospitals after treatment for COPD exacerbation ($n = 124$). The findings showed that after control for physiologic status (forced expiratory volume in 1 second, percentage predicted), the factors of anxiety, perceived health competence, daily functioning, and family emotional coping predicted depressed mood.

Wunderlich (2003) explored the relationship between physiological and psychological variables and their ability to predict successful weaning from mechanical ventilation. To conduct the study, the researcher further developed and tested the Psychological Observational Weaning Evaluation Rating Scale (POWERS), estimated the ability of the POWERS to predict successful weaning from the ventilator, determined the degree of association between the physiological variables as measured by the Weaning Readiness Assessment Scale (WRAS), examined effects of demographic information, and established the combination of study variables that best predicted the success of weaning from mechanical ventilation. Higher POWERS scores were associated with failure to wean. The model was effective at predicting successful weaning but was problematic in identifying possible failures to wean. This study lends support for the need of health care professionals to assess beyond physiological parameters and evaluate psychological status of patients weaning from mechanical ventilation.

A study by Chen et al. (2005) used a cross-sectional population to examine the goodness of fit exhibited by the proposed RAM-based framework of nutritional health for community-dwelling elders. Through the use of SEM both the links among the covert constructs and the relations among all the manifest indicators were tested. The researcher stated that theoretically, the results indicated that functional status, oral health, depressive symptoms, and satisfaction with support affected nutritional health directly. Oral health, depressive symptoms, functional status, and satisfaction with support mediated the effects of age, ethnicity, education, and the number of medications and chronic illnesses on nutritional health. Further, the model accounted for 35% of the variance in nutritional health and demonstrated a good fit with the data. The authors stated that future research needs to move beyond describing nutritional health and examining how cultural social factors relate, to how psychosocial factors may interact with biological processes longitudinally.

Toughill (2001) explored 141 women with incontinence. This study was based on the RAM precept that the person functions holistically with each mode related to and affected by others (Roy, 2009). For this study, urinary incontinence was conceptualized as the focal stimuli with changes in the physiological mode compounded by contextual and residual stimuli affecting the condition. Quality of life was conceptualized as a sense of well-being. Well-being stems from satisfaction or dissatisfaction with the areas of life important to the individual. This study examined the relationship between quality of life, age, adaptation, and severity of urinary incontinence. According to the researcher's framework, women used coping mechanisms to adapt to the focal stimulus of incontinence. Results of the regression analysis indicated that adaptation had the greatest impact on quality of life for the women. The other variables did not have significant impact on participants. Self-satisfaction was found to increase with quality of life.

In Levesque et al. (1998), the research team in nursing science from Montreal, Canada, consolidated their efforts to work on a program of research based on the RAM. The authors used data from five studies to elaborate on a theoretical model, to define the conceptual elements, and to formulate theoretical middle range propositions. Four groups of formal and informal caregivers and community-dwelling elders from five different studies ($n = 2,187$) were considered. Theoretical propositions derived from the RAM were supported by the LISREL VIII. The focal stimulus of perceived stress, the contextual stimulus of conflicts in the exchange of social support, and one component of the coping mechanisms were positively linked directly or indirectly with psychological distress, an indicator in the self-concept mode. The authors assert that the findings from this study should be considered in the further development of middle range theory.

Using a cross-sectional descriptive study, Rees (1995) investigated the existence of significant relationships among coronary artery disease (CAD), knowledge, anxiety, social support, self-efficacy, and adaptive health behaviors of diet, exercise, and smoking. The subjects were patients treated with percutaneous transluminal coronary angioplasty (PTCA). In this study the self-concept as represented by self-efficacy was influenced by the role-function mode represented by anxiety. Knowledge, anxiety, social support, and self-efficacy influenced one or more of the adaptive health behaviors of diet modification, exercise, and smoking. Self-efficacy was the single most predictive variable that was consistently related to adaptive behavior.

Lin's (2005) study assessed multiple role adaptation within maternal and student roles among female registered nurses (RNs) who had children and returned to school to obtain baccalaureate degrees. Lin explored relationships among demographic (number of children, age of youngest child, and employment status), physical (sleep quality, health perception, and activity), psychosocial factors (self-identity, role expectation, role involvement, and social support), and multiple-role adaptation (role accumulation). Results of this study showed positive correlations between role accumulation and the contextual variables of sleep quality, health perception, and activity. These findings suggested that mother-students who had better sleep quality, health perception, and activity levels had more effective multiple-role adaptation than those who did not report these behaviors.

Using a predictive design, Kan (2007, 2009), in a dissertation later published in a journal, examined the relationships among or combinations of adaptive behaviors (physical health, personal meaning, role function, and social support), age, and gender. The study explored the recovery of patients having CABG surgery for the first time using the four adaptive modes of the RAM. Analysis of variance was used to examine differences in the adaptive behaviors among certain demographic groups. The findings reported a correlation ($r = .32$, $p < .01$) between perceptions of recovery and role function. No statistically significant correlations were found among the other adaptive behaviors or perceptions of recovery. An important finding is that the adaptive behaviors of role function and social support were identified as contributors to the prediction of recovery.

Lu (2001) explored the relationship among caregiving stress, functional capability, and self-care behavior. The aim was to determine whether there is a mediating effect of functional capability on the relationship between caregiving stress and self-care behavior for elderly caregivers of persons with Alzheimer disease. The subjects were 99 caregivers over 50 years of age recruited from a registry. Depression and anxiety were strong mediator variables that accounted for most of the effect of care giving stress on actual self-care behavior.

The purpose of a study by Pecthprapai (2007) was to explore adaptation, determine factors associated with adaptation, and identify the predictors of adaptation among Thai adults who experienced MBTI. Subjects were Thai middle-age men who experienced MBTI in the previous 3 to 12 months ($n = 130$). The investigator reported the following findings: Quality of life was positively associated with social support but did not significantly correlate with other stimuli. The mediator effect of coping and depression symptoms was not supported. All stimuli together with coping and depressive symptoms significantly explained 15.8% of the variation of quality of life, with social support as the most powerful variable in the equation. However, all stimuli, coping, and depressive symptoms were not able to explain successfully the Glasgow Outcomes Scale Extended (GOSE). Despite the fact that coping and depressive symptoms were not supported as mediators in the original conceptual model, the interactions among coping, social support, and depressive symptoms could explain quality of life. This finding suggested that coping and depressive symptoms are the moderators of quality of life.

Another study in Thailand focused on primiparous postpartum mothers (*n* = 124). The aims of the study by Phahuwatanakorn (2004) were to examine the relationships among social support, maternal employment, postpartum anxiety, and maternal-role competencies in Thai primiparous mothers recruited in postpartum and well-baby clinics at a public hospital. The author reported findings that social support and employment had an effect on postpartum anxiety, but only social support had an effect on maternal competencies. Support from families and significant persons affected maternal competencies as evidenced by caring for the babies. Only social support could predict the level of postpartum anxiety.

Description of Studies Related to Stimuli

Roy describes focal stimuli as the degree of change that precipitated the behavior being observed. This focal stimulus is the one most immediately confronting the individual and the one to which the person must make an adaptive response. It may be an environmental change, a change in a relationship, or an internal change. Contextual stimuli are all those that contribute to the effect of the focal stimulus and residual stimuli may have an effect that is not yet determined. With stimuli the researcher can explain, predict, or prescribe the adaptive response. The researcher will construct efficient observations, formulate a hypothesis or hypotheses, collect data, and possibly develop new nursing interventions, adding to the body of knowledge of our profession.

Out of the 12 studies on stimuli, 8 studies (67 % of the total) were conducted in the United States. Three were implemented in Taiwan and one in Thailand. Studies were carried out in institutions or in the community. Institutional settings included hospitals; also studies were in mixed settings, and community households. The populations used in the studies included adult women, elderly Taiwanese adults, patients with cervical cancer, patients with arthritis, senior residents, adult care givers, and Taiwanese children ages 7 to 18 years (see Table 5.3).

Woods (1997) proposed a middle range theory synthesized from the RAM and linking the theoretic framework of PTSD to adaptation. The author examined adaptation and traumatic stress responses in abused (*n* = 53), formerly abused (*n* = 55), and nonabused women (*n* = 51). Hypotheses and research questions were derived from the proposed middle range theory. A predictive–comparative design was used to establish the relationships among patterns and severity of abuse, adaptation, and the occurrence and severity of features in battered women. Woods conceptualized the dependent variable to be the occurrence of the characteristic features of PTSD and the independent variables to include the focal, contextual,

TABLE 5.3

Studies That Explain, Predict, or Prescribe Related to Stimuli

Author(s) and Date	Purpose	Sample	Design	Findings
1. Woods (1997)	To test the empirical validity of two propositions of the Roy adaptation model (RAM) with a population of battered and formerly battered women, and to investigate the context, occurrence, and predictors of characteristic features of posttraumatic stress disorder in women in three different situational contexts (currently battered, formerly battered, and never battered)	Women who were abused (*n* = 53), post abuse (*n* = 55), and nonabused (*n* = 51)	Predictive	Strong evidence for direct relationships among physical, emotional, and/or sexual abuse as a traumatic event that produces the response of PTSD; PTSD was present in both abused and post abused women in this sample; women in abusive relationships are subject to chronic threat and injury as well as acute episodes of violence. Depression was the most important predictor of PTSD in this sample

(continued)

TABLE 5.3
Studies That Explain, Predict, or Prescribe Related to Stimuli (*continued*)

Author(s) and Date	Purpose	Sample	Design	Findings
2. Woods and Isenberg (2001)	To test the efficacy of a middle range theory of adaptation as a mediator of intimate abuse and traumatic stress in battered women	Women, 53 currently abused, 55 post abused, 52 nonabused women (*n* = 160)	Predictive— series of regression equations	• Abused women experienced significant risk of homicide • Significant correlations—focal stimuli of abuse and response of PTSD • Path between physiologic responses and each predictor variables of abuse is significant • Path between physiologic responses and PTSD is significant • Correlation of self-concept and each predictor of abuse is significant • Role function correlates significantly with physical abuse, but not with emotional abuse and risk of homicide, nor PTSD • Interdependent significant correlations with each predictor variable of abuse and with PTSD
3. Shyu, Lu, and Wu (2004)	To examine environmental barriers and mobility	Elderly Taiwanesse adults post hip-fracture (*n* = 87)	Explain–predict– prescribe, regression analysis	Prefracture condition accounted for 40% of the variance and environmental conditions accounted for 20% of the variance

Author	Purpose	Sample	Approach/Analysis	Findings
4. Sirapongam, Putwatana, Kitrungroj, and Piratchavet (2002)	To explore the severity of side effects, self-esteem, social support, and education on role adaptation	Patients with cervical cancer receiving radiation therapy in Bangkok (*n* = 86)	Explain–predict–prescribe, regression analysis	Role adaptation, social support, self-esteem, and severity of side effects accounted for 54% of the variance. Education did not contribute to role adaptation
5. Tsai, Tak, Moore, and Palencia (2003)	To test a middle range theory of chronic pain derived from the RAM	Older people with arthritis (*n* = 71)	Explain–predict–prescribe, path analysis	The direct effects of chronic pain, disability, social support, age, and gender accounted for 37% of variance in daily stress
6. Tsai (2005)	To test a theory of distress and depression in chronic pain, with financial hardship as a contextual stimulus	Older people with arthritis (*n* = 235)	Explain–predict–prescribe, path analysis	Disability and financial hardship predicted distress , whereas social support and age had a reverse effect. Disability, social support, financial hardship and age predicted distress, whereas pain, disability, and distress predicted depression
7. Han (2002)	To identify factors influencing anticipatory nausea and vomiting (ANV) in cancer patients	Adult patients with cancer hospitalized for chemotherapy, third cycle or above (*n* = 66)	Explain–predict–prescribe, regression analysis	Factors directly related to ANV were psychological symptoms and severity of postchemotherapy nausea and vomiting. Environmental cues related to ANV were awareness of hospital setting and sensory stimuli

(continued)

TABLE 5.3

Studies That Explain, Predict, or Prescribe Related to Stimuli (*continued*)

Author(s) and Date	Purpose	Sample	Design	Findings
8. Chen, Chang, Chung and McCorkle (2005)	To evaluate the dynamics of nutritional health within the context of RAM	Senior residents who lived in an inner-city public housing complex (n = 310)	Explain–predict–prescribe, structural equation modeling	The presence of depressive symptoms, oral health problems, lower functional status, and income less than $10K emerged as independent predictors of under nutrition, or compromised nutritional health
9. Nuamah, Cooley, Fawcett, and McCorkle (1999)	To test three propositions of the RAM related to quality of life (QOL) in cancer patients	Newly diagnosed post surgical cancer patients 60 years of age and over (n = 375)	Explain–predict–prescribe, structural equation modeling	Severity of illness and adjuvant cancer treatment were the strongest indicators of health-related quality of life (HRQOL). HRQOL was strongly defined by affective status, functional status, and physical symptoms, and less by social support. HRQOL at 3 months was significantly predicted by HRQOL at baseline
10. Yeh (2002)	To test the theory that environmental stimuli and communication influence biopsychosocial responses	Taiwanese children with cancer aged 7–18 years of age at the time of their cancer diagnosis and their parents (n = 116)	Explain–predict–prescribe, structure equation modeling	Severity of illness demonstrated an excellent fit with stage of illness, lab values, and total hospitalizations. Communication with others, severity of illness, and age were influenced by biopsychosocial responses

11. Hay (2005)	To test a theoretical path model of the effects of age, income, gender, education, time on dialysis, functional health status, spirituality, powerlessness, and depression on QOL of elderly end-stage renal disease patients	Patients over 65 years in center for hemodialysis (n = 79)	Explain–predict–prescribe, path analysis	Total functioning, depression, powerlessness, and spiritual coping all had significant direct effects on QOL. Powerlessness also had a significant indirect effect on QOL through total functioning
12. Tsai (1998)	To predict caregiver stress and its outcome from demographic characteristics, objective burden in caregiving, stressful life events, social support, and social roles	Adult caregivers of an elderly relative who were included in longitudinal survey data from (American Changing Lives) (n = 236 for Wave 1 and 271 for Wave 2)	Explain–predict–prescribe, structural equation modeling	Objective burden in caregiver stress and perceived stress were not the primary determinants of outcomes. Race, age, gender, and relationship with the care recipient played important roles in predicting focal, contextual stimuli, depression, and adaptive modes

and residual stimuli, and the reactions in the four adaptive modes. One of the strengths of this study was the power analysis performed to determine an adequate sample size. The sampling technique used in this study was a nonprobability quota. The analysis showed that the focal, contextual, and residual stimuli accounted for 62% of the explained variance in the occurrence and severity of PSTD in the sample. Woods stated that physical, emotional, and sexual abuses by an intimate partner were identified as stressors that would initiate a pattern of physiologic and psychological responses in the abused woman. She found positive relationships among physical, emotional abuse, and risk of homicide in intimate relationships in battered women. Woods found significant differences in self-esteem between women in the abuse and nonabuse situational context. The researcher reported that she also found moderate negative relationships between the stability with which one views the self and PSTD. Woods also reported that the findings of her study provide strong evidence of the presence of PTSD in both abused and post abuse women. Therefore, nurses will assess all women physically and emotionally in current or previous relationships of intimate partner violence.

Woods and Isenberg (2001), using a predictive design, examined adaptation as a mediator of traumatic stress in battered women. The outcome gives support to linking the theoretical framework of PTSD with Roy's conceptual model. Intimate partner abuse is a stressor that initiates a pattern of physiologic and psychologic posttraumatic stress responses in battered women. Woods and Isenberg's (2001) analysis included regression and path analytic procedures. The purpose of this research was to test one aspect of a proposed middle range theory synthesized from the RAM and linked with the framework of posttraumatic stress. Results indicated direct relationships between the focal stimuli of abuse and the response of PTSD, and adaptation in the physiologic, self-concept, and interdependence modes partially mediated the relationship between the focal stimulus of abuse and the response of PTSD in battered women. The researchers confirmed that adaptation is a partial mediator of PTSD. If so, this finding has an implication for nursing practice. If abuse in an intimate relationship is suspected or reported nurses need to assess for PTSD. Utilization of interventions directed toward assimilation and integration of traumatic events is needed to alleviate the distressful patterning of responses. Additionally, the authors identified a second intervention area related to the physiologic, self-concept, and interdependence adaptive modes. They stated that nurses can assist abused and postabused women by finding means to decrease their physiologic distress, increase their self-esteem, and learn how they can create and maintain intimate relationships.

Using regression analysis, Shyu, Liang, Lu, and Wu (2004) explored the relationship between environmental stimuli, specifically, barriers and the mobility of elderly persons with hip fracture after surgery. The follow-up study was conducted 3 months after hospital discharge. After controlling for prefracture conditions, findings showed that subjective environmental barriers related to reduced walking ability, self-care ability, and role performance of elderly persons with hip fractures. The researchers stated that their study systemically expands the use of RAM in the following ways. First, it supports the relationship of physical environmental stimuli on adaptive behaviors in two adaptive modes. Also, although the RAM was developed in the Western culture, it was useful in a Taiwanese study. Based on the findings of this study, nurses need to assess and intervene in the areas of the home environment that are subjective barriers for elderly persons with hip fractures in order to promote physical functioning, including mobility, activities of daily living (ADLs), and role function.

Sirapongam, Putwatana, Kitrungroj, and Piratchavet (2002) used regression analysis to investigate adaptation in the role-function mode. The aim was to determine the predictive power of severity of side effects, self-esteem, social support, and education on role adaptation of patients with cervical cancer receiving radiation therapy in Bangkok, Thailand. The study focused on roles of being a wife, worker, and the sick role. The focal stimulus was the external modification produced by the radiation therapy. In this study the physiological, self-concept, and interdependence modes were represented by empirical indicators that were severity of side effects, self-esteem, and social support, respectively. The mean score on role adaptation suggested that patients getting radiation had high levels of adaptation. As noted, role adaptation was viewed as the combination of adaptation to three subroles, including wife, work, and sick roles. The seven highest mean scores were in the sick-role adaptation and were explained by the social mechanisms within the role-function mode of the RAM. Education was the only predictor that was not significantly correlated with adaptation. The author stated that a possible reason could be that most subjects in this study were relatively homogenous with respect to education. Around 72% of the patients had primary school certificates, whereas only 12.79% of the patients had vocational or undergraduate education. Therefore, the combination of social support, self-esteem, and severity of side effects accounted for 54.8% of the variance in role adaptation of patients. The researchers concluded that nurses will consider the importance of enhancing effective adaptation. In doing so, factors influencing role adaptation should be assessed and followed by specific planned nursing interventions.

Using a secondary analysis, Tsai, Tak, Moore, and Palencia (2003) tested a middle range theory of chronic pain derived from the RAM. The original research used path analysis to explain the relationships among functional disability, chronic daily stress, social support, and depressive mood of elders with arthritis. The model was supported by data showing that pain, disability, and social support resulted in perceived daily stress that in turn predicted depression. Pain, disability, and social support, however, explained only 35% of the variance. This study was a first step in validating a middle range theory of chronic pain derived from the RAM in a sample of older people with arthritis. Findings supported that daily stress was an important factor leading to depression in older people with arthritis. To treat depression, health care providers need not only use antidepressants for symptom control but must try to understand the influence of daily stress for individuals. With this understanding the nurse can develop a strategy to minimize the impact of perceived daily stress.

A study by Tsai (2005) tested the theory of chronic pain with financial hardship added as an additional variable or contextual stimulus. The theory was tested using a secondary data-analysis strategy, and the study variables were constructed from the original data set. Pain was measured by one question: "On how many of the past 7 days have you had any sorts of aches and pains other than headache?" Responses were on an 8 point scale ranging from none to seven days, with higher scores reflecting more frequent pain. Physical disability was also measured; financial hardship was measured by three items asking respondents to rate the frequency of the following: having trouble paying the bills; not having enough money to buy food, clothes, and other household needs; and not having enough money to pay medical bills. In this study, disability, social support, financial hardship, and age resulted in distress, which in turn led to depression, although unexpectedly, chronic pain had no impact on distress. Interestingly, the data-derived model showed that although pain had no impact on distress, it had a direct impact on depression. A test of the theory suggested that pain, disability, and social support predict distress in elders with arthritis. Distress in turn has an impact on depression.

Han (2002), basing her research in the RAM, studied the factors of anticipatory nausea and vomiting in cancer patients. Her model views nausea and vomiting as responses to internal and external stimuli. The focal stimuli occurred from the anxiety about chemotherapy; contextual stimuli, included severity of postchemotherapy nausea and vomiting, physical and psychological symptoms, environmental factors, cancer type; and residual stimuli included age and motion sickness. The psychological symptoms and severity of postchemotherapy nausea and vomiting appeared prominent as the influencing factors on ANV in cancer patients accounting for 39.5% of the variance. As a focal stimulus, anxiety about chemotherapy was not discovered to be a significant factor for ANV. As contextual stimuli the previous experiences in chemotherapy and the postchemotherapy nausea and vomiting appeared to be major factors with which the ANV can be preassumed. The study attempted to manipulate anxiety about chemotherapy as focal stimuli; severity of postchemotherapy nausea and vomiting, physical and psychological symptoms, environmental factors and cancer type as contextual stimuli and age and motion sickness as residual stimuli; based on RAM. The focal, contextual, and residual stimuli divided by priority in RAM did not divide clearly and the results showed that all stimuli are related, influencing each other. The ANV is a phenomenon that cannot be explained with a specified source of stimulation based on RAM. Future studies can be designed using other variables that affect adaptation.

Chen et al. (2005) stated that the aim of their study was to examine the goodness of fit for the proposed RAM-based framework of nutritional health for community-dwelling elders. The authors noted that the success of nutrition care depends on careful identification of those elders at greatest risk for malnutrition. The RAM was used as a conceptual framework for a holistic understanding of nutritional health among community-dwelling elders. Using the standard error of the mean (SEM), the investigators analyzed both the links among the constructs and the strengths of the relationships among them. The results showed that functional status, oral health, depressive symptoms, and satisfaction with support affected nutritional health directly. Oral health, depressive symptoms, functional status, and satisfaction with support mediated the effects of age, ethnicity, education, the number of medications, and chronic illnesses on nutritional health. The model gives an explanation for 35% of the variance in nutritional health and demonstrates a good fit with the data. The framework tested by Chen and colleagues offers a theoretical and empirical roadmap for the development of nutritional interventions that promote adaptation, independence, and quality of life for community-dwelling elders.

A study by Nuamah et al. (1999) focused on focal stimuli of adjuvant cancer treatment and severity of the disease. Three propositions derived from the RAM that related to quality of life in cancer patients were tested with SEM. Severity of illness and adjuvant cancer treatment were the strongest indicators of health-related quality of life (HRQOL). HRQOL was strongly defined by affective status, functional status, and physical symptoms, and less by social support. HRQOL at 3 months was significantly predicted by HRQOL at baseline. The investigators noted that the major contribution of this study is that the multidimensionality of HRQOL can be accounted for simultaneously in a way that makes sense and that there is a conceptual fit between the HRQOL framework and the framework of a traditional nursing theory (RAM).

Yeh (2002) tested the RAM-based theory of HRQOL in Taiwanese children with cancer. The researcher postulated that the stimuli included severity of illness, age, gender, communication with others, and understanding of the illness. The severity of the illness was a latent variable construct, including the stage of illness, laboratory values, and number of hospitalizations. Yeh used biobehavioral responses, that is, HRQOL, as a latent variable that consisted of (1) physical function, (2) psychological function, (3) peer/school function, (4) treatment/disease symptoms, and (5) cognition functions. Study findings included that the stimuli of severity of illness, age, gender, understanding of illness, and communication with others influenced the biobehavioral responses of children with cancer. The four adaptive modes from RAM (physiologic, self-concept, interdependence, and role function), and five dimensions from HRQOL (physical, disease/symptom related, psychological, peer/school, and cognitive) are interrelated. The three most important findings were (1) the construct of severity of illness confirmed an excellent fit with stage of illness, (2) the HRQOL also confirmed good construct validity with five domains, and (3) the study supported the RAM-based proposition that stimuli influenced psychosocial responses.

A theoretical path model was tested by Hay (2005). The effects of age, income, gender, education, time on dialysis, functional health status, spirituality, powerlessness, and depression on QOL of elderly patients with ESRD was tested. Subjects were patients over the age of 65 years recruited in a center for hemodialysis ($n = 79$). Total functioning, depression, powerlessness, and spiritual coping all had significant direct effects on QOL. Powerlessness also had a significant indirect effect on QOL through total functioning.

Tsai (1998) derived the theory of caregiver stress from the RAM, to examine the relationships among stimuli, coping mechanisms, and adaptive modes. The researcher aimed to predict caregiver stress and its outcome from demographic characteristics, objective burden in caregiving, stressful life events, social support, and social roles. The author hypothesized that the concept of objective burden in caregiving could be the most important stimulus leading to perceived caregiver stress. She tested the hypothesis that higher perceived caregiver stress would result in ineffective responses (poor health function, lower self-esteem/mastery, role enjoyment, and marital satisfaction, and less ability to reciprocate). In addition, Tsai examined the role of depression and the function of contextual stimuli in the model. Analysis of the data did not support the initial theory. Based on that premise, the primary model was modified by reevaluating the relations among constructs in empirical data using SEM. The robustness of the final data-derived model was further partially cross-validated with another sample and was further simplified. Findings showed that (1) objective burden in caregiving and perceived caregiver stress were not the most important determinants of outcomes in the context of long-term caregiving; (2) perceived caregiver stress and depression are related yet different concepts in predicting caregivers' outcomes; (3) depression was the most easily aroused outcome of perceived caregiver stress; (4) contextual stimuli do not have either the main effect on perceived caregiver stress or a moderated effect on the relation between objective burden in caregiving and perceived caregiver stress, instead, they influenced caregivers' outcomes directly; (5) gender is the only residual stimulus that was found to predict perceived caregiver stress; and (6) there were no causal relationships among adaptive modes; instead, adaptive-mode variables were either predicted by depression, contextual stimuli, or residual stimuli.

CRITICAL ANALYSES OF STUDIES

As noted in the last two chapters, the critical analyses of the studies involved summarizing the results of the scored evaluation. Evaluations on each study were conducted by one or more members of the project team. In addition the authors of this chapter commented on the strengths and weaknesses of the studies designated as using the designs that explain, predict, and prescribe. The range of scores for the studies was from 20 (highest possible) to 16. A total of 16 out of the 44 studies earned the highest possible score of 20 points, meaning that they were rated as meeting the criteria for high-quality research in all of the four categories scored. Only two of the studies scored 16 (lowest possible for inclusion), which means that they had an acceptable level of 80% of the criteria met. All studies were deemed appropriate to be used for further knowledge development and evidence for practice.

The overall analysis of these studies shows that the majority of the research was related to middle range theory testing, evaluation of the dynamic relationships among variables derived within the context of the RAM, and testing of propositions derived from the RAM. In the majority of the studies, the samples were convenience samples, with few random samples. The designs of the studies largely aimed to explain and predict. The investigators discussed implications for practice or possible prescriptions for practice.

A number of researchers used multiple regression analyses to predict rather than determine differences in groups. This analysis is based on probability theory, which is in keeping with how nursing looks at empirical relationships. As with contemporary empiricism, the probability of a link between variables and the context of other variables is useful in understanding the phenomenon. Examples of studies using multiple regression are: Kittiwatanapaisan (2002); Corbett (1995); Jarczewski (1995); Shin, Park, and Kim (2006) Rees (1995); Lin (2005); Henderson, Fogel, and Edwards (2003); Kan (2007); Polichnowski (2008); Toughill (2001); Woods (1997); Shu, Liang, Lu, and Wu (2004), Sirapongam et al. (2002); and Han (2002).

On the other hand, other investigators used path analysis, a model-testing design. The model identifies all the paths expressing the relationships among the concepts. The purpose of the analyses is to test whether or not data are consistent with the model. Large homogeneous samples are needed, and sometimes the data are split into a set to determine the model and another to test the model. Through this approach it is possible to achieve richer understanding of the data. Some examples include the work of Kessenich (1996), Huang (2002), Robinson (1995), Hamner (1996), Burns (1997), Tsai (2005), Chen (2005), and Chen and Narsavage (2006). Tsai et al. (2003) also used path analysis to achieve richer understanding of the middle range theory of chronic pain derived from the RAM. SEM is a specific approach used with path analysis to test theories. Several researchers identified that they used this statistical procedure, including: Dunn (2001), Ducharme et al. (1998), Yeh (2003), Zbegner (2003), Chiou (1997), Wunderlich (2003), Dunn (2005), Chen (2005), Levesque et al. (1998), Chen, (2005), Tsai (1998), Yeh (2002), and Nuamah et al. (1999). The study by Tsai (1998) was a particularly diligent form of testing a model of caregiver stress. The author trimmed the model twice and used another sample to confirm the best fit.

The use of the RAM provided specificity concerning variables with predictable effectiveness, such as testing a middle range theory of chronic pain. The 11 studies that explained, predicted, or prescribed related to stimuli seem to have a high potential for implementation in practice since most had useful new knowledge about dealing with the factors affecting adaptation to common health issues. Many of the other studies provide a basis for continued knowledge development.

CONCLUSION

In this chapter we described and critiqued the large number of studies based on the RAM that used designs that provide for higher levels of understanding the phenomena being studied, that is, explaining, predicting, and prescribing. They show the difficulty and rewards in implementing complex designs that are closely linked to theory. They are rich with insights and provide clear direction for both practice and for further research. The number of studies using advanced statistics to explain and predict as well as evidence of programs of research is encouraging.

REFERENCES

Fawcett, J. (2010). Theory testing and theory evaluation. In J. Butts & K. Rich (Eds.), *Philosophies and theories for advanced nursing practice* (pp. 605–623). Sudbury, MA: Jones & Bartlett Learning.

Polit, D., & Beck, C. T. (2012). *Nursing research: Generating and assessing evidence for practice.* (9th ed.). Philadelphia, PA: Lippincott Williams & Wilkins.

Roy, C., & Roberts, S. (1981). *Theory construction in nursing: An adaptation model.* Engelwood Cliffs, NJ: Prentice-Hall.

Roy, C. (1988). An explication of the philosophical assumptions of the Roy adaptation model. *Nursing Science Quarterly, 1,* 26–34.

Roy, C. (2009). *The Roy adaptation model* (3rd ed.). Upper Saddle River, NJ: Prentice Hall Health.

Weiss, S. J. (1995). Contemporary empiricism. In A. Omery, C. E. Kasper, & G. G. Page (Eds.), *In search of nursing science* (pp. 13–26). Thousand Oaks, California: SAGE.

BIBLIOGRAPHY

Bournaki, M. (1997). Correlates of pain-related responses to venipunctures in school-age children. *Nursing Research, 46*(3), 147–154.

Burns, D. (1997). Coping with hemodialysis: A mid-range theory deduced from the Roy adaptation model (Doctoral dissertation, Wayne State University). *Dissertation Abstracts International, 58*(03B), 1206.

Chen, Y. (2005). *The influence of physiological factors, psychological factors, and informal social support on hospital readmission in discharged patients with COPD in Taiwan* (Doctoral dissertation, Case Western Reserve University).

Chen, C. C. H., Chang, C. K., Chyun, D. A., & McCorkle, R. (2005). Dynamics of nutritional health in a community sample of American elders: A multidimensional approach using Roy's Adaptation Model. *Advances in Nursing-Science, 28*(4), 376–389.

Chen, Y., & Narsavage, G. L. (2006). Factors related to chronic obstructive pulmonary disease readmission in Taiwan. *Western Journal of Nursing Research, 28*(1), 105–124.

Chiou, C. (1997). Correlates of functional status of hemodialysis patients in Taiwan (Doctoral dissertation, University of Pennsylvania). *Dissertation Abstracts International, 58*(11B), 5887.

Corbett, R. (1995). The relationships among trace elements, pica, social support, and infant birthweight (Doctoral dissertation, University of South Carolina). *Dissertation Abstracts International, 56*(06B), 3125.

Ducharme, F., Ricard, N., Duquette, A., Levesque, L., & Lachance, L. (1998). Empirical testing of a longitudinal model derived from the Roy adaptation model. *Nursing Science Quarterly, 11*(4), 149–159.

Dunn, K. S. (2001). *Adaptation to chronic pain: Religious and non-religious coping in Judeo-Christian elders* (Doctoral dissertation, Case Western Reserve University).

Dunn, K. S. (2005). Testing a middle-range theoretical model of adaptation to chronic pain. *Nursing Science Quarterly, 18*(2), 146–156.

Hamner, J. B. (1996). Preliminary testing of a proposition from the Roy adaptation model. *Image: Journal of Nursing Scholarship, 28*(3), 215–220.

Han, S. (2002). Factors of anticipatory nausea and vomiting in cancer patients. *Journal of Korean Academic Nursing, 32*(7), 977–985.

Hay, C. G. (2005). Predictors of quality of life of elderly end-stage renal disease patients: An application of Roy's model. *Georgia State University, 99.* Retrieved from http://proquest.umi.com/pqdweb?did=888859871&Fmt=6&clientId=7750&RQT=309&VName=PQD.

Henderson, P. D., Fogel, J., & Edwards, Q. T. (2003). Coping strategies among African American women with breast cancer. *Southern Online Journal of Nursing Research, 4*(3), 20–47.

Huang, C. (2002). *Sleep and daytime sleepiness in first-time mothers during early postpartum in Taiwan* (Doctoral dissertation, University of Texas at Austin).

Jarczewski, P. (1995). Social support, self-esteem, symptom distress, and anxiety of adults with acquired immune deficiency syndrome (Doctoral dissertation, University of Alabama at Birmingham). *Dissertation Abstracts International, 56*(04B), 1936.

Kan, E. Z. (2007). Adaptive behaviors and perceptions of recovery following coronary artery bypass graft surgery. *Pennsylvania: Widener University School of Nursing.* Retrieved from HYPERLINK "https://email.bc.edu/owa/redir.aspx?C=bkw2f-2RGUunDNuMoxw5SWZhfAB2T88Ivo_yY3AukVc-XFoS45QUDrP8iqnmsgHu7dHYv4TRKho.&URL=http%3a%2f%2fproquest.umi.com%2fpqdweb%3fdid%3d1390306701%26Fmt%3d6%26clientId%3d7750%26RQT%3d309%26VName%3dPQD" \t "_blank" http://proquest.umi.com/pqdweb?did=1390306701&Fmt=6&clientId=7750&RQT=309&VName=PQD

Kan, E. Z. (2009). Perceptions of recovery, physical health, personal meaning, role function, and social support after first-time coronary artery bypass graft surgery. *Dimensions of Critical Care Nursing, 28*(4), 189.

Kessenich, C. (1996). Quality of life of elderly women with spinal fractures secondary to osteoporosis (Doctoral dissertation, University of Alabama at Birmingham). *Dissertation Abstracts International, 57*(08B), 4976.

Kittiwatanapaisan, W. (2002). *Measurement of fatigue in myasthenia gravis patients* (Doctoral dissertation, University of Alabama at Birmingham).

Levesque, L., Ricard, N., Ducharme, F., Duquette, A., & Bonin, J. (1998). Empirical verification of a theoretical model derived from the Roy adaptation model: Findings from five studies. *Nursing Science Quarterly, 11*(1), 31–39.

Lin, L. (2005). Multiple role adaptation among women who have children and re-enter nursing school in Taiwan. *The Journal of Nursing Education, 44*(3), 116–123.

Lu, Y. (2001). *Caregiving stress effects on functional capability and self-care behavior for elderly caregivers of persons with Aizheimer's disease.* Cleveland, OH: Case Western Reserve University (Health Sciences). Retrieved from http://proquest.umi.com/pqdweb?index=54&did=728903191&SrchMode=1&sid=1&Fmt=2&VInst=PROD&VType=PQD&RQT=309&VName=PQD&TS=1224508512&clientID=7750

Narsavage, G. L., & Chen, Y. (2008). Factors related to depressed mood in adults with COPD after hospitalization. *Home Healthcare Nurse, 26*(8), 475–482.

Nuamah, I. F., Cooley, M. E., Fawcett, J., & McCorkle, R. (1999). Testing a theory for health-related quality of life in cancer patients: A structural equation approach. *Research in Nursing and Health, 22*(3), 231–242.

Pecthprapai, N. (2007). Adaptation to mild traumatic brain injury among Thai adults. *Ohio: Case Western Reserve University.* Retrieved from http://proquest.umi.com/pqdweb? did=1324382231&Fmt=6&clientId=7750&RQT=309&VName=PQD.

Phahuwatanakorn, W. (2004). The relationships between social support, maternal employment, postpartum anxiety, and maternal role competencies in Thai primiparous mothers. *District of Columbia: The Catholic University of America.* Retrieved from http://proquest.umi.com/pqdweb?did=765147751&Fmt=6&clie ntId=7750&RQT=309&VName=PQD.

Polichnowski, E. J. (2008). *Adaptation through spiritual well-being as a mediator or moderator of the relationship of the adverse psychological effects of dating violence in a sample of university students.* Johns Hopkins University, 211 pp. Retrieved from http://proquest.umi.com/pqdweb? did=1540415481&Fmt=6& clientId=7750&RQT=309&VName=PQD

Rees, B. (1995). Influences of coronary artery disease knowledge, anxiety, social support, and self-efficacy on adaptive health behaviors of patients treated with a percutaneous transluminal coronary angioplasty (Doctoral dissertation, University of Alabama at Birmingham). *Dissertation Abstracts International, 56*(07B), 3696.

Robinson, J. H. (1995). Grief responses, coping processes, and social support of widows: Research with Roy's Model. *Nursing Science Quarterly, 8*(4), 158–164.

Shin, H., Park, Y. J., & Kim, M. J. (2006). Predictors of maternal sensitivity during the early postpartum period. *Journal of Advanced Nursing, 55*(4), 425–434. doi:10.1111/j.1365-2648.2006.03943.x.

Shyu, Y. I. L., Liang, J., Lu, J. F. R., & Wu, C. C. (2004). Environmental barriers and mobility in Taiwan: Is the Roy adaptation model applicable? *Nursing Science Quarterly, 17*(2), 165–170.

Sirapongam, Y., Putwatana, P., Kitrungroj, L., & Piratchavet, V. (2002). Factors influencing role adaptation of patients with cervical cancer receiving radiation therapy. *Thai Journal of Nursing Research, 6*(4), 163–176.

Toughill, E. H. (2001). *Quality of life: The impact of age, severity of urinary incontinence and adaptation* (Doctoral dissertation, New York University).

Tsai, P. (1998). Development of a middle-range theory of caregiver stress from the Roy adaptation model (Doctoral dissertation, Wayne State University). *Dissertation Abstracts International, 60*(01B), 0133.

Tsai, P. F. (2005). Predictors of distress and depression in elders with arthritic pain. *Journal of Advanced Nursing, 51*(2), 158.

Tsai, P. F., Tak, S., Moore, C., & Palencia, I. (2003). Testing a theory of chronic pain. *Journal of Advanced Nursing, 43*(2), 158–169.

Woods, S. (1997). Predictors of traumatic stress in battered women: A test and explication of the Roy adaptation model (Doctoral dissertation, Wayne State University). *Dissertation Abstracts International, 58*(03B), 1220.

Woods, S. J., Isenberg, M. A. (2001). Adaptation as a mediator of intimate abuse and traumatic stress in battered women. *Nursing Science Quarterly, 14*(3), 215–221.

Wunderlich, R. J. (2003). *An exploratory study of physiological and psychological variables that predict weaning from mechanical ventilation* (Doctoral dissertation). St. Louis, MO: Saint Louis University.

Yeh, C. (2002). Health-related quality of life in pediatric patients with cancer. A structural equation approach with the Roy adaptation model. *Cancer Nursing, 25*(1), 74.

Yeh, C. (2003). Psychological distress: Testing hypotheses based on Roy's adaptation model. *Nursing Science Quarterly, 16*(3), 255–263.

Zbegner, D. K. (2003). *An exploratory retrospective study using the Roy adaptation model: The adaptive mode variables of physical energy level, self-esteem, marital satisfaction, and parenthood motivation as predictors of coping behaviors in infertile women* (Doctoral dissertation). Chester, PA: Widener University School of Nursing.

Zhang, W. (2004). *Factors influencing end-of-life decisions regarding the living will and durable power of attorney: An application of Roy's Adaptation Model* (Doctoral dissertation, Georgia State University).

6

Quantitative Studies:
Interventions Designs

KATHRYN LAUCHNER AND MARTHA V. WHETSELL

The purpose of nursing knowledge is to improve nursing practice. In the last three chapters the authors reported research that developed knowledge about how people deal with changing situations of health in studies that describe, delineate relationships, and explain or predict. This knowledge can be used to design interventions for nursing practice. Nursing interventions have been defined as "deliberative cognitive, physical or verbal activities performed with, or on behalf of, individuals and their families (that) are directed toward accomplishing particular therapeutic objectives relative to individuals' health and well-being" (Grobe, 1996, p. 50). Once a nursing intervention is designed, it is tested for its effect on the expected outcome. A number of study designs can be used to test interventions. The most common are the quasi-experimental and the experimental study. With a well-designed study, one can measure the effect of the intervention, the independent variable, or the dependent variable. The major terms used here are summarized in Box 6.1.

Research methodologists urge that the intervention be clearly described and designed whether it is an action at a given time, such as the method of tracheal suctioning of a patient or a protocol of approaches, including those that are educational, supportive, and psychomotor, as for example, working with a newly diagnosed person with diabetes. Further, it is necessary that the intervention is clearly linked to the outcome measures. The purpose of this chapter is to analyze intervention research using the Roy adaptation model (RAM) and to show what evidence it can provide for practice. Specific aims are to (a) describe the studies in this group, (b) critique the research, and (c) provide exemplars for change in practice based on research.

OVERVIEW OF STUDIES WITH INTERVENTION DESIGNS

In the category of studies with intervention designs the project team designated 25 studies. In Chapter 2 the main clusters of propositions from the RAM were described as a way to organize the presentation of the studies. Box 6.1 lists definitions for research using nursing interventions. In Box 6.2 the number of studies in the categories of internal coping processes of individuals, adaptive modes, stimuli, and nursing process are noted. The next section is on the studies related to interventions with internal coping processes.

BOX 6.1
KEY DEFINITIONS FOR RESEARCH WITH NURSING INTERVENTIONS

Nursing interventions—nursing activities that are expected to improve the outcomes of those who receive them.

Quasi-experimental and experimental designs—examine cause and effect under conditions in which it is possible to detect changes due to the intervention.

Independent variable—an intervention that is managed by the researcher to create an expected effect on the outcome measures.

Dependent variable—an outcome that is predicted and measured in the research design and presumed to be the result of the independent variable.

BOX 6.2
DESCRIPTIVE STUDIES BASED ON CATEGORIES OF RAM PROPOSITIONS ($n = 25$)

- Descriptive studies related to internal coping processes—individual ($n = 6$)
- Descriptive studies related to adaptive modes ($n = 11$)
- Descriptive studies related to stimuli ($n = 2$)
- Descriptive studies related to the nursing process ($n = 6$)

Description of Studies Related to Internal Coping Processes

In the six studies that examined individual internal coping processes, three studies (75%) were conducted in the United States and the other three were done in Puerto Rico (25%). The studies were conducted within institutions or in community settings. These settings included hospitals, mixed settings, community residence, and hemodialysis clinics. The populations of the studies included relatives of nursing home residents, women, caregivers of hemodialysis patients, Puerto Rican women with breast cancer, and staff nurses (see Table 6.1).

Blackmore et al. (1996) examined whether or not an invitation to have larger involvement in the nursing home care of relatives resulted in increased satisfaction in former caregivers. The researchers hypothesized that the intervention of an invitation would have an effect on the adaptation of family members to the institutionalization of a close friend or relative. The researchers used randomization to assign the subjects to two groups, one of which was invited to have increased care involvement. After 6 weeks there was no significant difference between the two groups, thereby not supporting the study's hypothesis. The results did call into question the amount of time needed for adaptation. Adaptation of family members to the institutionalization of a close friend or relative may not take place in 6 weeks. The time needed for adaptation was addressed in an earlier review of the RAM research. Similar studies may provide more useful results if adaptation is measured frequently over a longer period of time.

Fathima (2004) used a quasi-experimental one-group pretest and posttest design to examine the effects of an information-booklet intervention for caregivers of chronic renal failure patients undergoing hemodialysis. The researcher used purposive sampling ($n = 30$). She reported findings of a statistically significant improvement in caregivers' knowledge in the posttest with those who had the information booklet. Analysis of variance showed no correlations between the selected demographic variables with posttest knowledge.

In another quasi-experimental study Chorchado (2006) investigated the difference in mood state and self-concept in cancer patients undergoing breast surgery after receiving preparatory sensory information (PSI). The researcher used a non probability convenience sample and a t-test for data analysis. The author reported that treatment and control group means differed significantly on mood states. This was reported as showing that subjects in the treatment group had more postoperative affect balance than the control group. The t-test for the mean score of the self-concept posttest

TABLE 6.1

Intervention Studies Related to Internal Coping Processes—Individual

Author(s) and Date	Purpose	Sample	Design	Findings
1. Blackmore, Percival, and Toye (1996)	To discover whether satisfaction is increased when former caregivers are invited to have increased input into their relatives' care	Relatives of nursing home residents who were their former caregivers ($n = 31$)	Intervention, experimental	No significant difference was found between caregivers invited to have extra input into residents' care when compared with caregivers not invited to have extra input
2. Fathima (2004)	Examine the effects of an information booklet provided to caregivers of hemodialysis patients on knowledge of homecare management	Caregivers of hemodialysis patients ($n = 30$)	Intervention, single group pretest–posttest design	A statistically significant improvement existed in caregivers' knowledge in the posttest of those with the information booklet. Analysis of variance showed no correlation between the selected demographic variables with posttest knowledge scores
3. Corchado (2006)	To determine whether a difference exists in mood state and self-concept postsurgery in cancer patients after receiving preparatory sensory information	Puerto Rican women with a diagnosis of stage I, II, or III breast cancer who had breast conservative surgery or mastectomy ($n = 60$)	Intervention, repeated measures between subjects and within subjects	The intervention group had significantly higher postoperative self-concept and mood state scores. There were no relationships between age and the mood states or self-concept scores

Source	Purpose	Sample	Design	Findings
4. Uding, Jackson, and Hart (2002)	To determine staff nurse knowledge about diabetes management, and the usefulness of an educational intervention for enhancing knowledge	Staff nurses in a 400-bed suburban acute care facility that relied on staff nurses for diabetes education ($n = 72$)	Experimental, single group pretest–posttest control group	Teaching intervention significantly improved the experimental group's knowledge about diabetes
5. Flaugher (2002)	Test the effect of music on perception of chronic pain, depression, and anxiety using RAM combined with gate control theory of pain	$n = 67$ Ambulatory cancer patients ($n = 67$; 27 males, 40 females)	Three experimental groups: new-age music, self-selected music, no music	Music decreased the perception of chronic pain. Music had no effect on depression or anxiety
6. Serçekuş and Mete (2010)	To study the effects of antenatal education on prenatal and postpartum adaptation in a Turkish context	$n = 120$ nulliparous women participating in a study conducted between 2006 and 2008; two experimental groups received either group education or individual education; the control group received standard care	Quasi-experimental	Although there were statistically significant differences between the groups in terms of prenatal adaptation; no difference was found in postpartum adaptation. Post hoc analysis showed that women in the experimental groups (individual and group education) were better adapted in the prenatal period compared with those in the control group

185

measure demonstrated that the treatment group scores were significantly higher (M = 171.90, SD = 1.57 at p < .001 level) than the control group (M = 137.40, SD = 1717.03).

In both of these studies (Chorchado, 2006; Fathima, 2004), the authors conceptualized the intervention of providing information as the stimulus that influenced the process of adaptation in caregivers of hemodialysis patients and in cancer patients undergoing breast surgery. The influence as interpreted by the RAM is that the cognator processing of learning is activated.

Uding et al. (2002) recruited a convenience sample to research the level of diabetes-management knowledge of staff nurses. The study explored the usefulness of an educational intervention for enhancing the staff nurses' knowledge about diabetes. Uding et al. (2002) inferred that in order to guide positive patient outcomes, the nurse must frequently update knowledge to optimize her practice. The reported efficacy of the educational intervention included comparisons pre- and postinter-vention, measurement scores for experimental and control groups, and differences between the groups. Descriptive statistics were chosen to describe the sample. Comparative statistics, such as, a t-test for independent samples, Mann–Whitney U, and chi-square analyses determined no significant differences between the two groups or any of the demographic variables. The intervention significantly (p = .000) improved the experimental groups' knowledge. The results supported the use of teaching interventions to provide staff nurses with an opportunity to contribute to their own staff's development. While integrating the new knowledge into their current practice, staff nurses use new knowledge to innovate practice. Additionally the authors stated that improving the knowledge of nurses is the first step toward facilitating efficacy of patient education. The researchers also reported that their findings reflect a definite need for continued teaching and need of further research regarding nurses' knowledge.

In a three-group intervention, Flaugher (2002) tested the effect of three types of music on perception of chronic pain, depression, and anxiety. The sample was male and female ambulatory patients with cancer (n = 67). In general, the researcher reported that music decreased the perception of chronic pain. Still music had no effect on depression or anxiety. Cognator activity is involved in processing pain perception with different stimuli.

Serçekuş and Mete (2010) studied the effects of antenatal educa-tion on prenatal and postpartum adaptation in a Turkish context. Subjects were nulliparous women participating between 2006 and 2008 (n = 120). Two experimental groups received either group education or individual education, whereas the control group received standard care.

The researchers reported that there were statistically significant differences between the groups in terms of prenatal adaptation. However, no difference was found in postpartum adaptation. Post hoc analysis showed that women in the experimental groups (individual and group education) were better adapted in the prenatal period compared with those in the control group.

Description of Studies Related to Adaptive Modes

All 11 of the intervention studies (100%) assigned to the section on adaptive modes were conducted in the United States. The studies were carried out in institutions or in the community. Institutional settings included hospitals, long-term-care facilities, and community settings, which included schools, senior centers, and an asthma camp. The study populations included older adults in long-term-care facilities, adults diagnosed with cancer, women with stage IV metastatic breast cancer, women with stress urinary incontinence, preterm infants, preschool children, senior citizens, adolescents, and patients with kidney transplants (see Table 6.2).

Fitzsimmons (2001) examined the relationship between participation in a biking therapy program and the level of depression in older adults living in long-term-care facilities. The subjects were those with a diagnosis or symptoms of depression ($n = 40$). The design included a treatment and a control group with pretest and posttests. In this study the intervention of bike-therapy participation was to increase positive coping or cognator mechanisms through social interaction to reduce or eliminate depression as a measure of self-concept adaptation. Study results indicated that the level of depression in the treatment group decreased significantly, indicating an adaptive response to participation in the intervention of the biking program. The results of this study showed that the use of biking therapy was a positive nursing intervention in the treatment of depression.

Using nonprobability consecutive sampling, Headley et al. (2004) conducted a quasi-experimental study to examine the effects of a seated exercise program on fatigue and quality of life (QOL). The subjects were women with stage IV metastatic breast cancer beginning outpatient chemotherapy ($n = 38$). In this research the chemotherapy regime was viewed as the focal stimulus, which leads to ineffective responses (fatigue and decreased QOL) in this population. The exercise intervention was viewed as a way of managing input to the adaptive system. Descriptive statistics were used to examine the demographic data. Chi-square, Fisher exact, and analysis of variance were performed to assess differences between the groups based on demographic data. The researchers used a mixed

TABLE 6.2
Intervention Studies Related to Adaptive Modes

Author(s) and Date	Purpose	Sample	Design	Findings
1. Fitzsimmons (2001)	To determine whether participation in a therapy biking program had an effect on the degree of depression	Older adults in a long-term-care facility with a diagnosis or symptoms of depression ($n = 40$)	Intervention, experimental	The treatment groups' pretest means decreased significantly at the posttest, denoting a marked decrease in depression, indicating an adaptive response to participation in biking therapy
2. Headley, Ownby, and John (2004)	To examine the effects of a seated exercise program on fatigue and quality of life (QOL)	Women with stage IV metastatic breast cancer beginning outpatient chemotherapy ($n = 38$)	Intervention, nonequivalent control group and intervention group	Both groups demonstrated increased fatigue and decreased physical well-being. The intervention group experienced significantly less increase in fatigue and a lower decrease in physical well-being
3. Johnson (1997)	To compare the effects of a submaximal voluntary contraction exercise protocol with the effects of a near maximal voluntary contraction exercise to recondition the circumvaginal musculature to reduce incontinence	Women with stress urinary incontinence ($n = 32$)	Intervention, repeated measures	Significant improvements were found for total sample on endurance, mean maximal muscle strength, average contraction intensity, peak contraction intensity, perianal electromyographic amplitude, episodes of leakage, perceived severity of leakage, and quantity of urine loss during incontinent episodes

4. Modrcin-Talbott, Harrison, Groer, and Younger (2003)	To examine the physiological and behavioral effects of a gentle human touch (GHT) on preterm infants	Caucasian medically fragile preterm infants, 27 to 32 weeks gestational age admitted to the neonatal intensive care unit ($n = 20$)	Intervention, experimental	Infants in the experimental group showed significantly: • Less actual sleep time • Decreased frequency of motor activity • No change in heart rate or O_2 saturation • No behavioral distress cues • More quiet sleep • Drowsy state GHT is not aversive to fragile preterm infants
5. Sparks (1998)	To examine the effects of touch and distraction on injection pain in preschool children	Preschool children receiving immunizations in a metropolitan area ($n = 105$)	Intervention, nonequivalent control group and intervention group	Both distraction and touch significantly reduced the self-reported injection pain in this sample of preschool children
6. Flood and Scharer (2006)	To examine the relationships between creativity, functional performance, and successful aging	Senior citizens who attended senior centers in South Carolina ($n = 57$)	Intervention, experimental	No significant increase in creativity or successful aging between intervention and control groups. Black participants scored higher on creativity preintervention

(continued)

TABLE 6.2
Intervention Studies Related to Adaptive Modes (*continued*)

Author(s) and Date	Purpose	Sample	Design	Findings
7. Buckner et al. (2007)	To use the RAM modes to describe adolescent campers' adaptation during and after attending a Young Teen Asthma Camp and relate that adaptation to the acquisition of asthma responsibility	Adolescents between the ages of 12 and 15 attending asthma camp in 2003 and/or 2004 (*n* = 34)	Intervention, single group pretest and posttest	Improvements in self-efficacy supported adaptation in self-concept and role-function modes. Adolescents demonstrated maturing responsibility in asthma management in interdependence mode
8. Samarel, Tulman, and Fawcett (2002)	To find the most effective methods of obtaining social support for women diagnosed with breast cancer by testing the effectiveness of a telephone social support and education intervention	Women who were 2 to 4 weeks postsurgery for nonmetastatic breast cancer from Arkansas and New Jersey (*n* = 197)	Intervention, experimental	Arkansas experimental and control groups were not significantly different in benefit obtained related to mood disturbance, cancer-related worry, symptom distress, and relationships with significant others. New Jersey experimental group had better outcomes than control group
9. Zeigler, Smith, and Fawcett (2004)	To report findings of a program evaluation project that identified the experiences of both participants and	10 women with history of breast cancer (23 meetings of group) 2 nurses	Intervention, single group pretest and posttest	Larger % of responses adaptive posttest; Physiologic pretest 50% adaptive and posttest 60% adaptive; One measure of self-concept pretest 62.5% adaptive and posttest 60% adaptive;

	facilitators of a community hospital-sponsored breast cancer support group			Role all adaptive, pre and posttest; Interdependence—all adaptive pre and posttest; Nurses responses reflect adaptation in four adaptive modes
10. You, Chung, so, and Choi (2008)	Study the effect of the Dan Jeon Breathing Exercise Program (DJBEP) on QOL in patients after kidney transplantation	Volunteer patients from an outpatient clinic in Korea after kidney transplantation ($n = 29$)	Quasi-experimental with an experimental and nonequivalent control group and a pretest, posttest design	There were significant differences found between the experimental and the control groups, indicating the effectiveness of the DJBEP intervention on improving QOL, self-esteem, enhanced serum cholesterol and creatinine, and muscle strength, and decreasing stress level and level of uncertainty
11. Young-McCaughan et al. (2003)	Test the feasibility of an exercise program modeled on cardiac rehab to improve physiologic and psychological parameters	Adult patients diagnosed with cancer in the past 2 years ($n = 62$)	Prospective repeated measures	Significant improvement in: • Exercise duration and intensity • Self-reported energy level • QOL scores • Self-reported sleep difficulties • No significant improvement in objective sleep measures

model, multilevel approach similar to growth-curve analysis to interpret the intervention data. The authors concluded that women with advanced cancer who perform seated exercise had slower decline in physical well-being and less increase in fatigue.

Johnson (1997) compared the effects of a submaximal voluntary contraction exercise protocol with the effects of a near maximal voluntary contraction exercise protocol to recondition the circumvaginal musculature in women with stress urinary incontinence. Using a health provider referral network and newspaper advertisements, the investigator recruited the voluntary convenience sample. Subjects were women with stress urinary incontinence ($n = 32$). The investigator developed an experimental, repeated-measures design that tested measurements of endurance, strength, and muscle recruitment to promote training-induced changes in continence control. The researcher found that the intervention used over time produced significant improvements for the total sample on the following major study variables: endurance, mean maximal muscle strength, average contraction intensity, peak contraction intensity, perianal electromyography amplitude, episodes of leakage, perceived severity of leakage, and quantity of urine loss during incontinent episodes. The researcher found significant differences between the submaximal exercise protocol group and the near maximal voluntary contraction exercise protocol in training-induced mean maximal contraction strength and quantity of urine leakage during incontinent episodes on one-tailed independent t-tests. No significant differences were found between the groups on the other study variables. Findings of this study supported application of the principles of exercise physiology to recondition the circumvaginal musculature. Daily monitoring of training-induced changes provided information to adjust exercise contraction intensity as muscles changed in strength. Although statistical significance was not found in each group comparison, within-group improvements in incontinence would suggest that use of combined exercise regimens to benefit endurance and strength components of pelvic floor function is appropriate. The researcher stated that the findings support the use of biofeedback as an adjunctive therapy to promote compliance and record performance.

A team of investigators, Modrcin-Talbott et al. (2003), examined the physiological and behavioral effects of a gentle human touch on preterm infants. Subjects were Caucasian medically fragile preterm infants, 27 to 32 weeks gestational age admitted to the neonatal intensive care unit (NICU) ($n = 20$). Infants in the experimental group showed significantly less actual sleep time, decreased frequency of motor activity, and more quiet sleep. The findings of no change in heart rate or O_2 saturation and no behavioral distress cues indicated that GHT is not aversive to fragile preterm infants.

Sparks (1998) used a quasi-experimental design that examined the effects of touch and distraction on injection pain in preschool children. The sample consisted of 105 children who were randomly assigned to three different groups. After obtaining the results from the children's self-reported fear, she conducted analysis of variance (ANOVA) that yielded no significant difference between the interventions ($f = .08$, $p = .79$). However, the researcher found a significant difference between the intervention groups and the standard care group ($f = 6.48$, $p = .013$). Factorial ANOVA demonstrated a significant treatment main effect, but no significant interaction effect. Therefore, both distraction and touch reduced significantly the injection pain of this sample of children. The RAM provided the theoretical framework for this study by the interventions altering the environment to promote adaptation to injection pain experience. The researcher stated that all the children were administered the immunization, therefore the focal stimulus was not altered, but the contextual stimulus was manipulated through the use of distraction and touch with the outcome of better adaptation in the form of perception of pain.

Two researchers, Flood and Scharer (2006), investigated the relationships among functional performance, creativity, and successful aging within the context of the RAM. Using a pretest–posttest experimental design, the effects of a creativity-enhancement intervention in older adults was examined. In this study, the researchers hoped to influence the cognator subsystem, conceptualizing, perceptual and information processing, learning, judgment, and emotion, by involving research subjects in creative activities. Subjects were senior citizens in senior centers ($n = 57$). The researchers hypothesized that functional performance and creativity were coping processes that play vital roles in successful aging. Successful aging was the expected outcome in the adaptive modes. Study findings indicated that, although creativity did not significantly predict successful aging, functional performance was a statistically significant predictor of successful aging. Additionally, the researchers found some statistically significant results and findings about the possibilities for creativity enhancement. The researchers noted that interventions aimed at enhancing functional performance mechanisms have the potential to positively impact older adult's information processing, learning, and emotional health.

The purpose of the study by Buckner et al. (2007) was to describe adolescent asthma camp attendees' adaptation in each of the four adaptive modes and relate that adaptation to the acquisition of asthma responsibility. The researchers used a quasi-experimental pretest and posttest design. They investigated the ratings of self-efficacy and responsibility to describe adaptation in the RAM's four modes to establish the initial

effectiveness of the intervention in producing changes in adaptive outcomes. Improvements in self-efficacy supported adaptation in self-concept
and role function. Adolescents demonstrated maturing responsibility in
asthma management in the interdependence mode.

Samarel, Tulman, and Fawcett (2002) developed an education intervention for women with early-stage breast cancer using a three-group,
three-phase randomized clinical trial of 125 women. The study was
limited to examining the outcome variables that represented the self-
concept and interdependence modes. According to the researchers,
the experimental group received 13 months of combined individual
telephone and in-person group support and education. Control group
1 received 13 months of telephone-only individual support and education, and control group 2 received one-time mailed educational information. The findings did not support the overall hypothesized effects of
the interventions. However, the study findings did indicate group differences in mood disturbance, loneliness, and quality of a relationship with
a significant other. The authors noted that this suggests that individual
telephone support may provide an effective alternative to in-person
support groups.

Zeigler, Smith, and Fawcett (2004) reported findings of a project to
identify the experiences of both the participants in and facilitators of a
community-hospital-sponsored breast cancer support group. This study
used a repeated-measures survey methodology and qualitative data were
analyzed using content analysis. Themes extracted from the data were categorized, according to each of the four RAM modes. The results of this study
indicated that the combination of information and emotional and social support were effective in promotion adaptation. The researchers asserted that
nurses and other health professionals who establish community-based cancer support groups should consider formal evaluation of the outcomes, from
the perspectives of both participants and facilitators, and should publish the
results. The results were limited to one breast cancer support group with a
small number of female participants and two facilitators. Results cannot be
generalized to support groups for other types of cancer or to cancer support
groups for men.

Young-McCaughan et al. (2003) used a prospective, repeated-measures
design to investigate the feasibility of an exercise program patterned after
a phase II cardiac rehabilitation program to improve selected physiologic
and psychologic parameters of health in patients with cancer. The focal
stimuli for this study are the diagnosis and treatment of cancer with exercise as an intervention to facilitate positive adaptation. The exercise program was designed to facilitate an adaptive response to the focal stimuli of
cancer diagnosis and treatment. The independent variable was a 12-week

exercise program designed after an existing phase II cardiac rehabilitation program. The dependent variables were changes over time in exercise tolerance, activity and sleep patterns, and QOL. The researchers assert that the diversity of the sample in terms of cancer diagnosis, stage of cancer, cancer treatments, and time course of treatment were significant strengths of the study. However, the investigators also state that the constraints of the small sample size precluded an in-depth analysis of the role of these factors in determining outcomes. The authors reported that their findings indicated that patients with various types and stages of cancer can exercise safely using a cardiac rehabilitation model, with significant improvements in exercise tolerance, activity and sleep patterns, and QOL. Although standard exercise prescriptions can serve as a baseline, exercise prescriptions for patients with cancer, particularly those undergoing treatment, must be based on patient's current level of functional capacity and abilities.

Description of Studies Related to Stimuli

The two intervention studies categorized as related to stimuli were conducted in the United States. The populations of the studies included middle-age women with chronic illness and elderly individuals residing in a long-term-care facility (see Table 6.3).

Hill, Weinert, and Cudney (2006) used an experimental design to examine the effects of a computer-delivered intervention on measures of psychosocial health, such as, social support, self-esteem, empowerment, self-efficacy, depression, loneliness, and stress. The subjects were chronically ill rural women ($n = 100$), 35 to 65 years of age. The chronic illnesses included diabetes, rheumatoid condition, heart disease, cancer, and multiple sclerosis. The sample lived at least 25 miles outside an urbanized area (a city of 12,500) on a ranch, farm, or in a small town. Repeated-measures analysis of variance was conducted to evaluate the effects of the computerized intervention on changes in psychosocial outcomes of interest. Although statistically significant differences between intervention and control groups were found only for social support, self-esteem, and empowerment, all psychosocial indicators improved in the intervention group and declined or remained stable among controls.

Banks (1998) studied the effects of animal-assisted therapy in combating loneliness, and described the characteristics of individuals who selected to participate in her study. The investigator studied elderly individuals residing in long-term care facilities ($n = 45$). The researcher used power analysis and randomly assigned the sample into control and experimental groups.

TABLE 6.3
Intervention Studies Related to Stimuli

Author(s) and Dates	Purpose	Sample	Design	Findings
1. Hill, Weinert, and Cudney (2006)	To examine the effects of a computer-delivered intervention on measures of social support, self-esteem, empowerment, self-efficacy, depression, loneliness, and stress	Middle-aged women, with chronic illnesses who were living in rural areas ($n = 100$)	Intervention, experimental	Significant differences were found in women who participated in intervention group versus control group for improvements in self-esteem, social support, and empowerment
2. Banks (1998)	To determine the effects of animal-assisted therapy (AAT) and to describe the characteristics of the participants in AAT	Elderly individuals residing in long-term-care facilities ($n = 45$)	Intervention, single group pretest and posttest	AAT was associated with significant reduction in loneliness. Subjects who elected to participate in AAT had a history of pet ownership

Using the RAM as the theoretical framework, Banks (1998) focused on the concept of environmental stimuli as a factor influencing adaptation and the influence of the interdependence mode on the individual's response to the environment. Therefore, the use of the animal-assisted therapy (AAT) may be a positive contextual stimulus that helps with loneliness among the elderly. The results of this study demonstrated a statistically significant effect of AAT on loneliness in the elderly.

Description of Studies Related to the Nursing Process

Five of the six intervention studies assigned to the section on the nursing process were conducted in the United States (83%). One study was carried out in Finland. One researcher used a secondary analysis from a previous study by the principal investigator. Another study obtained data by telephone, three studies took place in suburban schools, and another was action research by nurses and patients. The population of the studies included adults with heart failure, women who were 2 to 4 weeks postsurgery for nonmetastatic breast cancer, fifth- and sixth-grade students attending suburban schools, and nursing home patients and their nurses (see Table 6.4).

Bakan and Akyol (2007) performed a secondary analysis from a randomized, parallel, controlled clinical trial that was conducted in 2005 with 43 patients, 21 in the intervention group and 22 in control. A booklet for patient training was given to those in the intervention group. Participants received a patient identification form, assessment form for physiological data, the Minnesota Living with Heart Failure Questionnaire, the Interpersonal Support Evaluation List, and the 6-Minute Walk Test. Results revealed that the patients in the intervention group adapted to their condition and that the four adaptive modes of the RAM were interrelated. Patients' QOL was enhanced, their functional capacities increased, and social support within the interdependence dimension improved in patients in the intervention group. In this study, the experimental adaptation program, social support, age, gender, and disease severity were the environmental stimuli of interest. In the present study, health-related QOL (HRQOL) was considered to be a latent variable that reflects overall response of the adaptive system to environmental stimuli. The components of HRQOL and social support were reflected in the four biobehavioral adaptive modes.

Coleman et al. (2005) examined the efficacy of a nursing intervention that involved telephone social support and education to encourage emotional and interpersonal adaptation to breast cancer. According to the authors, the study was designed to examine two variables of the RAM, self-concept and interdependence. No significant difference was found between participants who received telephone and in-person social support

TABLE 6.4

Intervention Studies Related to Nursing Process

Author(s) and Date	Purpose	Sample	Design	Findings
1. Bakan and Akyol (2007)	To examine the effects of an experimental education, exercise, and social support program on adaptation in persons with heart failure	Adults with heart failure (n = 43 with 21 intervention and 22 control patients)	Intervention, experimental with secondary data analysis	Intervention patients showed significant improvement in physical, emotional, and total dimensions when compared with the control group
2. Coleman, Tulman, Samarel, and Wilmoth (2005)	To find the most effective methods of providing social support for women diagnosed with breast cancer by testing the effectiveness of a telephone social support and education intervention	Women who were 2 to 4 weeks postsurgery for nonmetastatic breast cancer from Arkansas and New Jersey (n = 197)	Intervention, experimental	Arkansas experimental and control groups were not significantly different in benefit obtained related to mood disturbance, cancer-related worry, symptom distress, and relationships with significant others. New Jersey experimental group had better outcomes than control group

Author	Purpose	Sample	Type	Outcomes
3. Frame (2002)	To examine the effect of a support group on the perceptions of scholastic competence, social acceptance, and behavioral conduct	Preadolescents diagnosed with ADHD (n = 65)	Intervention, experimental	Significant increases for treatment group in perceptions of: • Social acceptance • Physical appearance • Athletic competence • Global self-worth
4. Frame, Kelly, and Bayley (2003)	To examine the effect of a support group on the perceptions of scholastic competence, social acceptance, and behavioral conduct	Preadolescents diagnosed with ADHD (n = 65)	Intervention, experimental	Significant increases for the treatment group in perceptions of: • Social acceptance • Athletic competence • Physical appearance • Global self-worth
5. Frame (2003)	To test the Frame Model of Preadolescent Empowerment as a means of enhancing the self-perception of children with attention deficit/hyperactivity disorder	Fifth-and sixth-grade students attending a suburban elementary school (n = 65)	Intervention, experimental	Participation in the support group greatly enhanced perceptions of social acceptance, physical appearance, athletic competence, and global self-worth in preadolescents with ADHD

(continued)

TABLE 6.4

Intervention Studies Related to Nursing Process (*continues*)

Author(s) and Date	Purpose	Sample	Design	Findings
6. Taival (1998)	To plan and evaluate effects of training home care nursing staff to use the Roy adaptation model on the patients' adaptation, on home visits, on nurses' views of adaptation, and to evaluate the training program content and feasibility	Home nursing patients =100 (interviews once each year for 3 years) Nurses visiting homes (visits observed = 30 over 3 years)	Action research intervention with repeated, before, during, and after change, mixed methods of measures	Patients in home nursing had adaptation problems that remained unchanged; feelings of not meeting role expectations and less to give to significant others worsened; self-concept improved, more satisfied with self and what has been achieved in life

and education and those who received only telephone social support and education. The authors noted that the findings suggested that telephone support could provide an effective alternative to in-person support groups.

In a dissertation study, Frame (2002) examined the effect of a support group on preadolescents who were diagnosed with attention deficit hyperactivity disorder (ADHD; $n = 65$). The outcome variables were perceptions of scholastic competence, social acceptance, and behavioral conduct. The researcher reported significant increases in the treatment group in perceptions of social acceptance, physical appearance, athletic competence, and global self-worth.

Frame, Kelly, and Bayley (2003) published a test of the effectiveness of a school-based, nurse-facilitated support group in increasing perceptions of scholastic competence, social acceptance, behavioral conduct, perceived athletic competence, perceived physical appearance, and perceived global self-worth in preadolescents diagnosed with attention deficit disorder (ADD) or ADHD. The research design was a quasi-experimental design with 65 preadolescents in an upper-middle-class community. The subjects were randomly assigned to either the experimental or control group. The authors stated that preadolescents with ADHD have to adapt to their environments and that those children need to learn strategies that will help them adapt. Successful adaptation strategies, which empower preadolescents, can lead to more favorable comparisons with their non-ADHD peers. As noted, findings showed significant increases in the treatment group in perceptions of social acceptance, physical appearance, athletic competence, and global self-worth.

In a later publication, Frame (2003) reported on a test of the Frame model of preadolescent empowerment as a means of enhancing the self-perception of children with ADHD. Students from the fifth and sixth grades in a suburban elementary school ($n = 65$) participated in the intervention study. Participation in the support group had greatly enhanced perceptions of social acceptance, physical appearance, athletic competence, and global self-worth in preadolescents with ADHD.

Taival (1998) planned and evaluated effects of training home care nursing staff to use the RAM on the patients' adaptation, on home visits, on nurses' views of adaptation, and to evaluate the training program content and feasibility. The subjects were home nursing patients in Finland ($n = 100$) who were interviewed once each year for 3 years and with a nurse doing home visits (visits observed = 30 over 3 years). The specialized intervention approach called action research was used with repeated mixed-methods measures that were used before, during and after change in the intervention. Findings showed that patients in home nursing had adaptation problems that remained unchanged, however, self-concept improved and subjects were more satisfied with self and what they achieved in life. For nurses there was an improvement in the atmosphere of the nursing process. However, nurses were not more holistic than in the beginning and they focused on physical needs. Nurses listened and gave encouragement. Nurses' descriptions exhibited humanistic features; health concepts grew wider, and patient well-being was seen as the goal of nursing, as was adaptation—more often than it had been before. The environment was less broadly understood and nurses appraised the model as a suitable framework for the nursing process.

CRITICAL ANALYSIS OF STUDIES

The process for critiquing the studies was described in Chapter 2 and illustrated in the other chapters of Part II. Basically we will present the results of the scored evaluations done by the project team on the studies assigned to this chapter and then comment on the strengths and weaknesses noted. Based on the criteria, scores could range from a high of 20 points to a low of 4 points. In addition to the four basic criteria for evaluating quantitative studies, there are additional considerations for the strength of intervention studies. For example, the randomized two-group clinical trial, with an intervention and a control group, is considered stronger evidence of the success of an intervention than a pretest and posttest given to a single group from a convenience sample.

Of the 25 quantitative studies classified as intervention studies, 8 (32%) were scored the top level of 20 points, indicating that they met the expected criteria for the research. One study, Blackmore et al. (1996), was scored at 14 points and was not considered for further knowledge development.

One strength of this set of studies was the number of investigators who randomized groups as intervention and control and who checked that the two groups were generally equivalent on major demographic or clinically relevant variables. Other strengths were the care taken with measurement; often the psychometric properties were given both from the literature and from the sample used. Other times the investigators noted that they may not have had an instrument sensitive to the outcome they were trying to measure. Some issues that reoccur with these studies can lead to weaknesses. For example, the length of time these studies take to access the number of subjects, conduct the intervention, and do posttesting can lead to threats to reliability such as consistency of treatment, including changes of research staff. Second, threats to validity such as history and maturation can occur. Some studies lasted 2 years or longer allowing for situations to change that could affect the outcome measures. For example, the study by Taival (1998) lasted 3 years, and the home care patients were aging during this time, which could affect their adaptation needs, which was also an outcome measure. In this case the investigator did not include any measures to minimize these threats to validity and reliability.

CONCLUSION

This chapter has presented and critiqued the 25 studies classified as quantitative intervention studies. A variety of approaches to intervention research were used from simple pretest–posttest designs with a convenience sample to studies with a control and one or more intervention groups. In general the studies were well-designed and offered a beginning or advanced level of testing an intervention. These studies can be used to design the next-level study to provide knowledge that is applied directly to practice. This is a significant beginning to intervention research using the RAM.

REFERENCE

Grobe, S. J. (1996). The nursing intervention lexicon and taxonomy: Implications for representing nursing care data in automated patient records. *Holistic Nursing Practice, 11*(1), 48–63.

BIBLIOGRAPHY

Bakan, G., & Akyol, A. D. (2007). Theory-guided interventions for adaptation to heart failure. *Journal of Advanced Nursing, 61*(6), 596–608.

Banks, M. (1998). The effects of animal-assisted therapy on loneliness in an elderly population in long-term care facilities (Doctoral dissertation, Louisiana State University Medical Center in New Orleans). *Dissertation Abstracts International, 59*(03B), 1043.

Blackmore, A., Percival, C., & Toye, P. (1996). Satisfaction with nursing home care of a relative: Does inviting great input make a difference? *Collegian, 3*(2), 4–6, 8–11.

Buckner, E. B., Simmons, S., Brakefield, J. A., Hawkins, A. K., Feeley, C., Kilgore, L. A., … Gibson, L. (2007). Maturing responsibility in young teens participating in an asthma camp: Adaptive mechanisms and outcomes. *Journal for Specialists in Pediatric Nursing, 12*(1), 24–36.

Chorchado, J. L. (2006). *The effects of preparatory sensory information on breast conservative and mastectomy cancer patient: Mood states and self-concept.* Chester, PA: Widener University School of Nursing.

Coleman, E., Tulman, L., Samuel, N., & Wilmoth, N. C. (2005). The effect of telephone social support and education on adaptation to breast cancer during the year following diagnosis. *Oncology Nursing Forum, 32*(4), 822–828.

Fathima, L. (2004). The effect of information booklet provided to caregivers of patients undergoing hemodialysis on knowledge of home care management. *Nursing Journal of India, 95*(4), 81–82.

Fitzsimmons, S. (2001). Easy rider wheelchair biking. A nursing-recreation therapy clinical trial for the treatment of depression. *Journal of Gerontological Nursing, 27*(5), 14–23.

Flaugher, M. (2002). The intervention of music on perceptions of chronic pain, depression, and anxiety in ambulatory individuals with cancer. *The University of Alabama at Birmingham 2002 D.S.N.*, 124. Retrieved from https://mail.bc.edu/Redirect/metaquest.bc.edu:4000/sfx_local?sid=SP:NU&id=pmid:&id=&issn=&isbn=978-0.

Flood, M., & Scharer, K. (2006). Creativity enhancement: Possibilities for successful aging. *Issues in Mental Health Nursing, 27*(9), 939.

Frame, K. (2002). *The effect of a support group on perceptions of scholastic competence, social acceptance and behavioral conduct in preadolescents diagnosed with attention deficit hyperactivity disorder.* Widener University School of Nursing, 183. Retrieved from https//mail.bc.edu/Redirect/metaquest.bc.edu:4000/sfx_local?sid=SP:NU&id=pmid:&id=&issn=&isbn=978-0

Frame, K. (2003). Empowering preadolescents with ADHD: Demons or delights. *Advances-in-Nursing-Science (ANS), 26*(2), 131–139.

Frame, K., Kelly, L., & Bayley, E. (2003). Increasing perceptions of self-worth in preadolescents diagnosed with ADHD. *Journal of Nursing Scholarship, 35*(3), 225–229.

Headley, J., Ownby, K. K., & John, L. D. (2004). The effect of seated exercise in fatigue and quality of life in women with breast cancer. *Oncology Nursing Forum, 31*(5), 977–983.

Hill, W., Weinert, C., & Cudney, S. (2006). Influence of a computer intervention on the psychological status of chronically ill rural women: Preliminary results. *Nursing Research, 55*(1), 34–42.

Johnson, V. (1997). Effects of submaximal exercise protocol to recondition the circumvaginal musculature in women with genuine stress urinary incontinence (Doctoral dissertation, University of Texas at San Antonio). *Dissertation Abstracts International, 58*(03B), 1213.

Modrcin-Talbott, M. A., Harrison, L. L., Groer, M. W., & Younger, M. S. (2003). The biobehavioral effects of gentle human touch on preterm infants. *Nursing Science Quarterly, 16*(1), 60.

Samarel, N., Tulman, L., & Fawcett, J. (2002). Effects of two types of social support and education on adaptation to early-stage breast cancer. *Research in Nursing Health, 25*(6), 459–470.

Serçekuş, P., & Mete, S. (2010). Effects of antenatal education on maternal prenatal and postpartum adaptation. *Journal of Advanced Nursing, 66*(5), 999–1010.

Sparks, L. (1998). A comparison of the effects of cutaneous stimulation and distraction on children's perceptions of injection pain (Doctoral dissertation, Saint Louis University). *Dissertation Abstracts International, 60*(04B), 1536.

Taival, A. (1998). The older person's adaptation and the promotion in home nursing care: Action research of the intervention through training based on the Roy Adaptation Model (elderly) (Doctoral dissertation, Tampereen Teknillinen Korkeakoulu, 1998). *Dissertation Abstracts International, 60*(01C), 0113.

Uding, J., Jackson, E., & Hart, A. L. (2002). Efficacy of a teaching intervention based on nurses' knowledge regarding diabetes. *Journal for Nurses in Staff Development, 18*(6), 297–303.

You, H. S., Chung, S. Y., So, H. S., Choi, S. J. (2008). Effect of a DanJeon breathing exercise program on the quality of life in patients with kidney transplants. *Transplantation Proceedings, 40*(7), 2324.

Young-McCaughan, S., Mays, M. Z., Arzola, S. M., Yoder, L. H., Dramiga, S. A., Leclerc, K. M., ... Nowlin, M. U. (2003). Change in exercise tolerance, activity and sleep patterns, and quality of life in patients with cancer participating in a structured exercise program. *Oncology Nursing Forum, 30*(3), 441–454.

Zeigler, L., Smith, P. A., & Fawcett, J. (2004). Breast cancer: Evaluation of the common journey breast cancer support group. *Journal of Clinical Nursing, 13*(4), 467–478.

III

Middle Range Theories Derived From Research

Nursing as a profession provides service to society based on specialized knowledge. Specialized knowledge is based on theory and research. In Chapter 1 we proposed the content and process of developing middle range theory backed by research as a significant way to develop knowledge for nursing practice. This book takes a particular approach to developing middle range theory for practice by capitalizing on a given nursing theory and a specific set of research reports. Theories in nursing can be classified based on the scope of the theory. Specificity and abstractness of concepts and propositions distinguish the levels. It is common to describe theory on four levels—meta-theory, grand theories, middle range theories, and practice theories. Meta-theory refers to the worldview of nursing and its philosophical perspectives. Grand theory is the level that is abstract and provides a perspective of the goals and structure of nursing practice. "Conceptual model" is another name given to grand theories. Walker and Avant (2011) list 20 representative grand theories published from the 1960s through the 1980s, including the Roy adaptation model of nursing first published in 1970 and the basis for the current project. Middle range theories differ from grand theories by focusing on given phenomena and having fewer, more concrete concepts. Practice theories generally involve a desired goal and prescriptions for nursing actions to reach the goal. They have the fewest number of concepts that are even more specific and concrete.

In recent years middle range theories have been broadly accepted as key to supporting nursing practice (McEwen, 2007). Although middle range theories were used in other disciplines since the 1960s, more recently nurse scholars have supported strongly the call for middle range theory development in nursing. The reasons for this movement lie in the nature of middle range theories. The limited number of concepts are closer to practice; some can be generalized across situations and sometimes clinical specialties; they can be tested in research since the concepts can be defined operationally; and most important, their relative simplicity leads to adoption in practice.

In creating middle range theories observations from various sources such as literature, clinical practice, or research studies are clustered together. From the related observations similarities are classified and major concepts identified. The concepts are discrete and observable, but at a level of abstraction that can be generalized across clinical situations that relate to the phenomenon of concern. The identified concepts are interrelated in theoretical statements. The concepts and statements are used to create the middle range theory, which can be depicted in a visual schema. Each approach to observations from different sources has been successful in creating middle range theories that are useful for practice. For example, Meleis' theory of experiencing transitions (Meleis, 2010) resulted from integrating the results of five research studies. Lenz (2007) described the common approach of literature reviews that are summarized and depicted in a diagram. The relationships depicted are then tested in research using a method such as path analysis. One example is Richmond's model of post-injury disability (Richmond, 1997). The chronic illness trajectory framework (Corbin & Strauss, 1991) combined numerous accounts of practice experiences by nurses in a series of grounded theory studies.

In the current project the innovative strategy for knowledge for practice is to use the distinct advantage of drawing on a body of research based on one grand theory, the Roy adaptation model, to derive the concepts to create middle range theories. Lenz (2007) noted that conceptual clarity is needed as a basis for theory development and also provides the vital step of measurement for research. However, she indicated that the value of concept-level work often is not realized. The concept-level work of the Roy adaptation model has developed over more than 40 years of published concepts with definitions and descriptive theoretical bases. The researchers of the 172 studies reported in Part II began with the grand theory developed by Roy. In designing studies, the investigators added their own clinical and literature observations. They created research questions that they answered with the research. The commonalities for cumulative knowledge of studies based on one conceptual framework are great. Useful cumulative knowledge is particularly realized in developing middle range theories that can change nursing practice. The team of researchers/authors on this project developed a six-step process for generating middle range theories as explained in Chapter 8.

Part III presents the middle range theories derived from studies grouped in content areas of great need in practice. Each demonstration of generating middle range theory follows the six-step process. In Chapter 7 Roy synthesized from research a general middle range theory of coping. For Chapter 8 she has selected studies that lead to a theory of adapting to life events. Dobratz focused on development of a middle range theory of loss in Chapter 9. For Chapter 10 Buckner and Hayden used selected studies to create middle range theories related to adapting to chronic health conditions. Finally, Hayden and Buckner bring together the Roy model-based studies on families to derive a new middle range theory of adapting families.

REFERENCES

Corbin, J. M., & Strauss, A. (1991). A nursing model for chronic illness management based upon the trajectory framework. *Scholarly Inquiry for Nursing Practice, 4,* 155–174.

Lenz, E. R. (2007). Mid-range theory: Impact on knowledge development and use in practice. In D.A. Jones & C. Roy (Eds.). *Nursing knowledge development and clinical practice* (pp. 61–77). New York, NY: Springer Publishing Company.

McEwen, M. (2007). Introduction to middle range nursing theories. In M. McEwen & E. Wills (Eds.), *Theoretical basis for nursing* (2nd ed.). Philadelphia, PA: Lippincott, Williams and Wilkins.

Meleis, A. I. (2010). *Transitions theory: Middle range and situation specific theories in research and practice.* New York, NY: Springer Publishing Company.

Richmond, T. S. (1997). An explanatory model of variables influencing post-injury disability. *Nursing Research, 46,* 262–267.

Roy, C. (1970). Adaptation: A conceptual framework for nursing. *Nursing Outlook, 18*(3), 43–45.

7

Synthesis of a Middle Range Theory of Coping

SISTER CALLISTA ROY

The main purpose of this project is to generate middle range theories (MRTs) for nursing and to derive evidence for practice. This approach is one way to synthesize research and build cumulative knowledge to impact changes in practice. This chapter builds on the analysis of studies in Part II to exemplify the process of generating a MRT of coping. MRT has been described as consisting of a set of concepts that are focused on a limited part of the reality the nurse meets in practice (Smith & Liehr, 2008); it is less abstract than grand theories, closer to practice, and has fewer concepts; the concepts can be related to propositions and can be operationally defined (McEwen & Wills, 2010). Walker and Avant (2011) noted that MRTs share some of the conceptual economy of grand theories but provide the specificity needed for usefulness in research and practice. As a result, MRTs have increased in importance in building knowledge for practice. In the introduction to Part III we clarified why MRTs are being recognized as significant for practice based on their characteristics. In Box 7.1 we summarize these key points.

A MRT identifies a fewer number of concepts and these are closer to practice because they are more concrete than the abstract concepts of the grand theory. For example, according to Roy's theoretical work, the grand theory describes four adaptive modes, including role function, as major concepts of the adapting person (Roy, 2009). The theorist created a MRT of

---

BOX 7.1

WHY MIDDLE RANGE THEORIES ARE SIGNIFICANT FOR DEVELOPING KNOWLEDGE FOR NURSING PRACTICE

- Have a limited number of concepts that are closer to practice
- Can be generalized across given situations and sometimes clinical specialties
- Can be tested in research because the concepts can be defined operationally
- Have a relative simplicity that leads to adoption in practice

---

the role function adaptive mode as a specific system (Roy & Roberts, 1981) based on the literature current at that time. The inputs of the role system are clarity of role cues and cultural norms, which include accuracy of perception and adequacy of social learning. This leads to a process of adequacy of role taking, which combines with internal and external validation. The outcome of the system processing is role mastery. MRT is derived from the exploration of specific instances of a phenomenon or experience, from research, literature, and/or practice. The synthesis of related concepts into knowledge can be generalized beyond a given situation and serve as the seeds of further knowledge development, including designing and testing interventions in nursing practice. If concepts of the theory look at human experiences, as with the adapting person, the theory can be generalized across clinical specialties because the grand theory proposes that the need to adapt is a common phenomenon experienced by all who encounter changes. Because the concepts are more concrete than in grand theories, they can also be operationally defined and tested in research. All of these characteristics of MRTs lend a simplicity that makes them easier to eventually implement in practice.

In each of the examples of generating MRT the team of authors for Chapters 7 through 11 demonstrate the significance for developing knowledge for nursing practice in a specific way. To select the foci of the middle-range theory development, the team reviewed the basics concepts of the Roy adaptation model (RAM) together with all studies identified from the literature to that time in the planning. This included more than half of the final 172 studies. Discussion centered on the central concepts of the RAM and the purpose and findings of the studies reviewed. According to the RAM the person or group is defined as an adaptive system with central coping processes that lead to adaptation and promote health. The goal of nursing practice is to promote adaptation with individuals and groups by assessing factors that influence adaptive abilities and intervening to help manage the environment and enhance coping processes (see Box 7.2 for glossary of terms related to RAM). The decision seemed clear that the studies lent themselves to developing MRTs of the core concepts of coping and adaptation.

Given a conviction about the significance of MRT, the project team set up a series of steps for developing MRTs. The steps were derived both from the literature and the unique approach of this project. In reducing a large body of information to units that are clear and understandable, the initial step is to cluster together units that are similar. In this project among the

---

BOX 7.2
GLOSSARY OF TERMS RELATED TO THE
ROY ADAPTATION MODEL

Persons and groups—Open adaptive systems that use central coping processes to maintain adaptation in a changing environment; can be viewed as four interrelated modes of adaptation—physiologic/physical, self-concept/group identity, role function, and interdependence.

Adaptation—The process and outcome whereby thinking and feeling people, as individuals or in groups, use conscious awareness and choice to create human and environmental integration.

Coping processes—Innate and acquired ways of responding to the environment to promote the goals of adaptation; for the individual these are called the cognator and the regulator and for the group the innovator and stabilizer.

Goals of adaptation—Survival, growth, reproduction, mastery, and human and environment transformations.

Coping capacity—The ability of the person based on his or her patterns of responding to changes in the environment that use his or her coping styles and new strategies to adapt effectively to changes that are challenging.

Goal of nursing practice—To promote adaptation for individuals and groups by assessing factors that influence adaptive abilities and intervening to help manage the environment and enhance coping processes and capacity.

Factors that influence adaptation—commonly known as stimuli; focal—most immediate, contextual—all other factors present in the situation that contribute to the affect of the focal stimuli, and residual—an environmental factor within or outside the person or group with affects in the situation that are unclear.

172 studies, initially we found five clusters of studies that had similar foci. For developing each MRT, step 1 is to describe the studies selected. The description was organized based on some commonalities among smaller groups of studies assuming that this would be useful to the reader in learning about the scope of the entire set of studies. For example, in Chapter 9 on adapting to loss, the author ordered the presentation of the selected studies by types of loss, that is, studies related to the death of a spouse; another about women who suffered loss of a stillborn infant; then the specific loss of a loved one through a sudden, violent death; and finally studies about persons or caregivers of persons diagnosed with terminal illness receiving hospice care or focused on the experience of persons who were at the end of life's continuum.

In step 2 the entire cluster of studies acted as a series of observations from which we identified concepts for that MRT. Pertinent concepts were those that provided insights into the broad concepts from the RAM described previously. Initial concepts identified were circulated among the team and we learned from each other how to select for both content and level of generality. In step 3, as noted above, we took care that the level of generality was discrete, observable, and generalizable. Often it took several critiques by the team to agree on an appropriate level of generalization of concepts. In step 4 we drew a pictorial schema of the interrelated concepts in the MRT. Because the studies were based on the RAM and were focused on the phenomena of coping and adaptation, factors that influence it and/or interventions to promote it, the schema of relationships among the concepts of the studies took a similar shape in each chapter. Still, the team repeatedly shared and critiqued work in progress. For step 5 the theoretical statements that linked the concepts together as propositions were synthesized from the findings of the selected studies. This process was repeated in each demonstration of generating a MRT. Finally in step 6, given the reservoir of research, the studies of a given cluster that lead to the MRT generation also provided findings to provide initial evidence to support the MRT. This does not mean that the MRT would not be further developed theoretically and tested in further research. Rather we are capitalizing on the accumulated research to provide evidence as a basis for claiming some evidence for practice. The six steps are summarized in Box 7.3.

Synthesizing research based on the RAM using this stepwise process for generating MRT can provide unique insights for nursing practice. There are many approaches to developing MRTs as noted in Chapter 1. However, research that used the same grand theory lends strength to the process as noted in how broader grand theory concepts guided selection of specific concepts from the studies. The work also provides the possibility of clarifying and adding to the development of the grand theory.

BOX 7.3
HOW MIDDLE RANGE THEORIES ARE GENERATED
FROM RELATED RESEARCH STUDIES

1. Studies are selected that cluster together by similarities.
2. The studies are used as observations, are classified, and major concepts identified.
3. The concepts are discrete and observable, but at a level of abstraction that can be generalized across clinical situations.
4. The concepts are used to draw a pictorial schema of the interrelated concepts.
5. The identified concepts are interrelated in theoretical statements or propositions.
6. The findings from the research are used to provide evidence to support the new MRT.

To exemplify this process, the first MRT generated is on a general approach to coping understood as a central concept in the RAM. The purpose of this chapter is to inductively create from the studies a new general middle range theory of coping. As a MRT the results will be more specific and thus amenable for use in practice by leading to deriving effective nursing interventions to be tested. The aims of this chapter are (a) to identify and define concepts of coping that address both person and environment, (b) to relate the concepts in a visual depiction of the MRT, (c) to identify relational propositions and show support for the propositions from the research analysis presented in Part II, and (d) to identify ways that knowledge from the MRT can change practice by identifying how to create effective interventions.

GENERATING A MIDDLE RANGE THEORY

The significance of MRT for nursing practice and the basic steps in the process of creating such theories were the beginning point for generating this particular MRT. I will follow the steps of creating a MRT by clustering similar observations together and identifying major concepts from a selection of studies. The concepts are expected to be discrete and observable, but also above the level of abstraction of the individual situation so that that they can be generalized across clinical situations. From the concepts a depiction of the MRT is derived. Theoretical statements are written based on linking the interrelated concepts as reflected in the research studies. The first step of MRT building is to select studies to use for the observations in this theory building; these are described next.

Studies Selected for Middle Range Theory Development—Step 1

Given that all of Part III is dedicated to deriving MRTs of coping and adapt-ing, it was a particular challenge to select studies for this chapter to derive an overall MRT of coping. The challenge was handled by looking at the aim in selecting studies. The aim was to find out what the RAM-based research could offer to intervention, particularly as there is a broad literature with little consensus about coping. Again, the advantage of studies based on one theory's use of concepts has some consistency in general under-standing and in the use of foundational terms. Synthesizing new insights based on the research studies can offer even more and perhaps more cohe-sive insights. Furthermore the work can address some of the issues such as multiple conceptualizations of coping, the separation of conceptualiza-tions and measurement and disagreements about whether coping is state or trait based (Schwarzer & Schwarzer, 1996). Traits are more enduring characteristics and states are more fleeting conditions. This distinction is important for designing nursing interventions.

Of particular interest were studies that focused specifically on cop-ing and had explicit identification of concepts and their relationships. Some publications were reports of multiple studies that derived models of coping that were also tested. These were selected as likely useful. Of particular value were two reports that included multiple studies over two points in time. All of the studies selected were evaluated as meeting the general criteria for standards of research adequacy and were authentically based on the RAM. The selection process resulted in five research reports covering 13 studies that could be helpful in synthesizing a MRT of cop-ing. Regardless of the differences in patient populations and their environ-ments, the persons and situations were used by the investigators to study in some way the coping of individual persons.

Dunn (2005) used a convenience sample of 200 Judeo-Christian com-munity-dwelling adults with chronic pain of at least 3 months duration to test her MRT of adaptation to chronic pain. Of note is that the author tested relationships among contextual variables such as age, gender, and race; the focal stimulus, total chronic pain intensity; compensatory life processes such as the use of religious and nonreligious coping strategies; and adap-tive responses. The design called for several coping scales and an analysis using structural equation modeling. The second study also used commu-nity-based elders and provided an intervention to examine the relation-ships between creativity and successful aging in the context of the RAM (Flood & Scharer, 2006).

The third study was a mixed-methods study by Raleigh, Robinson, Marold, and Jamison (2006) who explored how hospice supports family caregivers in their decision to provide care at home and in the caregiv-ing process. Another purpose of this work was to look at the relationships between hospice support and coping, and hospice support and spiritual well-being in bereaved caregivers. The latter purpose was particularly useful to this project because the researchers identified the focal stimuli as the terminal illness and death of a loved one; the contextual stimuli as hospice support, caregiver burden, and spiritual well-being, and the setting. They focused on cognator coping efficacy using the Jalowiec Coping Scale (1993) and then looked at the outcome of adaptive or ineffective ability and satisfaction or lack of it in their caregiving.

The last two reports are related because they used the same set of studies at two points in time. Levesque, Ricard, Ducharme, Duquette, and Bonin (1998) derived a model of psychological adaptation from the RAM and aimed to verify the model with data from five studies. The empirical data, including scores from coping scales, were pooled from studies exploring the same variables but involving different populations. The samples studied included: informal caregivers living with a demented relative ($n = 125$), informal primary caregivers of a psychiatrically ill relative admitted to a psychiatric hospital ($n = 200$) and the same caregivers during the remission period ($n = 163$), professional caregivers in geriatric long-term care ($n = 1564$), and community-dwelling elderly couples ($n = 135$) for a total of 2,187 participants. The report published by Ducharme, Ricard, Duquette, Levesque, and Lachance (1998) used these samples with a structural equation analysis at two points in time and an exploratory longitudinal analysis.

Concepts—Steps 2 and 3

Background

In approaching step 2, the key step of identifying concepts for a MRT of coping, it may be useful to first examine what we know about coping. "To cope" has been defined as to deal successfully with a difficult problem or situation. Nurses work with people in continually changing life situations, including many who are facing difficult problems or situations related to their health. Whether a middle-age person needs to lose 30 pounds to stay healthy, a teenager learns he has cancer, or a previously infertile couple conceives their first child, each person will be facing the difficulty of learning to cope with a changing situation. Nurses are the health care providers most often working with people during these changing situations, whether the person is returning to a community clinic and is seen by the same nurse or is a patient with the same nurse working a 12-hour acute care shift. The focus of nurses' knowledge is viewing people as a whole in their changing environments, and thus nurses are best prepared to help people deal with these changing situations. A MRT of coping can be helpful for nurses in all areas of practice.

The literature related to coping has grown significantly in recent decades. Aldwin (1994) described the literature in the field as "exploding" in 1994. In her more recent follow-up review she identified 37,000 additional articles on coping (Aldwin, 2007). The author noted that coping is recognized as the crucial variable in understanding the effect of stress on physical and mental health. As noted, the RAM defines the person or group as an adaptive system at the center of which are coping subsystems (see Figure 7.1) that deal with internal and external stimuli. In writings and research I have chosen to explore more deeply this part of the conceptual framework because the continuing interest in coping theory and research, as noted by Folkman and Moskowitz (2004), is both that it is an explanatory concept related to how people differ in response to stress, and that it also has potential as the basis for interventions. A number of issues in the literature and noted above are unresolved and learning more about them relates to how to plan effective interventions.

A MRT of coping includes concepts that are interrelated as derived from an understanding of the process of adaptation from the RAM. As early as 1981 Roy described adaptation as an interactional process with focal stimuli being mediated by contextual and residual factors to partially produce the interaction called stress. The other half of the interaction is the coping processes being triggered to produce adaptive or ineffective responses (Roy & Roberts, 1981). The concepts have specific meanings

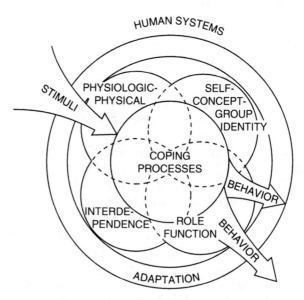

FIGURE 7.1 The Person or Group as Adaptive System

within the model (Roy, 2009; see Box 7.2). The focal stimulus is the internal or external stimulus most immediately confronting the person and has also been described as the amount of change taking place. Contextual stimuli are all other stimuli present to the person that contribute to the affect of the focal stimulus. The residual stimuli are environmental factors within or outside the human system that have unclear affects in the current situation.

Roy (2011) built on earlier work to describe coping strategies as behaviors whereby adaptation processing is carried out and adaptation processing is defined as the patterning of innate and acquired ways of taking in, handling, and responding to a changing environment in daily situations and in critical periods that direct behavior toward survival, growth, reproduction, mastery and transcendence. This interactional view of coping and adaptation is in keeping with the literature on coping. Specifically, there are recommendations that call for both an approach that views persons in interaction with the environment and for conceptualizing stress and adaptation together (Aldwin, 2007; Holahan, Moos, & Schaefer, 1996). The outcome, as noted in the definition of coping and adaptation processing, is adaptive or ineffective behavior that reach the goals of adaptation expressed in the four adaptive modes. Looking at outcomes as effective and as being expressed in multiple dimensions as in the adaptive modes is congruent with the multidimensional approaches noted as most promising in the coping literature (Frydenberg, 2002).

For step 2, the main concepts of this MRT were identified as the stimuli, the coping processes, and the outcomes, based on both an understanding of the grand theory and the analysis of the studies selected. For this chapter the stimuli are synthesized from the studies as focal, contextual, and residual. Although the definitions of these terms are spelled out in the grand theory, they can also be seen in the studies under consideration. The studies presented a variety of situations, still when looking at the studies the investigators had identified the characteristics under differing circumstances. The coping processes are the coping strategies combined from the five project reports. Finally, the outcomes identified by the investigators are expressed in synthesized middle range outcomes that are related to the stimuli and the strategies. Step 3 is a major part of the process as each concept is synthesized at the required level of generality.

Concept 1—Stimuli

Within the studies selected the focal stimuli can be identified with three phrases: chronic pain, stress of caregiving, and illness and death of a loved one. Within these selected studies I identified stimuli that represent some of the major changes that people face and that nurses are called on to help people with in the effort to cope with these changes. They are long-term changes, indicate significant challenges, and demand major coping efforts. In one selected study Flood and Scharer (2006) noted the growing importance of assisting people with successful aging in the United States, yet they indicate the lack of practical guidelines on how to promote this process. The authors designed and tested an intervention to deal with the generalized changes of aging. Unless interrupted by an early death, all people will deal with the experience of aging and the growing numbers of persons in the United States over 65 years and over 85 years is well documented. As the investigators noted, efforts are made to understand the experience but little research has focused on how to deal with the stimulus of aging and to age successfully. This stimulus is coupled in the MRT with chronic pain, the focal stimulus studied by Dunn (2005). Although aging does not necessarily involve chronic pain, the synthesis seems justified in the two studies. Flood and Scharer used the Arthritis Impact Management Scale to measure functional status. With arthritis, whether osteo- or rheumatoid, pain is often a feature. Dunn used the definition of chronic pain as of at least 3 months duration. In both studies the sample was community-dwelling elders, $n = 57$ for Flood and Scharer and $n = 200$ for Dunn. For Flood the contextual stimuli included demographic variables and functional performance. For Dunn gender and race were the contextual stimuli identified.

Eleven of the studies deal with the perceived stress of caregiving. In the series of five studies reported by Leveque et al. (1998) and five by Ducharme et al. (1998), the focal stimulus included in the informal caregiver studies was the variable of perceived feeling of being stressed or upset by the dysfunctional behaviors of the ill person. For professional caregivers' studies, the stimulus was the perceived feeling of being stressed or upset by the severe or terminal illness. Finally, in the aged-spouses study, the focal stimulus was perceived stress associated with situations occurring during the aging process. Contextual stimuli for all study samples included: available or enacted social support, conflicts in the exchange of social support, and gender. The studies reported in these two publications included a total of 2,187 participants in groups ranging between $n = 125$ and $n = 1564$.

The caregivers in the study by Raleigh et al. (2006) were 21 recently bereaved family caregivers from whom data were obtained during a follow-up visit 4 to 6 weeks after the death of a loved one. The focal stimulus was the terminal illness and death of a loved one. The contextual stimuli were external environmental factors of hospice support, caregiver burden, requests of the patient, desire to help, and the setting, and also the internal factor of spiritual well-being.

Concept 2—Coping Processes

As noted the studies were selected because they focused on coping strategies and although there are some variations in how these concepts are named and measured, they are rooted in the understanding given by the RAM and described earlier. Flood and Scharer (2006) were interested in intervening to promote successful aging. The investigators aimed to influence the cognator subsystem, targeting perceptual and information processing, learning, judgment, and emotion. They proposed that functional performance mechanisms and creativity were coping processes that can lead to successful aging. Dunn (2005) specifically called the processes compensatory life processes. Roy (2009) defines compensatory adaption levels as those in which the cognator and regulator are activated by a challenge. Recognizing some of the ethnic variations in responses to pain, Dunn chose to use religious coping and nonreligious coping as her coping-process variables. The processes for coping were simply labeled "coping strategies" and included active coping nonreligious and passive/avoidance in the studies reported by Levesque et al. (1998) and by Duchane et al. (1998). For Raleigh et al. (2006) the processes were identified as coping efficiency, that is, cognitive and emotive ways of processing the environmental factors. The findings of these studies will be used to create the common propositions of the MRT being derived.

Concept 3—Outcomes

An important component of any MRT is outcomes. In particular, the literature calls for looking at coping from the perspective of effective outcomes. As noted, the RAM defines outcomes of coping processes as adaptive or ineffective behaviors that reach the goals of adaptation and are expressed in the four adaptive modes. The researchers of the studies being considered each selected specific ways to look at the multidimensional outcomes within the RAM. Dunn (2005) hypothesized outcomes in the role function and self-concept modes as functional ability, depression, and spiritual well-being. Flood and Shearer (2006) assumed that successful aging can be considered evidence of integrated adaptation levels and their framework for the intervention study looked at successful aging as measured by two self-concept dimensions: life satisfaction and purpose in life. In Raleigh et al.'s (2006) work the outcome concepts were adaptive and ineffective responses specified as the ability and satisfaction in caring for one's loved one at home or the inability and lack of satisfaction in caring for one's loved one at home. In the series of studies reported by Levesque et al. (1998) and by Ducharme et al. (1998), the outcome was viewed in the self-concept adaptive mode and was identified as the level of psychological distress. In the study by Flood and Shearer, self-concept was an outcome variable in the form of life satisfaction.

Pictorial Schema—Step 4

Diagramming related concepts is a way to communicate economically some complex theoretical ideas. For example, in teaching language a popular strategy used until about 30 years ago was diagraming sentences. In this process the subject and verb of the sentence were selected and other parts of speech added on lines in a way that had consistent meaning. This approach to analyzing a sentence and depicting its structure with a predetermined visual scheme was thought to be helpful, particularly for beginners in a language such as young children and nonnative speakers. Similarly, theorists regularly present their work in a visual scheme. The complexity of where words are placed and how lines are used will vary depending on the stage of knowledge development and the purpose of the depiction. The outcomes of path analysis can be very complex with a place for central and related concepts depicted with the statistical weights of their influence indicated. For MRTs it is common to use a simple schema that depicts the major concepts and uses lines with arrows to show the relationships among the concepts (Peterson & Bredow, 2009). Step 4 in the process of generating an MRT is creating a schema and for this MRT of coping the pictorial schema is depicted in Figure 7.2. The figure shows the three broad concepts: stimuli, coping strategies, and outcomes at the top, with bracketed concepts under them. Categories of concepts are bracketed and the relationships among concepts are shown by arrows.

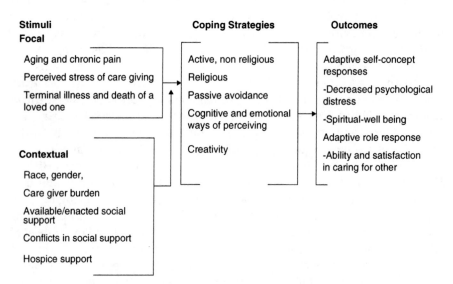

FIGURE 7.2   Schema of Middle Range Theory of Coping

Specific concepts under focal stimuli include aging and chronic pain, perceived stress of caregiving, and terminal illness and death of a loved one. Coping strategies identified in the MRT are active, nonreligious coping, passive avoidance, cognitive and emotional ways of perceiving, religious coping, and creativity. Outcomes include adaptive self-concept responses; specifically, decreased psychological distress, depression, and spiritual well-being; adaptive role responses include the ability and satisfaction of caring for others.

Propositions—Step 5

In constructing a MRT, synthesizing the relational statements among the concepts is a major step. Walker and Avant (2011) referred to statement synthesis as the point at which the theory builder starts to bring clarity and direction to the understanding of the phenomena of interest. The synthesis is aimed at specifying relationships between two or more concepts based on evidence. For purposes of this approach to knowledge development the evidence is provided by the results of the studies being used in the MRT development. The theory builder takes into account the strengths and weaknesses of the studies and carefully reviews the findings for common themes that were supported among the hypothesized relationships. "Proposition" is the name given to relational statements within the MRT. Some of the selected studies included models of relationships among their variables, however, where indicated the researchers revised the models based on findings. These findings provide the evidence for the propositions of this MRT on coping.

TABLE 7.1
Propositions of Middle Range Theory of Coping

1. Active coping strategies led to changes in the stimulus of perceived stress and to adaptation manifested by less psychological distress
2. Passive/avoidance coping strategies are related to the negative outcome of psychological distress, but over time to an increase in active coping strategies leading to adaptation
3. Cognitive coping of important decision making is helped by support of health providers
4. Religious coping used by those in chronic pain leads to positive self-concept affects of less depression and psychological distress; spirituality is a strategy used to cope with bereavement and to adapt effectively
5. Religious and nonreligious coping strategies are used by elders to handle higher pain intensities

(continued)

TABLE 7.1
Propositions of Middle Range Theory of Coping (*continued*)

6. Stronger stimuli lead to increased coping strategies as in greater perceived stress of caregiving and higher levels of chronic pain
7. The pooled effect of stimuli such as patient request and desire to be with and help the patient influence caregiver coping adequacy and an adaptive response
8. Support such as hospice leads to adaptation to care for the dying—although fewer coping strategies are used, they are more effective and similarly available; to enact social support for caregivers has a direct effect on active coping
9. Conflicts in social support among caregivers relates to passive/avoidance coping strategies and to greater psychological distress
10. Demographic backgrounds do not have as much influence on some outcomes as reported, for example, the level of self-reported pain intensity in elders was not related to age, gender, culture, or race
11. Gender and race had some effect in that women and non-White participants reported using religious coping strategies more often than did men and White participants
12. Race has some effect on creativity as in a sample from senior centers in which Black participants scored higher on creativity preintervention and postintervention in both the control and intervention group when the effort was to improve successful aging by increasing creativity

The propositions begin with statements derived from this set of studies that relate the coping strategies with adaptation outcomes (see Table 7.1). The five studies analyzed separately by Levesque et al. (1998) and Ducharme et al. (1998) as noted used a total of 2,187 participants in various caregiver roles. When the original model was not a good fit an exploratory search for a model that would fit the data better was done by modifying the indexes of the LISEREL program for each study. The authors explained that the RAM allows for reciprocal relationships and system feedback. Pathways not originally hypothesized, but theoretically relevant, were revealed. Proposition 1 states that active coping strategies lead to changes in the stimulus of perceived stress and to adaptation manifested by less psychological distress. The new linkages found by Levesque et al. were observed by Ducharme et al. at a later time indicating that the model is relatively stable over time. The revised models described by the investigators explained 32% and 47% of the variance of the outcome of psychological distress. Proposition 2 notes that passive/avoidance coping strategies are related to the negative outcome of psychological distress, but over time to an increase in active coping strategies leading to adaptation. This is an important statement because it takes time into account, showing how a person can change strategies when one approach is not working and also how coping varies with the stimuli. Ducharme et al. noted the meaning of this proposition as indicating that people who use active strategies such as problem solving at time 2 may have first used passive/avoidance strategies such as denial in the fact of stress at time 1. Studying the samples at different time points allows findings that emphasize the importance of the fit among the type of stressors, such as acute, chronic, and daily living, and the coping strategies that will be effective.

In a mixed-methods study, Raleigh et al. supported proposition 3 that cognitive coping of important decision making is helped by support of health providers. Specifically in this study a person can make the decision to care for a dying loved one at home when helped by hospice support. In proposition 4, it is noted that religious coping used by those in chronic pain leads to positive self-concept effects of less depression and psychological distress; spirituality is a strategy used to cope with bereavement and to adapt effectively. As supported by Dunn, the author found that elders with chronic pain who used religious coping strategies had positive self-concept outcomes manifested by less depression and psychological distress. Similarly in the study by Raleigh et al. spirituality was a coping strategy used by caregivers that helped their ability to cope with bereavement and to adapt effectively. Proposition 5 states that religious and nonreligious coping strategies are used by elders to handle higher pain intensities. Also in Dunn's study there was support for proposition 5. In the well-designed study of 200 community-dwelling elders, Dunn pointed out that findings suggested these elders appraised their pain as amenable to change. They are more likely to use problem solving and report the pain to a doctor or nurse, to take medication, and to use diversion and exercise. This finding differs from previous research that suggested that older adults use more passive, emotion-focused coping strategies and less information-seeking strategies.

In synthesizing the concepts of stimuli used in these studies, we derived an additional seven propositions. Proposition 6 notes, as predicted by the RAM, stronger stimuli lead to increased coping strategies as in greater perceived stress of caregiving and higher levels of chronic pain. This was the case in the samples of caregivers used by Levesque et al. and by Ducharme et al. in which the greater the perceived stress the greater the increase in coping strategies. Similarly Dunn found increasing coping strategies with higher levels of chronic pain. Proposition 7 notes that the pooled effect of stimuli such as patient request, desire to be with and help the patient influence caregiver coping adequacy and adaptive responses. This proposition follows a similar principle to earlier ones about stimuli, but deals with the pooled effect of stimuli. In Raleigh et al.'s study of those who chose to be caregivers of a dying loved one, the pooled effect of stimuli that influenced caregiver adequacy and an adaptive response included patient request and the caregiver's desire to be with and desire to help the patient.

Proposition 8 states that support such as hospice leads to adaptation to care for the dying—although fewer coping strategies are used, they are more effective and similarly available enacted social support for caregivers has a direct effect on active coping. Support is derived from findings of the study by Raleigh et al. and partly also from studies by Levesque et al. and by Ducharme et al. The findings across studies clarify some of the relationships about support. Support from professionals such as hospice workers leads to adaptation to care for the dying. This adaptation comes about by using fewer but more effective coping strategies. Optimistic and confrontive coping styles were the most frequently used though the authors report that scores were not very high relative to the possible scores. Similarly, the sets of studies about a variety of caregivers showed that when social support is enacted for caregivers it has a direct effect on active coping. In proposition 9 it is noted that conflicts in social support among caregivers relate to passive/avoidance coping strategies and to greater psychological distress. The groups of studies reported by Levesque and Ducharme and their colleagues with varying large samples and more than one time frame had findings that supported this new insight into social support. In general positive support leads to positive outcomes, but conflicts related to support do not lead to adaptive outcomes.

The stimuli of the last three propositions are related to demographic factors. Proposition 10 states that demographic backgrounds do not have as much influence on some outcomes as reported, for example, the level of self-reported pain intensity in elders was not related to age, gender, culture, or race. These generalizations are synthesized from Dunn's (2005) study of pain in elders where the level of self-reported pain intensity was not related to age, gender, culture, or race. In this study of 200 community-dwelling older adults the author pointed out that most reported findings indicate the opposite. It is often assumed that greater pain comes with greater age, that culture can influence perceptions and expressions of pain, and that women report more pain than men. The findings from this study clearly suggest that regardless of racial background, whether the person is a man or a woman and whatever age, elders reported similar chronic pain intensities. In proposition 11 it is noted that gender and race had some effect in that women and non-White participants reported using religious coping strategies more often than did men and White participants. These were also findings from the study by Dunn.

In the intervention study by Flood and Scharer (2006) to promote successful aging, the main hypothesis about increasing creativity by group interventions was not supported. However, the authors described some unexpected findings synthesized in proposition 12 that states that race has some effect on creativity as in a sample from senior centers, Black participants scored higher on creativity preintervention and postintervention in both the control and intervention group when the effort was to improve successful aging by increasing creativity. The authors provided two possible reasons for the unexpected findings. First, likely the dose of creativity intervention was not strong enough or of long enough duration (1-hour sessions for 8 weeks) to make a difference and there may have been too many types of creativity activities (eight different activities). The authors noted that related to race, during the study, Black participants talked about how racial tensions had improved during their lives and gave descriptions of their experiences of discrimination. The suggestion is made and seems reasonable that perhaps Black participants had experienced greater numbers of life crises and these stressors had a bearing on present purpose in life and life satisfaction, the measures of successful aging mediated by creativity. No differences in aging by race are noted in the literature and the authors recommend that this finding is important to investigate further.

In looking at each study and across studies, the findings provide the basis for synthesizing the propositions of the MRT of coping. The desired outcome of clear statements of relationships between and among concepts (Walker & Avant, 2011) is reached. The theorist is pulling together and organizing the patterns of relationships reflected in the selected studies. Evidence of some form is required but statements will vary as to how much evidence supports different statements. Walker and Avant noted that improvements in measurement and other approaches to rigor may occur that permit preliminary "discovery" observations to be tested in a later stage of scientific refinement.

Evidence—Step 6

The MRT of coping derived from the selected studies is made up of 12 propositional statements about coping strategies and their outcomes and the focal and contextual stimuli that effect coping strategies and their outcomes. As noted some of the propositions inferred from the findings of these studies were different than originally hypothesized by the investigators. The investigators revised their original conceptual models. These new insights are useful in addressing the major issues in the literature on coping about how to design effective interventions. There is a long-time debate about whether coping lies more with the person or with the environment, that is, the issue of trait, a more enduring characteristic versus state, a more temporary condition. Does the person have personality traits that makes one tend to use some coping strategies and not others? Or is the state of the situation such that it has more influence on coping strategies selected? Answers to these questions are important in designing nursing interventions to promote coping.

Some findings from the selected studies lend some evidence of how to look at this issue. Dunn found that elders with greater reported pain intensity used more problem-solving coping and attributed this to their belief in change, a state situation. Still Dunn found that gender and race affected types of coping strategies in that women and non-White elders reported using religious coping strategies more often than men and White participants. In one case the stimuli led to one type of coping yet person traits such as gender and race affect the coping. Ducharme et al. showed that people could match their strategies based on whether the stress was acute, chronic, or part of daily living. The study by Raleigh et al. found that decision making to care for a loved one who was dying was helped by support from hospice nurses and further that these caregivers used fewer but more effective coping strategies with ongoing support.

This evidence is consistent with an unpublished study in which Roy, with colleague McCurry, did an initial exploration of state versus trait in coping using the Coping and Adaptation Processing Scale (CAPS; Roy, 2011). The study compared total coping scores and subscale coping scores for two groups that varied by acuity of illness. One sample was adults living in the community with stable neurological deficits (N = 349). The second was adults undergoing a surgical procedure at an ambulatory surgery center who completed the CAPS prior to surgery (N = 75) and 1 week following surgery (N = 30). In analyzing the findings, Roy and McCurry had some preliminary findings that tend to provide an interpretation for the findings of studies noted above on this important issue. T-tests for independent samples showed significant differences in total CAPS scores and for all subscale scores between the group with stable deficits and those facing same-day surgery (p < .000–.003). T-tests of difference (paired sample, two-tailed test) from presurgery to 1 week after surgery on total CAPS scores and all subscale scores showed no significant differences. However, when the group of surgical patients is divided into those who received a nurse-coaching intervention for symptom management and those who did not, there is a tendency for increased CAPS scores after intervention. Scores for the control group stayed essentially the same, whereas the experimental group had a mean of 3 points higher, which was close to statistically significant and this was the case even when the numbers at time 2 declined.

The investigators suggested that the best interpretation of their data is that coping is a trait, but that the coping and adaptation processing can be activated by an acute challenge. Further the effectiveness of coping and adaptation processing can be enhanced by nursing intervention. This interpretation also is supported by the study published in Spanish by Gonzalez (2007) and discussed in Chapter 13. In this study following a nursing intervention aimed at cognitive coping of patients postcardiac event, the experimental group had significantly greater changes in coping scores than the control group.

At this stage the derived MRT, including the propositions, provide understanding about coping that can direct knowledge for nursing practice. The interpretation coming from the exploratory work lends significant meaning to the propositions highlighted from those derived in this MRT. In the Dunn study, across the sample person traits such as gender and race had some influence on coping strategies used, that is, religious coping. However, with higher levels of pain, a new state situation was created and coping strategies changed to problem solving, likely aimed at the change. Ducharme et al. also showed that people could change their strategies based on the acuity of the situation. Finally, Raleigh et al. showed how coping in initial decision making and in carrying out care of a loved one who was dying was enhanced by the intervention of hospice nurses. The conclusion is that it is important to planning a nursing intervention to understand coping as a trait but that given more acute states, the coping and adaptation process can be activated within that state and other strategies used that better fit to reach successful adaptation. Further, the effectiveness of coping and adaptation processing can be enhanced by nursing intervention.

TRANSLATIONS FOR PRACTICE AND POLICY

One concern that led to proposing the development of this approach to knowledge is the recognized gap between nursing knowledge development and knowledge used in practice. Accumulating studies based on a common theoretical framework of nursing provides the possibility of synthesizing concepts and propositions into MRTs. With the concepts applied to specific research participants, they are closer to the practice level. The syntheses derived provide the opportunity to create new knowledge for practice that can be generalized across populations. An important concept for practice at a broad theoretical level is Roy's description of nursing intervention approaches as promoting adaptation by changing stimuli or strengthening the adaptive coping processes. With new insights on coping strategies at the heart of this MRT we can now demonstrate how this knowledge can be integrated into practice and bring about changes in policy.

Recommendation for Practice

Within the general MRT of coping we provided some clarity to the unsolved issue of whether coping is more person based as a trait or more situation based as a state. The answer lies in an understanding of people as having trait-based preferences for coping yet changes in their situations or new states bring about the opportunity for changing coping strategies. Nurses can use this understanding both to strengthen persons' preferred coping abilities and also to help with changes in coping strategies to handle changes in their lives, including health changes. We propose the development and widespread use of patient teaching tools on coping with this two-part understanding. Electronic format applications can be created that lead persons to recognize their preferred coping traits. With embedded videos the person can identify the cases most like themselves and receive prompts that provide understanding of these approaches and how to use them effectively. Second, they can learn about using new strategies in times of change and be prompted to contact their nurse coach to make changes in coping and to receive the support they need at this time.

This recommendation is supported by many approaches to health promotion. New tools are being developed to promote healthy behavior change (Leddy, 2005). Just as there are public programs that encourage physical exercise to promote health, there can be enthusiasm for a proposed electronic application (app) called *Exercising Your Ability to Handle Life and Change*. Nurses collaborate with health psychologists and health educators to create these user-friendly tools based on nursing knowledge of coping and adaptation strategies and how people can use them most effectively.

Exemplar for Policy Change

The importance of nursing knowledge related to this general MRT of coping calls for broad policy changes in how health care is delivered. The system needs to reposition the focus on health promotion and provide public access with nursing support to make the recognized significance of health promotion a reality. The 2011 strategic plan of the National Institute of Nursing Research (NINR) lists as their first priority "Enhance health promotion and disease prevention" (NINR, 2012, p. 5). The authors of the statement noted that health care professionals, policy leaders, and others in the health care arena have long recognized the place of health promotion in handling the problem of chronic illness. Further, the emphasis is that successful strategies for health promotion involve more than just educating individuals on healthy living habits. Scientists are challenged to determine the collective social and physical behaviors that lead to making healthy lifestyle choices. Health promotion requires a thorough exploration of behavior at multiple levels of society, including that of individuals, families, clinicians, health care organizations, communities, and populations. To focus on using the knowledge we have developed, we can imagine a time when health promotion for all has its rightful place and nurses are the providers that make the system work.

We can envision a time when the health-promotion application *Exercising Your Ability to Handle Life and Change*, and other health-promotion apps are readily available to all at public kiosks. These are located in grocery stores, pharmacies, shopping malls, places of entertainment, beauty salons, barber shops, churches, centers of transportation, and at delivery points for mail services. On a broad scale the distribution of goods and services will be linked to health care needs. This app will locate the nearest nurse with times of availability for coaching on coping. One can project that with effective coping skills, each individual, family, and community can better promote health for individuals and for groups.

CONCLUSION

This chapter served to introduce the key step in our approach to knowledge development for nursing practice. The process of generating MRT is articulated and exemplified in developing an MRT of general coping. The findings of the 13 studies provide evidence and insights about designing nursing interventions to promote coping. Coping is seen as a key step in health promotion. Understanding the basic principles of the successful use of coping and finding ways to implement these in practice can have a profound impact on the health of generations to come.

REFERENCES

Aldwin, C. (2007). *Stress, coping, and development* (2nd ed.). New York, NY: Guilford Press.

Ducharme, F., Ricard, N., Duquette, A., Levesque, L., & Lachance, L. (1998). Empirical testing of a longitudinal model derived from the Roy Adaptation Model. *Nursing Science Quarterly, 11*(4), 149–159.

Dunn, K. S. (2005). Testing a middle-range theoretical model of adaptation to chronic pain. *Nursing Science Quarterly, 18*(2), 146–156.

Flood, M., & Scharer, K. (2006). Creativity enhancement: Possibilities for successful aging. *Issues in Mental Health Nursing, 27*(9), 939.

Folkman, S., & Moskowitz, J. T. (2004). Coping: Pitfalls and promise. *Annual Review of Psychology, 55*, 745–774.

Frydenberg, E. (Ed.). (2002). *Beyond coping: Meeting goals, vision, and challenges.* London: Oxford University Press.

Gonzalez, Y. (2007). Efficacy of two interventions based on the theory of coping and adaptation processing. *Roy Adaptation Association Review, 11*(1), 4.

Holahan, C. J., Moos, R. H., & Schaefer, J. A. (1996). Coping, stress resistance, and growth: Conceptualizing adaptive functioning. In M. Zeidner & N. Endler (Eds.), *Handbook of coping: Theory, research and application* (pp. 24–43). New York, NY: Wiley.

Jalowiec, A. (1993). Coping with illness: Synthesis and critique of the nursing coping literature from 1980–1990. In J. S. Barnfather & B. L. Lyon (Eds.), *Stress and coping: State of the science and implications for nursing theory, research and practice* (pp. 65–83). (Sigma Theta Tau International Monograph No. 93). Indianapolis, IN: Center Nursing Press.

Leddy, S. (2005). *Integrative health promotion: Conceptual bases for nursing practice* (2nd ed.). Sudbury, MA: Jones and Bartlett.

Levesque, L., Ricard, N., Ducharme, F., Duquette, A., & Bonin, J. (1998). Empirical verification of a theoretical model derived from the Roy adaptation model: Findings from five studies. *Nursing Science Quarterly, 11*(1), 31–39.

McEwen, M., & Wills, E. M. (2010). *Theoretical basis for nursing* (3rd ed.). Philadelphia, PA: Lippincott Williams & Wilkins.

National Institute of Nursing Research website. (2012). Retrieved from http://www.ninr.nih.gov

Peterson, S., & Bedrow, T. (2009). *Middle range theories.* Philadelphia, PA: Wolters Kluwer/Lippincott Williams & Wilkins.

Raleigh, E. D. H., Robinson, J. H., Marold, K., & Jamison, M. T. (2006). Family caregiver perception of hospice support. *Journal of Hospice and Palliative Nursing, 8*(1), 25–33.

Roy, C. (2009). *The Roy adaptation model* (3rd ed.). Upper Saddle River, NJ: Prentice Hall Health.

Roy, C. (2011). Extending the Roy adaptation model to meet changing global needs. *Nursing Science Quarterly, 24*(4), 345–351.

Roy, C., & Roberts, S. (1981). *Theory construction in nursing: An adaptation model.* Englewood Cliffs, NJ: Prentice-Hall.

Schwarzer, R., & Schwarzer, C. (1996). A critical survey of coping instruments. In M. Zeidner & N. S. Endler (Eds.), *Handbook of coping: Theory, research, applications* (pp. 107–132). New York, NY: John Wiley & Sons, Inc.

Smith, M. J., & Liehr, P. (2008). *Middle range theory for nursing.* New York, NY: Springer Publishing Company.

Walker, L., & Avant, K. (2011). *Strategies for theory construction in nursing* (5th ed.). Upper Saddle River, NJ: Prentice Hall.

8

Synthesis of Middle Range Theory of Adapting to Life Events

SISTER CALLISTA ROY

Middle range theory (MRT) is recognized as a significant development in nursing knowledge. Among the arguments for this position is the notion that since MRTs are created with concepts closer to practice, they provide the promise of decreasing the gap between the acquisition of new knowledge and its use in initiating changes in nursing practice (see Box 7.1). We have introduced an innovative way to derive and use MRTs with the aim of creating knowledge that impacts nursing practice. Each chapter of this section applies a six-step approach to generating MRTs from research studies (see Box 7.3). As explained in Chapter 7, the team of authors developed the approach both from literature on MRT and by refining the process in working together to carry out this unique project. We know from the literature that many approaches have been used to derive MRTs and found to be useful (Meleis, 2007). Research projects, literature reviews, and clinical practice have all helped to derive new theories of the middle range. This project was unique in that the team could build on the advantages of having a large body of research based on one nursing grand theory (also referred to as a conceptual nursing model). Because the investigators of the studies located in the review and described in Part II used the Roy adaptation model as a conceptual framework, the concepts within the studies have similar derivations and meanings from the years of publication on the Roy adaptation model.

The researchers, working independently, had an understanding of persons and groups as open adaptive systems (see Box 7.2). The human system uses central coping processes to maintain adaptation in a changing environment. The system is affected by both internal and external changes within given contexts. The model refers to these as focal, contextual, and residual stimuli. For purposes of clinical or research analysis the system output can be viewed as four interrelated modes of adaptation—physiologic/physical, self-concept/group identity, role function, and interdependence. In keeping with the philosophical and scientific assumptions of the model, adaptation is described as the process and outcome whereby thinking and feeling people, as individuals or in groups, use conscious awareness and choice to create human and environmental integration. Adaptation is effective or ineffective in relation to meeting the person or groups goals. General goals of adaptation include survival, growth, reproduction, mastery, and human and environment transformations. The central coping processes are what lead to adaptation and eventually health. Coping processes are defined as innate and acquired ways of responding to the environment to promote the goals of adaptation. Within the model, for the individual the highest level abstraction of coping processes are called the cognator and the regulator and for the group the innovator and stabilizer. When dealing with MRT, we deal with concepts at a level of abstraction that is closer to practice. For example, the cognator may include coping strategies such as selective attention or problem solving.

The six steps of this unique approach developed by the team facilitate the synthesis of the findings of the studies. This approach is discussed in Chapter 7 and outlined in Box 7.3. In this chapter the process is used with selected studies related to coping with life events. In step 1, the selection of related studies, for this chapter, I selected 12 studies from those reviewed in Part II to create a MRT of adapting to life events. The studies included nurses dealing with difficult experiences in particular settings where they work. The process of adapting used by nurses has commonalities with strategies used by adults to deal with commonly occurring life events and by mothers or children who handle common and less common life experiences. As noted in the steps outlined earlier, the 12 studies are used as observations to select and define concepts that are interrelated in a MRT. The purposes of the chapter are (a) to identify and define concepts related to coping with life events, (b) to relate the concepts and depict the theory in a visual diagram, (c) to derive propositions from the interrelationships identified from the analysis of the research, (d) to demonstrate how the research-supported theory provides evidence for practice in clinical situations, and (e) to illustrate how knowledge from the MRT can change practice in an area of high-need priority.

GENERATING A MIDDLE RANGE THEORY

The 12 studies identified in step 1 are described briefly. Then I complete the remaining steps of generating MRT with these studies beginning with the important step of identifying the common concepts at the middle range level. The concepts are interrelated in a visual depiction of the synthesized MRT, in this case a two-part MRT of coping with life events. Theoretical statements, also called propositions, are derived from the studies and their findings and provide the evidence for the new MRT.

Studies Selected for Middle Range Theory Development—Step 1

In carrying out step 1, I evaluated from the review in Part II that all studies selected met the general criteria in the analytic phase of this work, that is, the standards of research adequacy and were based on the Roy adaptation model. Further the studies selected provided the possibility for insights into the concepts and relationships of an MRT of adapting to life events. In relation to this criteria, the 12 studies were selected because regardless of the population each showed that the human adaptive system responds to challenges that face people while adapting to a changing environment. In some cases these changes are experienced by a large percentage of the population, such as a child receiving an injection or a woman experiencing menopause. In other cases the adaptation that was studied is not a challenge for a broad population, such as perioperative nurses handling verbal abuse of physicians or college students experiencing dating violence, but the studies disclosed common coping processes to achieve adaptation.

Three of the studies related to nurses. Cook, Green, and Topp (2001) explored the incidence and impact of physician verbal abuse on perioperative nurses. This was a descriptive exploratory study of 78 perioperative nurses using a verbal abuse scale. In a qualitative, phenomenological study, Wright (2007) described the experience of five emergency nurses who routinely handle traumatic and violent events. Hanna (2005) used a modified phenomenology to redefine moral distress as conscious reflexibility, also called lived consciousness, in 10 registered nurses of various persuasions who were involved in assisting with abortions.

In the adult population, two studies related to dealing with dating or intimate partner violence and one study to decision making about advance directives. Polichnowski's (2008) study looked at adaptation to dating violence through spiritual well-being. This was a predictive, correlational study in which a convenience sample of 444 college students answered the relevant surveys by e-mail. In the next study Woods and Isenberg (2001) tested a MRT of adaptation as a mediator of intimate abuse and traumatic stress in battered women. The sample of 160 women was divided into 53 currently abused, 55 postabused, and 52 nonabused women. Survey data were used in a predictive, correlational study with data analyzed in a series of regression equations. A public data set was available to Zhang (2004) to test a model of decision-making responses related to advance directives. A total of 938 aging subjects were included and items extracted and scales constructed from survey questions that were analyzed using causal modeling and path analysis.

The remaining studies dealt with women and children in situations that included the common events of menopause, postpartum experiences, and having an injection and the less common, but too often shared experiences of a mother dealing with her child's health, that is, an infant in the neonatal intensive care unit (NICU), a child with severe cerebral palsy, and a child with cancer. In a descriptive correlational study Taylor (1997) included 194 postmenopausal women to determine the relationships among coping, attitude toward menopause, self-esteem, and demographic variables. A descriptive survey was conducted by Martin (1995) with 300 women to identify common postpartum problems and adaptation strategies to cope with these problems during the first 2 to 8 weeks following delivery of full-term healthy newborns. Sparks (1999) conducted an intervention study with 105 preschool children having immunization injections. The aim was to examine the effects of distraction and cutaneous stimulation on the pain of having the injection.

Lazenby (2001) used a phenomenological approach to study five Mexican mothers who had infants in the NICU. The aim was to explore the stressors and adaptation of these mothers using 10 open-ended questions categorized with the structure of the Roy adaptation model. Also using phenomenology, Moore (2005) interviewed five participants to explore the lived experience of being a mother of a child with severe cerebral palsy. Clark (2001) used a similar approach in interviewing three mothers to investigate the lived experience of mothers coping with their children's diagnoses of cancer.

Concepts—Steps 2 and 3

Moving to the important work of theorizing by identifying concepts for the middle range level we cover step 2, identifying the main concepts of the theory and step 3, synthesizing the concepts at the required level of generality, that is, discrete and generalizable, which are at the middle range level. The concepts of the MRT are of three types. First, the stimuli across the 12 studies were categorized into major types. Then coping strategies identified within the studies were synthesized, and finally the outcomes found by the investigators were similarly combined into mid-range categories. The concepts are related in a two-part schema depicted in Figures 8.1 and 8.2. For the stimuli categories, similar concepts are identified. Second, related coping strategies are synthesized. These are then conceptually connected to the outcomes. The development of each concept in the schema is described below and the derivations of the relationships among the concepts are shown in discussing the propositions.

Concept 1—Stimuli

The major conceptual categories of life events identified for this theory are as follows:

- *Developmental events* that are expected and may be related to internal or external changes (see Figure 8.1, column 1)
- *Situational events* that are unexpected and may be related to specific occurrences or to health challenges (see Figure 8.2, column 1)

The four studies in the first category of *developmental events* included postpartum problems, menopause, signing advance directives, and receiving injections by preschoolers. The *specific occurrences of situational events*

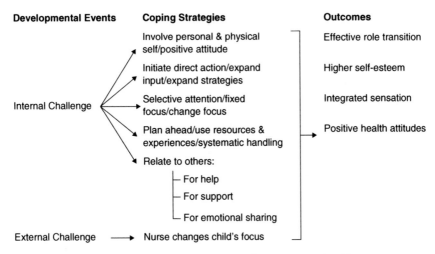

FIGURE 8.1   Middle Range Theory of Coping With Life Events, Developmental Events

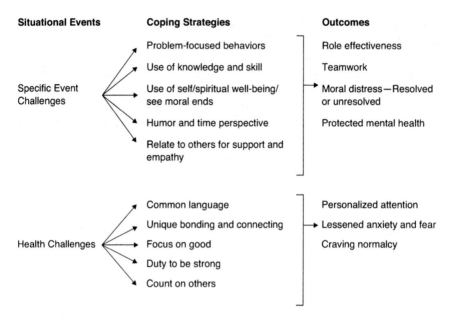

FIGURE 8.2   Middle Range Theory of Coping With Life Events, Situational Events

were studies of effects of physician verbal abuse on perioperative nurses, of emergency nurses exposed to traumatic and violent events, of nurses with different beliefs who participated in elective abortions, of college students and dating violence and women coping with intimate partner abuse. Situational events had a second conceptual category of *health challenges* and included Mexican mothers with an infant in the NICU, mothers who had children with severe cerebral palsy, and mothers of children with cancer.

Concept 2—Coping Strategies

The middle term of the emerging MRT is coping strategies. According to the Roy adaptation model, as noted, coping strategies act to promote adaptation. Adaptation can take many forms but is the outcome of the person or group as an adaptive system using coping strategies to handle the stimuli. Some researchers specifically aimed to identify coping strategies. Others, however, using an adaptation framework made it possible to identify coping strategies across the samples of research participants even if that was not the specific aim of the study. Again the effort is to identify the concepts at a middle range level. In Figures 8.1 and 8.2 the middle columns show the coping strategies synthesized for the two types of life events, developmental and situational. Five strategies were identified across the four studies related to the concept of *developmental events*. For example, when Martin (1995) surveyed 300 women to identify common postpartum problems, the author also identified the strategies these mothers used to cope with the identified problems during the first 2 to 8 weeks following delivery. By considering the MRT of coping by Roy (2011), discussed in Chapter 7, it was possible to synthesize these from discrete behaviors to conceptual categories of strategies of cognitive-emotional coping.

These conceptual categories also represented coping by other participants dealing with different developmental events. For example, Martin noted that women during early postpartum who identified getting chores done as a problem used a range of ways to cope with the problem. These included doing chores daily, which was called direct action, or ignoring them, called selective attention because the mothers chose to focus on their babies instead. The mothers also used direct action when the problem was loss of income and they returned to work. Selective attention includes a change of focus and for the preschoolers in the study by Sparks (1999) both distraction and light touch significantly reduced reports of pain from immunization injections. It is possible to infer that for the children to report less pain, the nurses promoted coping by efforts to change focus of attention of the children.

In the *situational events*, the first conceptual group is specific event challenges and six coping strategies were identified in the five studies selected (see Figure 8.2, column 2). Nurses were the participants in three studies, college students in one, and women who were abused in the fifth. Participants were dealing with difficult event challenges. Still, strong coping strategies were noted such as problem-focused behaviors and use of knowledge and skill. The personal self, particularly the spiritual self, is used for coping. For example, Hanna (2005) found that nurses who participated in elective abortions could see moral ends and have a time perspective in their processes of coping. Polichnowski (2008) reported that spiritual well-being was a moderator of coping with dating violence for college students. Adaptation in three of the adaptive modes was identified as a mediator between abuse and posttraumatic stress disorder in the research of Woods and Isenberg (2001).

Health challenges is the second conceptual group of situational events. Three studies of mothers dealing with children's health provided five additional categories of coping strategies (see Figure 8.2, column 2). It was Lazenby's (2001) finding of the effect of nurses not having a common language with the Mexican mothers of infants in a NICU that lead to inferring that a common language would be a coping strategy. It is interesting to note that the strategy of *relate to others* takes on a different meaning among the life challenges. For example, in Clark's (2001) study of mothers coping with their child's cancer the author identified the theme that there is a need to have others to count on and Moore's (2005) study of mothers of children with severe cerebral palsy noted that support from others is appreciated, but not always received. In developmental life *events*, the category of "relate to others" is for help, support, and emotional sharing, whereas in specific situational events in addition to relating to others for support there is also the coping strategy of relating for empathy. Further research can indicate whether these categories will remain distinct or might be combined for this MRT.

Concept 3—Outcomes

An important part of devising a MRT of adapting to life events is to look at the outcomes of the coping strategies. Outcomes for the theory were derived by looking across studies within each conceptual category of life events (see Figure 8.1, column 3). For developmental events, that is, studies of mothers in the early postpartum period, women adjusting to menopause, adults completing advance directives, and preschoolers receiving immunization injections, four outcomes were derived. These were named effective role transitions, higher self-esteem, integrated sensation, and positive health attitudes. The concepts are stated as adaptive outcomes within or across adaptive modes. This is expected since the use of the Roy adaptation model defines adaptive outcomes as integrated functioning in the adaptive modes and this understanding likely guided the researchers' choice of outcomes to analyze.

For the five studies labeled *specific situational events*, three of which related to nurses dealing with challenging events, four outcomes were derived (see Figure 8.2, column 3). These related to both role and self-concept and were given the concept names of role effectiveness, teamwork, moral distress (resolved or unresolved), and protected mental health. The second type of situational event was the *health challenges* and the three studies included mothers dealing with children with health issues. Three outcomes were derived and stated as personalized attention, lessened anxiety and fear, and craving normalcy (see Figure 8.2, column 3).

To create the theory, these terms are named as positive adaptation. However, this was derived by assuming given strategies could lead to a positive outcome. For example, Lazenby (2001) found that although Mexican mothers may experience the same stressors as Caucasian mothers, their inability to communicate with their babies' caregivers increased their anxiety. The lack of common language requires more personalized attention from the nurse. Thus these are put in positive terms and relate to the findings by Clark (2001) that a theme noted in mothers of children with cancer is a life plagued with fears. In this theory we assume that if coping strategies are effective, the outcome could be lessening of the anxiety and fear of mothers facing these health challenges for their children.

Craving for normalcy was a specific finding by Clark and seemed an important concept to include as an ongoing experience for these mothers. One can propose that this is present for mothers in the other two studies, although the researchers' methods were not planned to identify these findings as an ongoing outcome.

Pictorial Schema of Middle Range Theory—Step 4

In deriving an MRT of adapting to life events unique insights are noted. The coping strategies and outcomes take on specific nuances based on whether the life event is developmental or situational and whether it is a health challenge. Thus it seems useful at this stage of development to describe this as a two-part related MRT. In developing theories, as noted, diagramming the related concepts is a way to communicate economically some complex theoretical ideas. Two diagrams are presented as pictorial schema of MRT of adapting to life events in Figures 8.1 and 8.2. The figures were used in the preceding section to describe the identification of related concepts from the studies at the middle range level. In addition the relationships between the concepts were discussed.

Propositions and Evidence—Steps 5 and 6

In theory building, theoretical statements hold a particular place. A statement of a relationship between two or more concepts is central to science. "Proposition" is the general term used for relational statements. Such statements can vary in their empirical validation. The terms used are a matter of degree and circumstances. If a pattern of relationships is found in a number of empirical studies, the statement can be referred to as an empirical generalization. An empirical generalization might be considered a law when it receives wide acceptance and the data provide confidence in its validity. Few laws have been well developed in the human sciences. If a proposition is yet to be tested, the statement is called a hypothesis. Propositions are considered structural components of theories, that is, what the theory is made of (Meleis, 2007). A proposition tells us how one concept or idea is related to another and how they influence each other in looking at a given phenomenon. The assumption is that the concepts are defined in a way that fits the understanding of the theory being considered.

In a discussion about the synthesis of statements of relationships, Walker and Avant (2011) noted that in this process, "the theory builder starts to bring clarity and direction to the understanding of phenomena of interest" (p. 119). These authors identified conditions when statement synthesis can be a useful strategy. The condition most relevant to our work is what the authors describe as the situation in which there are several published research studies on a phenomenon of interest, but the information contained in them has not been organized together or integrated. This work requires thought and creativity because as Walker and Avant explained in this stage the theorist is "moving from evidence to inferences, and then generalizing from specific inferences to more abstract ones" (2011, p. 119). In our project the studies are our observations and our data. We use them to create the general statements or propositions of our mid-range theory of adapting to life events and each statement has the evidence from the studies behind it. The propositions for the MRT of adapting to life events are listed in Table 8.1 as referred to earlier in introducing the concepts. As noted, the task of syntheses of the MRT propositions is facilitated by an understanding of the grand theory that was the framework for all the selected studies. The studies provided multiple data points from which the more discrete concepts and propositions of the MRT can be synthesized.

The propositions begin with those that relate to strategies of regulator and cognator processing. Derived from the data across the studies, we can now specify that specific cognator processes result in given adaptive responses. In both developmental and situational life changes, as noted in proposition 1, taking direct action, planning ahead, handling issues systematically, and using resources and experience can affect adaptive responses across the adaptive modes and in general. The adaptive outcomes noted with life changes included adaptive responses in self-esteem, role transition, integrated sensation, and healthy attitudes. This was the case when women in menopause used resources and experiences and had healthy attitudes that promoted positive adaptation. Similarly, mothers in the postpartum period found that planning ahead helped with their role transition. In the next two propositions there is a divergence of what is effective cognator activity based on characteristics of the life event. Proposition 2 notes that in new role development or an unexpected role event, expanding input can lead to effective role transition or role effectiveness. Some situations call for expanding input such as with new role development as in becoming a mother and an unexpected role event, for example, an ill child. However, proposition 3 states that when life event or health challenges involve too many or unfamiliar challenges selective attention can help integrate the experience. The data of the studies clarify that when life events or health challenges involve too many or unfamiliar challenges, the more effective strategy is to focus in and use selective attention. For example, some new mothers found it useful to ignore chores and focus on the infant, preschoolers could integrate the experience of receiving an immunization injection better, that is, report less pain, when they received the nursing intervention of distraction or light touch.

TABLE 8.1
Propositions of Middle Range Theory of Coping With Life Events

1. Cognator processes of taking direct action, planning ahead, handling systematic use of resources and experience can affect adaptive responses in self-esteem, role transition, sensation, and health attitudes
2. In new role development or an unexpected role event expanding input can lead to effective role transition or role effectiveness
3. When life event or health challenges involve too many or unfamiliar challenges, selective attention can help integrate the experience
4. For nurses facing specific event challenges, problem-focused behaviors, use of knowledge and skill and humor can lead to role effectiveness, teamwork, and protected mental health
5. Time perspective can be useful in resolving moral distress
6. Use of personal and spiritual self, particularly seeing moral ends can protect mental health
7. Relating to others during developmental challenges is used for help, support, and emotional sharing
8. Relating to others during life challenges is used for support and empathy
9. Relating to others in health challenges is needed but may be lacking, leaving the person with a duty to be strong
10. The use of a common language between those dealing with health challenges and the nurse can lessen anxiety and fear
11. The pooled effect of contextual stimuli such as context, age, and socioeconomic status and residual stimuli such as childhood abuse and witness of violence affect the mental health outcomes of abuse
12. The unique bonding and connecting of mothers of ill children does not eliminate the craving for normalcy

Proposition 4 is the synthesized statement that for nurses facing specific event challenges, problem-focused behaviors, use of knowledge and skill, and humor can lead to role effectiveness, teamwork, and protected mental health. The statement was derived from the studies and adds some nuances to the use of cognator strategies. Nurses' coping goes from problem-focused behaviors and the use of their specific knowledge and skill to the more diffuse strategy of humor. These strategies lead to effectiveness in their roles, being able to work together to handle the specific event challenge of seeing trauma, or facing physician verbal abuse. Less stress and lessened depression are adaptive outcomes of these specific event challenges. Proposition 5 is similar to the generic proposition of the Roy adaptation model that notes that regulator and cognator processing affect adaptation over time. Proposition 5 states that time perspective can be useful in resolving moral distress. For nurses who were involved in elective abortions, taking a long-view perspective was useful in resolving the accumulated moral distress. Proposition 6 notes that the use of personal and spiritual self, particularly seeing moral ends, can protect mental health. We see here across studies other uses for self in coping. For these nurses and for college students dealing with dating violence, the use of personal and spiritual-self protected them from depression and from posttraumatic stress syndrome (PTSD). The finding that the nurses particularly used seeing moral ends in a positive way is consistent with the philosophical assumptions of the Roy adaptation model.

Propositions 7 through 10 address relating to others in the interdependence adaptive mode. There is a broad literature on social support yet some new insights emerge when synthesizing the studies under consideration. Slight differences in the data are worth noting when the life event is developmental or situational. Proposition 7 states that relating to others during developmental challenges is used for help, support, and emotional sharing. This was a strong finding for the mothers during the postpartum period and for women dealing with menopause. Proposition 8 notes that relating to others during life challenges is used for support and empathy. In situation-specific challenges, relation to others is used for support but includes the emotional aspect of empathy. When facing a situational challenge, the person wants those who relate to them to understand what they are going through and to feel with them. The nurses in difficult situations felt this way as reported by the researchers.

Proposition 9 states that relating to others in health challenges is needed but may be lacking, leaving the person with a duty to be strong. It was the study of mothers dealing with the health challenge of caring for a child with cancer that highlighted the finding summarized. Too often the mother is left alone and feeling the duty to be strong. Likely this could be the case in other health challenges, particularly when the health challenge is prolonged or when it is uncomfortable for people to be around as in the case of a child with cancer. This seems an important part of a MRT of adapting to life events since relating to others is a significant human need as described in the interdependence mode of the Roy adaptation model (Roy, 2009). This need can be difficult to meet during health challenges, and nurses are aware of this altered context and consider how they may enhance ways to meet interdependence needs. Proposition 10 states that a common language between those dealing with health challenges and the nurse can lessen anxiety and fear. The terms of this proposition are somewhat similar, however, the relationship is stated in the positive. In those dealing with health challenges the use of a common language is important so that the person can relate to the nurse and lessen the anxiety and fear of the situation. The Mexican mothers who had an infant in the NICU particularly needed contact with those who spoke their language to be able to understand the health condition and to handle it. In a multicultural society such as the United States, made up of waves of immigrants from different countries, and using different languages, such a basic need to facilitate adapting during a health care challenge is magnified and important for nurses to address.

Proposition 11 states the paradoxical situation that the unique bonding and connecting of mothers of children who are ill does not eliminate the craving for normalcy. The study by Clark (2001) had a small sample of mothers coping with their children's cancer. They had handled this health challenge for more than a year and the theme of craving for normalcy was clear and believable. It seems likely that this could apply to minor or major health challenges. We might consider a mother whose child wakes up complaining of a sore throat and the mother is immediately connected and responding to the child's discomfort. Still quietly she wishes it were a normal morning so she could get the child to school and be on time for a work commitment. Moore (2005) described that mothers of children with severe cerebral palsy from 4 to 11 years old create unique ways of bonding and connecting with their child. Another finding in this study was that the child's diagnosis of cerebral palsy is a lifelong journey of recurrent adversity eliciting a series of individualized responses. A reasonable inference, as described by Walker and Avant (2011) in the process of creating theoretical statements, is to say that the unique bond does not negate the craving for normalcy. This is not something the nurse can change but can sensitively acknowledge.

Proposition 12 is a middle range level of the higher level propositions of the Roy adaptation model listed in Chapter 2. Specifically, behavior in the adaptive modes determines adaptation levels and adaptation levels reflect the integration of the person with the environment. The proposition states that the pooled effects of contextual stimuli such as context, age, and socioeconomic status and residual stimuli such as childhood abuse and witness of violence affect the mental health outcomes of abuse. Woods and Isenberg (2001) used a sample of 160 women divided into three groups, 53 currently abused, 55 postabused, and 52 nonabused women to test adaptation in all four adaptive modes as mediators of the relationship between intimate partner abuse and PTSD. Each measurement of physiologic, self-concept, and interdependence separately acted as a mediator and the effect on adaptation in these three modes was additive. The authors reported that overall role function did not have the predicted effect on the relationship between each predictor variable and the outcome variable. They noted, however, that this relationship requires further study because there were correlations between abuse and several role subscales. As often is the case when findings are not as predicted, in considering new knowledge the question is raised as to whether the concept was adequately measured. Another consideration is whether the situation requires further theoretical development.

For example, do women who suffer abuse from an intimate partner see their roles differently and therefore need new definition and measurement when studying this life event?

The substantive structure of this MRT of adaptation to life events is made up of 12 propositional statements about coping with developmental and situational challenges. Based on the concepts of categories of stimuli or challenges, coping strategies, and adaptation outcomes derived from the selected studies, the propositions were synthesized. The derived MRT and the propositions in particular provide understandings of adapting to life events that are useful for nursing practice given the level of support from the studies selected. Further testing of the propositions is another proposed phase of knowledge development for practice.

TRANSLATIONS FOR PRACTICE AND POLICY

In Chapter 1 we examined the long-standing problem of a gap between nursing knowledge development and knowledge used in practice. As noted in a recent review of literature to identify current trends in nursing theories, Im and Chang (2012) identified theory being integrated into practice as a major theme. However, the authors interpreted their data as only the beginning of long overdue efforts to link theory to practice as a basis for nursing care. The effort of this research team is to move this link forward by showing the innovative approach to developing knowledge for nursing practice generating MRT from research based on one grand theory. As noted, MRTs are closer to practice than grand theories because the MRT concepts can be observed and tested. Further, when they are derived from research based on one grand theory, the Roy adaptation model, it is possible to cumulate the findings of diverse studies in areas significant for practice. In this chapter we developed knowledge about people adapting to life events both developmental and situational. What remains is to link this MRT to impact on practice in such a way that changes in practice can be realized.

Recommendation for Practice

Within the MRT of adapting to life events, many coping strategies were derived from the selected studies and it was noted that the adaptive effectiveness of given strategies varies with particular situations. We propose that a major responsibility for every nurse in practice is to coach each patient in the use of that person's own effective coping strategies to promote adaptation; which strategy to use under which circumstances? When to use one and when another; what coping strategies work best for them in a given situation and what situations call for learning new strategies. Nurses in outpatient, home care, and acute care settings will be aware of the need for coping with developmental challenges whether in pediatrics or with care of the elderly. Similarly, when patients across the life span are dealing with health challenges, they also can be dealing with situational life events. Looked at through the perspective of the MRT of adapting to life events, the nurse can be more effective in providing care.

This approach is supported by the position taken by the National Institute of Nursing Research (NINR, 2012, retrieved from http://www .ninr.nih.gov) that nurses study the behavior of systems that promote the development of personalized interventions. Focusing on coping strategies of the person toward adaptation is a valuable approach to individualizing care. Similarly, professional statements provide additional support for this recommendation. *Nursing's Social Policy Statement* (American Nurses Association, 2010) includes as an essential feature of the definition of professional nursing "attention to the range of human experience and responses to health and illness within physical and social environments" (p. 9). Provision 1 of the *Code of Ethics for Nurses* (American Nurses Association, 2001) notes that the nurse "practices with compassion and respect for the inherent dignity, worth and uniqueness of every individual" (p. 7). Focusing on helping patients to identify their own coping strategies and use them effectively to adapt is a way to give attention to the range of human experiences and responses and to practice with respect for the inherent dignity, worth, and uniqueness of every individual. It is the patient's own abilities and strengths in adapting that the nurse uses in the approach recommended as coaching each patient in the use of the patient's strengths.

Example From Practice

Consider a teenage single mother, Jamie W., who is challenged by the developmental event of becoming a mother. The nurse is providing home care for Jamie who was referred for postpartum follow up as a possible at-risk new mother. The nurse immediately identifies that Jamie has spent time and effort to learn all she can to care for her infant daughter. She uses some Internet sites she was given at the prenatal clinic to get information on everything from daily care to finding out about growth and development. Jamie is close to an older cousin who has two children and she often consults with her by phone and text messaging with small questions. In addition, Jamie is using what she learned in a health and first aid class in high school to keep a safe environment for her infant. The nurse talks with Jamie about how well she is adapting to being a mother and how the coping strategies of expanding her input and using resources and experience are helping her. Jamie says that she is really happy that her baby is doing well and she likes being a mother.

The nurse asks Jamie to talk about what is not working as well for her. Jamie says that her mother has been really helpful by letting her stay at home, helping with the baby, and even talking about how Jamie might return to school. However, Jamie says that what she really would like from her mother is more support and emotional sharing. The nurse affirms Jamie's desire as common and realistic. Together they begin to strategize how she can change this part of relating to her mother. Jamie decides she will start with a positive attitude and her gratitude to her mother. She will point out something specific that the baby is doing and ask her mother if she has noticed this too. Jamie hopes she can convey that it is really fun for her to share this part of the experience with her mother. The nurse agrees to return to visit Jamie the following week to see how the approach is going to expand the relating to her mother to include support and emotional sharing as well as practical help. The nurse is aware that this additional strategy can add to the effective role transition and self-esteem of the young mother and give her one more coping strategy as she continues adapting to the ongoing challenges of the new-mother role.

This is a simple example but the principles can be used by nurses in many settings for patients with developmental and life-event challenges. This recommendation can be supported by policy changes that enhance the ability of nurses to use nursing knowledge in collaborative practice and redesign of the health care system.

Exemplar for Practice Policy Change

An important report was released in October 2010 titled *The Future of Nursing: Leading Change, Advancing Health* (Committee on the Robert Wood Johnson Foundation Initiative on the Future of Nursing, at the Institute of Medicine of the National Academies, 2010). Since that time there have been extensive efforts to develop action teams in every state to implement the recommendations in the report. Yet the four key messages of the report are relevant to the unique generating knowledge for nursing practice being articulated and illustrated in this text. Major projects across the United States are looking at nurse credentialing, educational ladders, collaboration across systems, and information infrastructure. However, real change in nursing practice and thus in increased quality of health care is based on nursing knowledge and knowledge used in practice. Nurses can be taught MRTs of adaptation and in particular adaptation to developmental and situational life events. Nurses can be convinced of the need and their expertise in coaching each patient in the use of coping strategies aimed at adaptation as central to nursing practice. However, this approach calls for changes in practice policies in settings to support nurses in implementing care based on this new MRT.

An exemplar for policy change in a practice setting is: *Add a nurse-discharge planner for every inpatient unit.* This nurse would not be concerned primarily with finding long-term placements for patients across many settings. Rather the nurse in this redefined role would work with the primary care nurses on a given unit from the time the patient is admitted to plan for coordinating the patient's ability to adapt to their life events across settings. Recently, I visited a poster session in which a group of staff nurses were convinced that the broadly defined position of discharge nurse was absolutely essential on their unit. They planned the unit staffing to free one nurse to take on this role and were presenting the success of their project at the poster session. In conjunction with the example for practice described above, let us consider that the postpartum unit from which Jamie was discharged had a nurse with this special role in place. It was that nurse who identified that although Jamie was doing well initially, because of her age and unknown extent of resources, she might be at risk. This nurse used the electronic system in place to communicate with nurses in the community to make the referral that brought the nurse to Jamie's home to help her continue developing her strategies to cope with adapting to the developmental challenge of becoming a mother.

CONCLUSION

In this chapter selected studies based on the Roy adaptation model were used in a six-step approach to generate a new MRT of adapting to life events. This knowledge includes propositional statements supported by the research that are at a level that can be applied to practice. This new knowledge-based practice leads to envisioning changes in practice for the individual nurse and for the policies within practice settings.

REFERENCES

American Nurses Association. (2001). *Code for nurses with interpretive statements.* Washington, DC: Author.

American Nurses Association. (2010). *Nursing's social policy statement: The essence of the professional* (3rd ed.). Silver Spring, MD: Author.

Clark, E. D. (2001). *The lived experience of mothers with their child's cancer.* Toledo, OH: Medical College of Ohio at Toledo, Retrieved from http://proquest.umi.com/pqdweb?index=60&did=729283541&SrchMode=1&sid=1&Fmt=2&VInst=PROD&VType=PQD&RQT=309&VName=PQD&TS=1224510743&clientId=7750.

Cook, J. K., Green, M., & Topp, R. V. (2001). Exploring the impact of physician verbal abuse on perioperative nurses. *AORN Journal, 74*(3), 317–318, 320, 322–327.

Hanna, D. R. (2005). The lived experience of moral distress: Nurses who assisted with elective abortions. *Research Theory Nursing Practice, 19*(1), 95–124.

Im, E. O., & Chang, S. (2012). Current trends in nursing theories. *Journal of Nursing Scholarship, 44*(2), 156–164.

Institute of Medicine of the National Academies, Committee on the Robert Wood Johnson Foundation Initiative on the Future of Nursing. (2010). *The future of nursing: Leading change, advancing health.* Washington, DC: The National Academies Press.

Lazenby, L. M. (2001). *The experiences of Mexican mothers in a neonatal intensive care nursery.* University of Nevada, Reno, Retrieved from http://proquest.umi.com/pqdweb? index=59&did=727205361&SrchMode=1&sid=1&Fmt=2&VInst=PROD&VType=PQD&RQT=309&VName=PQD&TS=1224508512&clientId=7750.

Martin, B. (1995). An analysis of common post partum problems and adaptation strategies used by women during the first two to eight weeks following delivery of a fullterm health newborn (Doctoral dissertation, University of Mississippi). *Dissertation Abstracts International, 56*(06B), 3128.

Meleis, A. (2007). *Theoretical nursing, revised reprint: Development and progress* (4th ed.). Philadelphia, PA: Wolters Kluwer/Lippincott Williams & Wilkins.

Moore, L. A. (2005). *The lived experience of being a mother of a child with severe cerebral palsy.* Toledo, OH: Medical College of Ohio, Retrieved from http://proquest.umi.com/pqdweb?did=932417851&Fmt=6&clientId=7750&RQT=309&VName=PQD.

National Institute of Nursing Research. (2012). Retrieved from http://www.ninr.nih.gov

Polichnowski, E. J. (2008). *Adaptation through spiritual well-being as a mediator or moderator of the relationship of the adverse psychological effects of dating violence in a sample of university students.* Baltimore, MD: The Johns Hopkins University. Retrieved from http://proquest.umi.com/pqdweb?did=1540415481&Fmt=6&clientId=7750&RQT=309&VName=PQD.

Roy, C. (2009). *The Roy adaptation model* (3rd ed.). Upper Saddle River, NJ: Prentice Hall Health.

Roy, C. (2011). Extending the Roy adaptation model to meet changing global needs. *Nursing Science Quarterly, 24*(4), 345–351.

Sparks, L. (1999). A comparison of the effects of cutaneous stimulation and distraction on children's perceptions of injection pain (Doctoral dissertation, Saint Louis University). *Dissertation Abstracts International, 60*(04B), 1536.

Taylor, H. (1997). Self-esteem, coping and attitude toward menopause among older rural Southern women (Doctoral dissertation, University of Alabama at Birmingham). *Dissertation Abstracts International, 58*(05B), 2359.

Walker, L., & Avant, K. (2011). *Strategies for theory construction in nursing* (5th ed.). Upper Saddle River, NJ: Prentice Hall.

Woods, S. J., & Isenberg, M. A. (2001). Adaptation as a mediator of intimate abuse and traumatic stress in battered women. *Nursing Science Quarterly, 14*(3), 215–221.

Wright, R. R. (2007). *Experiences of emergency room nurses: What has been learned from traumatic and violent events?* New York, NY: Teachers College, Columbia University. Retrieved from http://proquest.umi.com/pqdweb?did=1390306751& Fmt=6&clientId=7750&RQT=309&VName=PQD.

Zhang, W. (2004). *Factors influencing end-of-life decisions regarding the living will and durable power of attorney: An application of Roy's Adaptation Model.* Atlanta, GA: Georgia State University.

9

Synthesis of Middle Range
Theory of Adapting to Loss

MARJORIE C. DOBRATZ

During the course of one's lifetime, an individual may experience multiple losses. As noted by Cassell (1983), the capacity of the human spirit to overcome loss is "wonderful beyond words" (p. 522). Yet, the loss of a loved one, or the impending forfeiture of one's own life, can result in a profound emotional and physical experience that is often explained as, or termed, "suffering". In his classic work, Cassell (1983) noted that suffering "refers to all the possible dimensions of an individual" (p. 522). These aspects include an individual's social relationships, work and social roles, body image, and spiritual life, along with physical symptoms. Thus, the Roy adaptation model (RAM) with its four adaptive modes provides the ideal structure in which to examine research that focused on loss. The purpose of this chapter is to review selected studies from the larger data-base and identify the common concepts that are associated with loss, then construct a middle range theory (MRT) from these specified concepts, and to provide an exemplar for impact on practice.

GENERATING A MIDDLE RANGE THEORY

In Chapter 7 the author provided a rationale for the importance of MRTs in building knowledge for practice. The characteristics of MRT make them important links between grand theory and practice-level theory. They have fewer concepts that are more concrete. This simplicity leads to MRT being more easily tested in research and applied in practice (see Box 7.1). In that chapter the six-step process for generating MRTs from related research studies was outlined and explained. This process is followed for the issue of adapting to loss. All of the studies that were selected for this chapter involved individuals who experienced a significant loss, such as the death of a long-term spouse, a stillborn infant, the loss of a loved one through violent death, and included those who faced the ultimate loss—that of life itself.

Studies Selected for Middle Range Theory Development—Step 1

It is the opinion of this author that loss and suffering are intertwined, inseparable concepts. This writer also holds the belief that individuals who experience a major loss are visited by suffering and grief. For this reason, professional intervention is the key as to whether or not a person's loss turns into chronic sorrow, long-term pathological grief, or results in a good death. To highlight professional interventions and to accomplish the goals of this chapter, eight studies that were framed within the structure of the RAM and that explored a significant loss were reviewed. Loss crosses the whole human spectrum and suffering and grief cut through all practice areas. The relevant studies for this chapter researched spousal loss (Martin, 2003; Robinson, 1995; Smith, 2001), mothers who experienced the loss of a stillborn infant (Short, 2004), the loss of a loved one due to sudden death (Watson, 2006), and the loss of life itself through terminal illness (Dobratz, 2002, 2004; Gandy, 2003). The participants who took part in these eight studies described the impact of a major loss on their lives. They also accounted for the contextual or environmental stimuli that helped them adapt to their loss. As determined by the initial reviewers, all of the eight studies met the criteria for research adequacy, and they were all framed within the structure of the RAM.

Three studies that were reviewed for this chapter related to the death of a spouse. With inclusion criteria of 65 years or older, Martin's (2003) qualitative study explored the lived experience of five aging (four women and one man) persons who were in the second year of their bereavement. The participants in Martin's study ranged from 71 to 87 years of age. Robinson (1995) chose the same time frame in her descriptive, correlational study of 65 grieving widows (range 45 to 84 years). These participants were too in the second year of bereavement that followed the deaths of their husbands. Robinson studied contextual stimuli of social support, social network, spiritual beliefs, and demographics, which were linked to an adaptive outcome of coping processes and grief responses. The final study by Smith (2001) approached spousal bereavement by exploring the lived experience of working men who had lost their wives through death. With a wide range in the time that had passed since their spouses' deaths (7 months to 26 years), Smith described grief from a predominantly male perspective.

Short (2004) approached loss from the other end of the life spectrum, when she described the experiences of five women who suffered the untimely death and loss of a stillborn infant. To capture the experiences of mothers who lost infants from 18 to 40 weeks of gestation, Short's qualitative, phenomenological study included both an initial and a follow-up interview. Similarly, Watson (2006) conducted face-to-face interviews with five participants who had lost a loved one through a sudden, violent death. The five women who participated in Watson's study were four siblings who had a lost brother or a sister and one individual who had lost her mother. The causes of the violent deaths were two murders, one suicide, one involuntary manslaughter (sister hit by drunk driver), and one vehicular death.

With similar participants who were diagnosed with terminal illness and who were supported with hospice care, another three studies explored the experience of persons who were at the end of life's continuum. Although Gandy's (2003) sample of two hospice patients was small, the data were clarified by a second interview, and there was sufficient data to emerge the themes. Dobratz (2002) studied home hospice patients when she detected the pattern of the becoming-self in 15 of a sample of 97 subjects who took part in a combined causal model and grounded theory study. In a secondary analysis of this same population, Dobratz (2004) extracted references to spirituality in 44 of these 97 subjects. The themes from the latter study on end-of-life spirituality were confirmed by an expert in qualitative methods. The concepts that emerged from the above eight studies and their relatedness to the RAM's framework is now described in the section that follows.

Concepts—Step 2

In their order of presentation, starting with the loss of a spouse, to the loss of a stillborn infant, to the loss of a loved one through sudden death, and then to life's final loss—death, the concepts that came forth in these studies showed striking similarities. As described in the translations section of this chapter, the findings can be supported by other theoretical writings, which lend credence to the RAM's well-designed framework. First, Martin (2003) detected six themes and the most common theme described by bereaved spouses was that of being lonely. The bereaved individuals in Martin's study oscillated back and forth between being grateful for the comfort that their lost spouses had given them and for the amount of time that they had been able to spend with their lost spouses, but they also struggled to overcome regrets, and they tried to resign themselves to the fact that life had to go on without their lost husbands or wife. This was an intense emotional response that called forth or induced feelings of loneliness. Nonetheless, for those around, which included family and others, they tried to be "strong" in their emotional adjustment.

Although it was not the intent of Martin (2003) and although it was not an inclusion criterion, all of the participants in her study were married for 50 years or longer. When asked the question: "Tell me what it has been like for you since your spouse died," all but one of the participants also experienced declining health. Despite the presence of supportive family members, all expressed profound, pervasive loneliness. Although they found comfort in church and other spiritual activities, participants spoke of the void that was left in lives by not being able to share their "spiritual space" with their significant other. Still, the importance of spirituality was noted in their lives. One widow said, "I know that we need to trust God, no matter what." Another replied, "You just ask the Lord for strength and He's right there ready to give you strength right away." In terms of the RAM framework, Martin reported that the concept of spousal loss impacted both of the two coping subsystems: cognator and regulator, and that it crossed all four of the RAM's adaptive modes: physiologic, self-concept, role function, and interdependence.

After having endured long spousal relationships, as supported by declining health, the surviving spouses in Martin's (2003) study experienced such intense, emotional stimuli that physiologic integrity was impacted. Furthermore, as seen by Martin, the loss of the spousal relationship, the "spiritual vacuum" that was created, and the loneliness that ensued were tied to both the interdependence and self-concept modes. Role transition from that of being a married person to that of being a widow or widower was related to the role mode. The often overwhelming emotions and life changes that surviving spouses in Martin's study had to endure cut across all four modes and came together in what is commonly called grief. Roy and Andrews (1999) noted that "when one considers the recurring nature of the stimuli that must be processed through the cognator" (p. 8), it is no wonder that adapting to life without a long-term spouse was a major impact. With psychic integrity and the self-concept mode dependent on "the need to know who one is so that one can be or exist with a sense of unity" (Roy, 2009, p. 44), knowing who one is as a widow or widower instead of a married individual takes place in stages, over a period of time, and does not occur overnight. Yet, in spite of the magnitude of their losses, the grieving widows and widower in Martin's study did attain some grief resolution. They were able to reintegrate to their new situations, and they were able to adjust emotionally or adapt to their loss event. The participants in Martin's research recounted the support of family members as being instrumental in their adaptive process and how their family's support helped them overcome feelings of loneliness.

Robinson (1995) too found that social support was related to adaptive coping in widows after the deaths of their husbands. Although spiritual beliefs were not a significant finding in Robinson's causal model study, she posited that the low reliability of the tool used to measure this concept ($r = .55$) may have impacted this variable. With the cognator's responses related to four cognitive–emotive channels: "perceptual and information processing, learning, judgment, and emotion" (Roy, 2009, p. 41), Robinson's work supported the impact of this coping subsystem on an outcome of adaptive grief response. In addition to social support being related to adaptive responses, the subjects in this study noted that they tried to stay busy and to keep active. To help them resolve their grief, these bereaved women talked about making frequent visits to the cemetery. Although Robinson found that individuals with higher coping scores (cognator) had lower grief response scores and higher role function scores, her study did not measure the effect of the grief response on the regulator or address cross-modal relationships.

The next loss study involved women who gave birth to stillborn infants who died from asphyxia, severe eclampsia, a twin who died in utero, an auto accident, and an unknown cause. In researching the lived experience of five women who lost infants from 18 to 40 weeks of gestation, Short (2004) described the experience of losing a stillborn as a profound, emotionally difficult event. In addition to this being a very difficult, emotional event in their lives, the loss of an infant was further compounded by feelings that they couldn't understand. One mother stated, "I felt as if someone had reached into my chest and stolen my soul." Although their losses occurred over a range of time, from 2 to 10 years, the women in Short's study felt an intense need to feel connected to their infants and to think of them as being real, live babies. They created memories of their lost child, used their babies' names in conversations with others, they celebrated their birthdays, and they made frequent visits to the cemetery so that they could still feel connected to them. These grieving mothers spoke about their being offended when others minimized or didn't recognize the magnitude of their losses. One said, "If you haven't lost a baby, people don't understand." Another said, "Every now and then I would get, 'are you over this yet?', and no I am not." Nevertheless, in spite of the negative communication, the importance of receiving social support from others was an expressed theme.

These grieving mothers talked about their desire to reach out to supportive others (spouses, groups). They all attended a local support group that was structured for women who had similar losses. With the interdependence mode focused on "interactions related to the giving and receiving of love, respect, and value (Roy, 2009, p. 45), Short (2004) described the importance of health care workers who recognized the depth of their pain. As reported by Short, health care professionals helped by "establishing trust, listening, and allowing the bereaved couple to express their grief" (p. 78). The importance of spirituality in helping these women overcome the losses of their infants was also noted. One woman noted that when she first learned that her baby was dead, it felt like God's arms were around her. She said, "It was like, you know arms went right around me and held me," and she then prayed for grace to help her overcome the loss of her infant.

As with Martin (2003), Short (2004) found that the intense suffering that these women endured impacted all four adaptive modes and cross-modal relationships were noted. Stimuli from their internal and external environments "acted as inputs through the senses to the nervous system" (Roy, 2009, p. 41), as they spoke of the physical changes that occurred in their bodies by way of the physiologic mode. In questioning the cause of their infants' deaths, they spoke about feelings of guilt, which relate to the moral–ethical part of the self-concept mode. As evident by their desire for connectedness to and their want for a real relationship with their lost babies, these grieving women talked about the stillborns as real, live infants, and of their need to give meaning to their loss by treating their lost infants the same as one of their living children. They placed mementos of the birth and photographs of their stillborn infants around the house, and celebrated their infants' birthdays. They also described the agonizing loss of the maternal role and how difficult it was for them to see another pregnant woman or one with a real, live infant. Likewise, as with Martin's (2003) finding, adapting to the loss of a stillborn infant was a complex phenomenon; one that occurred over time. With the exception of only one woman who was unable to conceive again, all of the other women in Short's study were able to give birth to a live infant after the death of their stillborn. Although they celebrated the birth of this new child, as well as the gift of being able to deliver a viable, live infant, these women never forgot the child they lost.

In another sample of five individuals, Watson (2006) researched the loss of a loved one to a violent, sudden death. Although the interval of the participants' losses ranged from 1 year and 7 months to 36 years, regardless of the time frame, the traumatic nature of their loved ones' deaths left a lasting impact and remained as long-term stimuli for these survivors. A common theme that came forth in Watson's study was the intense need of these individuals to find some kind of meaning in their loss. Watson recorded that all five of the participants in her study spoke about one or more events that occurred around the time of their loved one's death that held personal meaning for them. One woman whose brother was murdered said, "God makes you go through this because somewhere down the line, I'm gonna have to help somebody with a similar loss." Another participant whose sibling was killed by a drunk driver joined Mothers' Against Drunk Drivers (MADD). Although those who were able to find meaning in their loss seemed to have less difficulty overcoming the traumatic event, still, the sudden, violent nature of the deaths was very hard to overcome.

In Watson's (2006) study, two of the five participants had to resort to professional counseling, another two persons continued to struggle with their loss, and only one participant felt that she had resolved her loss. For this last individual, her mother's death by suicide ended a lifelong struggle with mental illness and she felt relief at her passing. As with the mothers who lost stillborn infants (Short, 2004), the survivors in Watson's research felt a need to feel their lost loved ones' "presence." They too wanted to know that they were doing alright in their new life form. As with the other loss studies, interactions with other persons in their lives and connectedness to other individuals influenced how these survivors adapted to losing a loved one through violent death.

These grieving individuals became angry when insensitive remarks were made, and they were hurt when others minimized, ignored, or seemed to place little value on the worth of the individual whom they had lost. One woman said that she was told, "Well, you need to forgive" (the man who murdered her brother). Another was told, "There's a reason for his death." In response to this latter remark, she replied, "That really made me angry because I couldn't see a reason for it." Unlike the support that the women of stillborn infants felt that they received from their health care professionals (Short, 2004), those who were bereaved by violent deaths mentioned the lack of support that they received from hospital and law enforcement personnel. Similar to Short's finding, even though the traumatic death of a loved one ranged from 1 year and 7 months ago to over 36 years, this group of participants noted that the sudden, unplanned nature of the losses remained with them as a long-term context. Still, in spite of the violent nature of the deaths that they experienced, these grieving survivors affirmed the "human need for meaning and purpose" (Roy, 2009, p. 28).

Difficulty in coping with loss was a common theme that also emerged in Smith's (2001) study on spousal grief in working men who were employed in a factory in one of the Midwestern states. In exploring spousal loss from this perspective, Smith found that the participants' grief was profound and lasting. One man replied, "It just felt like somebody cut your heart in half." Another said, "People tell me well you'll get over this. I haven't yet. When she died she took me with her." And so, unable to "promote the integrity of the human system" (Roy, 2009, p. 39), a focal stimulus of overwhelming grief resulted in compromised adaptation for the five widowers who took part in Smith's research. In describing the time after their wives' deaths, they sought refuge from grief by working overtime, drinking excessively, and increasing their smoking. One man had a 55-pound weight loss and another had a significant increase in his blood pressure. Instead of seeking counseling, they tended to hide their feelings and none sought professional counseling. To calm his nerves, one person sought medication from his physician and only one stayed connected to his church group. As evidenced by their behavioral responses and their perceptions of their situations, Smith described the difficult period that followed these men's losses as one of compromised adaptation. According to Roy (2009), this is defined as a time in which adaptive responses are not integrated and "when both integrated and compensatory processes are inadequate" (p. 37); one that leads to an adaptation problem.

As with the bereaved in Watson's (2006) study, working men who had lost their wives were ambivalent about receiving support and they perceived support in a more negative way. Although they felt that their families were being supportive in helping them care for their children, they perceived that they were overlooked and that less support was offered to them. Yet, in spite of the magnitude of their losses, with the main function of the role mode the need of individuals to maintain social integrity or "to know who one is in relation so that one can act" (Roy, 2009, p. 44), with the exception of the one man who had just lost his wife 7 months ago, all had remarried, and of the four participants, two had additional children with their new spouses. Although they spoke about the severity of, and about the long-term effects that resulted from their losses, these men attempted to resume their previous role of being a married man. In light of Smith's finding of compromised adaptation in working men who suffered spousal loss, and the long-term context of violent death as emerged in Watson's (2006) study, how do individuals adapt to the ultimate, total loss of one's own life through death?

Three end-of-life studies that were conducted with dying persons addressed the above question. Gandy (2003) recognized five themes emerging from the question that she asked in her study: What are the experiences that you've encountered since you were told that you have a terminal illness? The two participants (a male and a female, ages 74 and 91, respectively) in Gandy's study related their "lived experience" of being in hospice care. The one elderly woman was connected with family members who lived in the eastern part of the United States and, with the exception of neighbors, a few friends, and hospice supports, she was basically alone. For this participant, her biggest fears were loss of independence and loneliness. Nonetheless, in spite of these fears, she said, "It is not that I am afraid to die. I look forward to seeing my family and husband on the other side." The younger male participant, with the exception of a daughter and niece who both lived out of state, also had few family connections. Although his main source of support was a hospice nurse, he expressed the strength that came from his being connected to nature. Gandy (2003) linked the themes that came forth in her study to three of the RAM's adaptive modes: overwhelming loneliness to the interdependence mode, being homebound to physical decline to the physiologic mode, and their loss of independence to the role mode. Although a theme of showing "strength" was present in both participants, Gandy concluded that, before this concept could be linked to the self-concept mode, it required further clarification. Nevertheless, the importance of the self-concept mode in adapting to death and dying was present in the other two end-of-life studies that were reviewed.

When faced with one's ultimate death, the need of dying persons to find meaning from and to make sense out of their loss was emerged by Dobratz (2002). She described a pattern of dying that was named the becoming-self. In this pattern of dying, 15 individuals reintegrated their self-concept and adapted to the impending loss of their known earthly life. For these dying persons, they used "conscious awareness and choice to create human integration" (Roy, 1997, p. 44) by deliberately repressing negative feelings, sustaining themselves with prayer, focusing on life's meanings, and moving beyond the finite to the eternal. One dying person remarked, "I've got a perfect situation, I consider myself blessed." Another said, "When the time comes, I'm going to a better place." As with Watson's (2006) study, the becoming-self was framed within the philosophic assumptions of the RAM.

Within the philosophic principle of veritivity: "a common purposefulness of human existence" (Roy, 2009, p. 28), the becoming-self created meaning and purpose from the earthly stay. Within the philosophic principle of humanism: "the individual and subjective dimensions of the human experience as central to knowing and valuing" (Roy, p. 28), dying individuals in this pattern aimed toward integrity and they valued relationship with others. By accepting the end of one's earthly existence, they embraced "final reunion with God the creator" (Roy, 1988, p. 30) as they "reached beyond the boundaries of human existence" (Dobratz, 2002, p. 139).

The final study on end-of-life loss was a secondary analysis by Dobratz (2004) in which she explored the responses of 44 dying person who referenced spirituality. A core theme of believing emerged as the central theme of this study. Through their spirituality, dying individuals found comfort, released earthly concerns, created meanings, and reached toward the eternal. As with the becoming-self (Dobratz, 2002), these dying persons also described psychic and spiritual integrity, which is a part of the self-concept mode's "need to know who one is so that one can be or exist with a sense of unity, meaning, and purposefulness in the universe" (Roy, 2009, p. 88). This latter study also affirmed the RAM's philosophic assumptions with the core theme of believing connected to "human meaning in an omega point convergence of the universe" (Roy & Andrews, 1999, p. 35). In spite of the overwhelming physical impact of terminal illness, these hospice participants spoke openly about the importance of their spiritual beliefs and values when faced with end-of-life situations. The common concepts and themes that emerged in the eight studies just described are now brought together to build an MRT on adapting to loss.

Concepts and Themes to Synthesize Pictorial Schema of MRT—Steps 3 and 4

In synthesizing a MRT of adapting to loss, common themes were extracted from the findings. The themes provided the approach to identify categories at the middle range and to relate concepts, steps 3 and 4 of the process, for synthesizing MRTs used in this project. Roy (2009) defined the focal stimulus as "the internal or external stimulus most confronting the individual" (pg. 26). For the participants in these studies the immense work that was required of the cognator and regulator to process the suffering, pain, loneliness, and emptiness that resulted from the deaths of significant others was far deeper than any of the bereaved survivors expected (Martin, 2003; Short, 2004; Smith, 2001; Watson, 2006). The focal stimulus of losing a spouse, stillborn infant, or a loved one to sudden death, was said to be a profound emotional experience. Table 9.1 depicts the concepts and themes that emerged to synthesize an MRT of adapting to loss. Loss is the focal stimulus and its linkage to both the cognator and regulator are shown in the table.

As supported in the selected studies, and as noted in the table, the complex process of adaptation that occurs after a significant loss is related to all four adaptive modes. With contextual stimuli "all other stimuli present in the situation that contribute to the affect of the focal stimulus" (Roy, 2009, p. 26), *social support* and *spirituality* emerged as the two significant concepts that impacted loss (Dobratz, 2002, 2004; Martin, 2003; Robinson, 1995; Short, 2004; Watson, 2006). Along with the support given by others, these bereaved, grief-stricken participants found comfort in being with others and they expressed their need for *connecting to others* who remained in their lives. These others included the spouses of the grieving women who had lost their infants, support groups, family members, faith communities, friends, and professionals. There was also an expressed need to connect to their lost loved ones by visiting the cemetery and by *creating memories* (Robinson, 1995; Short, 2004). The loss of relationship and the void that was left by the death of a significant other is linked to the interdependence mode. Thus, the themes or subconcepts of *remaining connected* and

TABLE 9.1
Concepts for Synthesizing a Middle Range Theory of
Adapting to Loss

Stimuli	Coping Processes	Adaptive Outcomes
Focal	Regulator—Subsystem	Physiologic
Loss, a profound	Cognator—Subsystem	Declining health
emotional experience	Self-reintegrating	Self-concept
Contextual	to loss (resolving/	Finding/constructing
Social support	resigning to loss,	meaning
Spirituality	overcoming loneliness)	Going forward
Residual	(oscillating, complex	Being strong
Time of enduring	processing from	Finding strength
	grieving to resolving)	Forcing self to go on
		Role
		Relinquishing previous
		roles
		Assuming previous roles
		Interdependence
		Creating memories
		Remaining connected
		Connecting to others/
		Higher Power
		Forming new
		relationships

creating memories are attached to this mode as it is associated with "relational integrity or the feeling of security in nurturing relationships" (Roy, 2009, p. 450).

A diagnosis of terminal illness, or the impending loss of life itself, called on the cognator to actively process this overwhelming information. The desire of dying individuals to make sense of their time on Earth and for *constructing meaning* beyond death was apparent in the end-of-life studies by Dobratz (2002, 2004). Gandy (2003) too noted that the participants in her study displayed "adaptation of the self-concept mode by coming to terms with their life and the dying process through their strengths" (p. 48). Hence, adapting to end- of-life loss involved a "reorganized self-concept, life meaning and goals" (Knight & Emmanuel, 2007, p. 1194). For the participants in these life-ending studies, the participants' responses depicted that they had attained an adaptive state. Those individuals who had lost a loved one through violent death also spoke about their need for *finding meaning* within the brutal nature of their loved one's deaths (Watson, 2006). With the behaviors of the RAM's self-concept mode aligned with an individual's ability to maintain psychic integrity, the themes of *constructing* and *finding meaning*, and *finding strength* support the incredible capacity of humankind to adapt to loss. These emerged themes or sub concepts relate to the self-concept mode as depicted in Table 9.1.

The impact of *spirituality* was another common concept that came forth in the loss studies. Along with social support, this main concept was expressed as being most helpful in overcoming the loss of a spouse (Martin, 2003), a stillborn infant (Short, 2004) and one's own impending death (Dobratz, 2002, 2004). Along with the basic need of the self-concept mode to establish psychic equilibrium, the other requisite of this entity is "the need to exist with a sense of unity" (Roy, 2009, p. 45). As defined in adaptation nursing theory, existing with a sense of unity is considered spiritual integrity. Therefore, the contextual stimuli of spirituality that emerged supported the significance of this concept in adapting to actual or impending loss. Furthermore, as dying individuals disengaged from life, the spiritual dimension assumed an even greater importance as persons dealt with their mounting losses. These losses include all relationships and roles in life, along with the death of the physical-self. Thus, *connecting to a Higher Power* (Dobratz, 2004) and *connecting to others* were concepts that came forth in the studies of individuals who faced the loss of life through terminal illness. In spite of actual or impending loss, participants expressed their need for *being strong* and *going forward* (Martin, 2003), *finding strength* (Gandy, 2003), and *forcing oneself to go on* (Martin). These themes speak to expressed psychic and spiritual unity that is linked to the self-concept mode as shown in Table 9.1.

The passage of time that individuals required to process and resolve their losses by way of the cognator subsystem was another recurrent theme that surfaced in the loss investigations. Martin (2003) ably captured the meaning inherent within this concept when she reported that "grieving takes place in stages and that losses are resolved in time is supported when one considers the persistent recurring nature of the stimuli that must be processed through the cognator" (p. 8). Martin also noted that no assumptions could be made on the temporal limitations of grief, or on the time that an individual needs to emerge from one's loss experience as an adaptive whole. Because the time persons require to adapt to a significant loss remains unknown, it is designated as a residual stimulus. A residual stimulus is "an environmental factor within or outside the human system with affects in the current situation that are unclear" (Roy, 2009, p. 27). Hence, *time of enduring* is depicted in the MRT as a residual stimulus. Whatever the outcome, or whatever the time that it takes for a bereaved person to endure or adapt to a significant loss, there is a sense that some degree of adaptation or reintegration will occur.

An adaptive outcome is the result of the interplay of both coping subsystems: the cognator and regulator. The complex adaptation processes that take place in a loss experience crosses all four adaptive modes.

As noted, Martin (2003) reported that all but one of the surviving spouses suffered physical decline. Thus, *declining health* is a concept that is linked to the physiologic mode in the MRT model on adapting to loss. Gandy (2003) found that the effects of terminal illness on physical loss or declining health impacted not only the physiologic, but also the role of interdependence, and possibly the self-concept modes. The cross-modal impact of the loss studies was evident.

The responses of grieving individuals described links to the independence mode as found in the theme or subconcept of *connecting to others*. Also, as related to the interdependence mode, working-class men in Smith's (2001) study spoke about marrying again and of *forming new relationships*. In terms of the role mode, these same men talked about *assuming previous roles* of fathering additional children. All but one of the women who had lost stillborn infants conceived again, subsequently giving birth to live infants, and assumed a previously anticipated role: that of being a new mother again. The relationships of these themes and concepts to both the role and interdependence mode are depicted in Table 9.1.

When the concepts and themes were identified in Table 9.1, it was possible to synthesize the interrelatedness of the concepts and themes in a schema of the MRT of adapting to loss. This depiction is shown in Figure 9.1. In this format the major ideas derived from the selected studies provide an insightful picture of the process called "adapting to loss." As the findings from these eight studies show, grief and loss is a very complex phenomenon that cross all four adaptive modes, one that takes place over time, and one that moves in a back and forth, oscillating motion. Moreover, grief and loss are grounded in the philosophic assumptions that humans are purposeful and find meaning and value even when faced with the profound, emotional experience of loss.

Propositions—Step 5

On the basis of the above findings, the following propositions can be derived regarding adapting to loss. Because of their ability to be applied in a variety of practice settings across a wide spectrum of patient populations, these propositions have broad translation. Table 9.2 shows the propositions that were developed from the studies on adapting to loss. The propositions are sentences stating the relationships identified in steps 3 and 4, that is, the concepts, themes, and their pictorial schema. An important part of an MRT is the statement of the propositions.

Proposition 1 states simply that adapting to loss is a profound experience and this focal stimulus impacts both coping processes: cognator and regulator. This statement has been a key observation

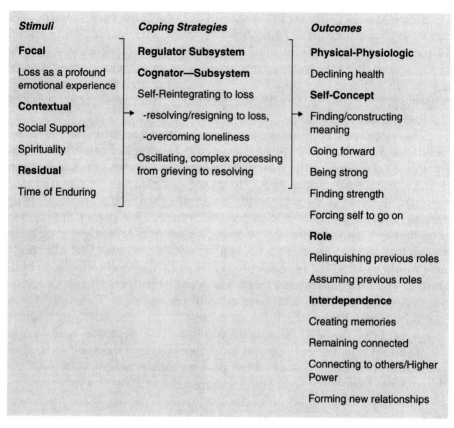

FIGURE 9.1   Middle Range Theory of Adapting to Loss

TABLE 9.2
Propositions for Middle Range Theory of Adapting to Loss

1. Adapting to loss is a profound experience and this focal stimulus impacts both coping processes: cognator and regulator
2. Adapting to loss is purposeful and the responses of bereaved individuals cross all four adaptive modes
3. Adapting to loss is influenced by the contextual stimuli of social support and spirituality
4. Enduring through loss, or the time that is required to adapt to loss, is unknown and remains a residual stimulus
5. Adapting to loss involves connecting to others and a Higher Power, going on or moving forward, and finding meaning in the loss
6. Adapting to loss takes place in stages in a back-and-forth motion, oscillating from grieving to resolving
7. Reintegrating one's self involves relinquishing old roles, learning new roles, and forming new relationships

throughout describing the selected studies and going through the process of identifying and relating concepts from the studies on loss. Proposition 2 notes that adapting to loss is purposeful and the responses of bereaved individuals cross all four adaptive modes. This summarized statement was identified across the selected studies. Proposition 3 is a specific synthesis of the findings of these studies and states that adapting to loss is influenced by the contextual stimuli of social support and spirituality. Proposition 4 summarizes that enduring loss, or the time that is required to adapt to loss, is unknown and remains a residual stimulus. This is an important proposition to include in any theory of loss and more and more evidence mounts about this important factor in adapting to loss. Proposition 5 makes the statement that adapting to loss involves connecting to others and a Higher Power, going on or moving forward, and finding meaning in the loss. In the set of studies based on the RAM, this was a strong finding, perhaps related to the philosophical assumptions of the model.

Proposition 6 notes that adapting to loss takes place in stages in a back-and-forth motion or oscillating movement from grieving to resolving. This proposition is a corollary to proposition 4. Just as we do not know the time it takes to adapt to loss, we do not always know the shape of adaptation; we only know from the studies that it does not take place in one continuous direction or slope. Those dealing with people who suffer loss can expect the oscillating motion of adapting. Proposition 7 states that reintegrating one's self involves relinquishing old roles, learning new roles, and forming new relationships. This statement is derived from the studies and makes logical sense in understanding role development and role taking, as described by Roy (2009).

Evidence—Step 6

Debates about the contributions of different kinds of evidence have resulted in positions that are less rigid than those held previously. Polit and Beck (2012) provide a pyramid of the levels of evidence regarding the effectiveness of an intervention that goes from the base of level VII of opinions of authorities and expert committees to level I of systematic review of randomized clinical trials. Still, the authors noted that the evidence hierarchy is not universally appropriate. For many important questions the hierarchy is not relevant. The authors give the example of the question: What is the experience of pain like for patients with cancer? Hearing from patients is likely the most relevant evidence. For the knowledge developed in this chapter, a broad view of evidence rather than a hierarchical one is highly relevant.

In dealing with the profound human experience of adapting to loss, it is not surprising that 9 of the 10 studies selected for this review used qualitative methods. Four studies were designed according to a form of phenomenology, those by Martin, Smith, Short, and Watson. One author of two studies used grounded theory, both studies by Dobratz, and Gandy's used content analysis. Only one author, Robinson, used a quantitative design for a descriptive correlational study. Differing philosophical perspectives are behind beliefs about the usefulness of different kinds of evidence. In the postmodern era nurses, among other scholars, emphasize the inherent complexity of people and their experience particularly in situations of health. People can shape reality by interpreting their experience. The appropriate methods used for nurses to learn about these experiences are qualitative research methods based on the interpretive traditions.

The description of the 10 selected studies provided rich data for deriving key concepts. The further discussion showed coherent themes from the studies. Finally, a promising MRT with clear propositions of both depth and breadth were derived from the studies. This process in itself has provided evidence for the theory.

TRANSLATIONS FOR PRACTICE AND POLICY

In exploring loss, these studies point to professionals' need for sensitive interactions with bereaved individuals. This may lead to changes in practice and in health policy. As described by these participants, they became angry when other individuals minimized the overwhelming magnitude of their loss (Short, 2004), focused on other family members (Smith, 2001), or avoided addressing their loss (Watson, 2006). Watson reported on the isolation that survivors felt following the sudden, violent deaths of their loved ones. In the "empty spaces" that were left by the loss of beloved spouses, anticipated infants, and of facing one's own death, these eight studies identified a common theme of bereaved individuals' needing to talk about their life-changing event.

Recommendation for Practice

The literature supports these observations and a recommendation for *consistent awareness and sensitive response in all areas of nursing practice to the needs of those suffering loss, both male and female.* As noted by one author, "death in most instances is perceived by those who grieve as a shattering experience" (Beder, 2005, p. 256). The responses of the participants in these studies poignantly verified this perception. One study brought to light the need for emotional social support by husbands who suffered the death of a wife. Together the findings of the studies confirmed the need for the varied participants to have someone to talk to, or for someone to listen to them. As described by Morse (2001), a suffering or bereaved person "will talk to whomever will listen, repeating the story of the loss over and over" (p. 51). The participants in this study spoke about their frustrations when others didn't want to hear their tale of grief, avoided this painful topic, or turned the other way. Beder (2005) noted that a significant loss "harkens back to our own most primitive need for attachment and love" (p. 257). At such times, when family and friends are unable to fill this void, then professionals may be the only ones to whom suffering, bereaved individuals can turn. Given that declining health is an outcome feature of the derived MRT of loss, nurses will meet those who have suffered loss in all areas of nursing practice.

Kim (2009) noted that professionals should act as couriers along a bereaved person's journey and stated that "support from others had to guide the bereaved, so as to make some sense of and or find benefit in the death" (p. 42). Although grief-stricken individuals search for their own meanings, Holtslander, Bally, and Steeves (2011) found that the greatest fear of bereaved spouses was that of "losing balance." During the difficult period that follows the loss, professionals should gently guide and support bereaved individuals, listen to their grief stories, and help them maintain a sense of balance or equilibrium.

The findings of the studies that were used to generate this MRT confirmed that bereaved individuals swung back and forth between responses that suppressed their feelings (*forcing themselves to go on*) and expressed emotions, such as anger, frustration, and other adaptive responses. Morse (2001) described an emotional state of *enduring* as a response to a threat to one's self-integrity that helps suffering individuals function in their day-to-day activities. This response state also allows suffering individuals to function in the present rather than deal with the past or future. Holtslander et al. (2011) described that bereaved caregivers whose spouses died from cancer, walked a "fine line" between deep grieving and moving forward. Thus, adaptive responses of suppression and expression are part of a bereaved person's journey as he or she attempts to move forward toward an adaptive outcome of resolution and reintegration. Through emotional suffering an individual ultimately becomes aware of the magnitude of one's loss, makes some sense out of and meaning from one's loss, and comes to the realization that life as previously lived is forever changed. Yang, Staps, and Hijmans (2010) stressed the important point that during interactions with grieving individuals, health care professionals should not assume their usual professional stance, but that they should interact with bereaved persons as a fellow human being; one who senses their pain and suffering and one who acknowledges their grief.

Exemplar for Policy Change in Practice

Although the importance of communication with professionals and others is supported, little is known about the time that a suffering, grieving individual needs to adapt to loss, or how long it takes for a person to pass through emotional suffering and reintegrate one's self into a new life without their loved one being present. The major policy change that comes from this understanding is to look differently at hospice care and all contact by nurses with those suffering loss. The exemplar for policy change in a practice setting is: *That the nursing diagnosis of grief or any form of dealing with loss be given a reimbursement code that does not place a limit on the length of a given visit or of the time frame for visits for those suffering loss.*

Yang et al. (2010) pointed out that individuals have to proceed through their difficulties within their own time frame and at their own speed. Thus, it is most important that professionals allow grieving individuals the time that they want to move at their own pace and not give advice as to where they should be at any particular point in time in resolving their loss. The participants in Short's (2004) study noted their frustration with others who expected that their loss should be resolved, and with those who had set their own time frame, not the grieving person's one. As described in these studies, professionals should also be aware of those individuals who are most vulnerable to loss: those who lose a loved one through violent death; those who are unable to express feelings about their loss (working men); those who are unable to seek counseling, support, or reach out to others; and those who are unable to assume a previous role, such as the woman who was unable to conceive again. The payment policies need to support the nursing vigilance for a very basic health need for a large percentage of the population.

In addition to implementing change based on our current level of knowledge, nursing scholars and those in practice will continue to develop knowledge and to find new ways to apply knowledge related to adapting to loss. As these studies showed, social support was a crucial stimulus that helped bereaved individuals navigate through difficult periods of rapidly oscillating and changing feelings, and ending their loss journey as an intact, reintegrated person. Although much remains to be known regarding the type of social support that is most effective following a loss, the bereaved mothers who lost stillborn infants reached out to their spouses and they felt that they were supported by a group of women who had experienced a similar loss. With the exception of the working men, bereaved spouses connected with family members and maintained their church affiliations. Beder (2005) noted the need of bereaved individuals to feel that they still remain connected to their loved ones. Thus, frequent trips were made to the cemetery so that grieving persons could still feel connected to their loved ones. Although much still needs to be known about the impact of social support on the self-reintegration process, it is known that the processing of emotions, feelings, and fears that takes place through the cognator subsystem occurs over time and that it is impacted by supportive others.

The process of how one disengages from a loss and reintegrates a new self-concept is, for the most part, unknown. In adjusting to end-of-life loss, Knight and Emanuel (2007) described a conceptual framework for reintegration that included three stages: (1) comprehension, that is, actively processing information and coming to the final realization that death is imminent; (2) creative adaptation, or the disengaging from life's losses, reflecting and adapting to the situation; and (3) reintegration, understanding oneself in a new way (p. 1191). Knight and Emanuel's reintegration model crosses four domains: physical, psychological, social, and spiritual, which overlap with the RAM's four adaptive modes. Although this framework was validated with end-of-life populations, it could be that this same process occurs in other loss resolution. Nevertheless, the studies that were reviewed for this MRT supported the impact of loss across all four of the adaptive modes. Therefore, professionals must be aware of ineffective responses as supported by declining health and weight loss and excessive drinking and smoking and assess components of the physiologic adaptive mode, as well as the effect on the psychosocial–spiritual components.

Although much still remains to be known about the interventions needed to support dying persons' existential and spiritual concerns, when faced with the loss of lives, the participants in Dobratz's (2002, 2004) studies expressed their need for a loving relationship with God and with significant others who were close to them. Murata (2003) noted that spiritual care for dying individuals is concerned with helping them recover a future beyond death, assisting them to look forward to seeing others beyond death, and providing them the opportunities to believe in the value of their autonomy. As autonomous beings, dying persons are given "freedom of self-determination and self-control in all dimensions of perceiving/thinking/speaking/doing" (Murata, p. 20). The dimensions that professionals can help dying persons adapt to are linked to the cognator's four cognitive–emotive channels: "perceptual and information processing, learning, judgment and emotion" (Roy, 2009, p. 41). Hence, at all times, dying persons must be approached as thinking, feeling, and emotional beings who are capable of making their own decisions. To fully support a dying person's autonomy, Murata noted that spiritual care involves the person being in relationship with others, and these others include health care professionals. At the same time, to be involved fully in spiritual care, health care professionals should understand the meaning of this complex concept.

In their concept analysis of spirituality, Sessanna, Finnell, and Jezewski (2007), identified four main themes: (1) spirituality as religious systems of beliefs and values; (2) spirituality as life meaning, purpose, and connection with others; (3) spirituality as nonreligious systems of beliefs and values; and (4) spirituality as metaphysical or transcendental phenomena (p. 252). Those who faced terminal illness and who approached death in these eight selected studies supported the fit of spirituality within these four themes. The man in hospice care in Gandy's (2003) study was connected with nature (a nonreligious value). Dying persons in Dobratz's (2002, 2004) research also spoke of religious beliefs and values, life meaning and purpose, and transcendence toward the eternal. Further analysis of the participants' spiritual responses in life-closing situations confirmed these four themes (Dobratz, 2013). The importance of spirituality as a contextual stimulus was also described by the participants in the other studies. They spoke of their need to find meaning, purpose, and connect with others, as well as the importance of their religious activities and belief systems. Nevertheless, not only with the dying, but also with the bereaved individuals who are left behind to grieve, it is important that health care professionals ascertain the beliefs, values, and spiritual meanings for individuals. Yang et al. (2010) reported on professionals' need to acknowledge what patients are going through and to be "knowledgeable about existential crisis" (p. 67). Clearly, the losses described by the participants in these eight reviewed studies point to the fact that loss is a profound experience that impacts the moral–ethical–spiritual self of the self-concept mode.

Furthermore, the individuals in these studies who did not receive the social or professional support that they needed and who were unable to draw on spiritual resources may be prone to long-term chronic sorrow or pathological grief. Parents who lacked social support and who did not receive intervention were prone to depression (Gordon, 2009). Aging spouses who lost a loved one through hospice care and who did not resolve their losses had higher depressive symptoms and less psychological well-being in the 18 months that followed their loss (Torgas, Stewart, & Nolen-Hoekesma, 2008). In comparison, Davis and Nolen-Hoeksema (1988) reported that bereaved individuals who made sense of their loss reported less distress 1 year after the event. Those in professional roles can help bereaved individuals to explore the meaning of their loss and assist each person to move forward (Martin, 2003). As noted by Henoch and Danielson (2009), the end-point of professional interventions will be a "sense of meaning and peace of mind" (p. 231).

CONCLUSION

To summarize, as professionals the gift of oneself and the offering of one's "presence" to those who experience loss provides comfort and allows the bereaved the time that they need to reintegrate from their loss. With its physical, spiritual, emotional, and social components, the RAM provides a meaningful framework for addressing the needs of those who incur loss. Although each suffering individual has his or her own specific set of stimuli for dealing with loss, to move forward, the person needs to reconstruct a new self-concept, re-create his or her known world into a new reality, and then learn who one is in relation to this new self and world. In the words of Cassell (1983), individuals "continue to suffer until they no longer believe the disruptions to be enduring, come to see the possibility of being whole again, or believe themselves to be total, intact persons, despite the loss of some aspect of themselves or their function" (p. 522). As confirmed by the bereaved and suffering individuals in these studies, in order to adapt they want to share their experience and need the warmth and caring of others before they can become whole again.

With descriptions of physical decline, loss of previous roles, and significant others, a focal stimulus of loss impacted all four modes. This focal stimulus was impacted greatly by contextual stimuli of social support and spirituality, and the time required to adapt to loss remains unknown. One hope is that, a review of these studies and the concepts that came forth to build an MRT of adapting to loss will provide insight and add knowledge as to how professionals can intervene to help bereaved individuals build a new self-concept and re-create a new world.

REFERENCES

Beder, J. (2005). Loss of the assumptive world—how we deal with death and loss. *Omega, 50*(4), 255–265.

Cassell, E. J. (1983). The relief of suffering. *Archives in Internal Medicine, 143,* 522–523.

Davis, C. G., & Nolen-Hoeksema, S. (1988). Making sense of loss and benefiting from the experiences: Two construals of meaning. *Journal of Personality and Social Psychology, 75*(2), 561–574.

Dobratz, M. C. (2002). The pattern of the becoming-self in death and dying. *Nursing Science Quarterly, 15*(2), 137–142.

Dobratz, M. C. (2004). Life closing spirituality and the philosophic assumptions of the Roy adaptation model. *Nursing Science Quarterly, 17*(4), 335–338.

Dobratz, M. C. (2013). "All my saints are within me": Expressions of end-of-life spirituality. *Palliative & Supportive Care, 11*(3), 191–198.

Gandy, L. L. (2003). *Through the voices of the dying.* Reno, NV: University of Nevada. Retrieved from http://proquest.umi.com/pqdweb? index=47&did=766450981&

SrchMode=1&sid=1&Fmt=2&VInst=PROD&VType=PQD&RQT=309&VName=
PQD&TS=1224509768&clientId=7750.

Gordon, J. (2009). An evidence-based approach for supporting parents experiencing chronic sorrow. *Pediatric Nursing, 35*(2), 115–119.

Henoch, I., & Danielson, E. (2009). Existential concerns among patients with cancer and interactions to meet them: An integrative literature review. *Psycho-Oncology, 18,* 225–236.

Holtslander, L. F., Bally, J. M. G., & Steeves, M. L. (2011). Walking a fine line: An exploration of finding balance for older persons bereaved after caregiving for a spouse with advanced cancer. *European Journal of Oncology Nursing, 15,* 254–259.

Kim, S. H. (2009). The influence of finding meaning and worldview of accepting death on anger among bereaved older spouses. *Aging and Mental Health, 13*(1), 38–45.

Knight, S. J., & Emanuel, L. (2007). Processes of adjustment to end-of-life losses: A reintegration model. *Journal of Pallliative Medicine, 10*(5), 1190–1198.

Martin, J. L. (2003). *Spousal grief in older adults: The lived experience of surviving spouses during the second year of bereavement.* Toledo, OH: Medical College of Ohio. Retrieved from http://proquest.umi.com/pqdweb?index=46&did=766679731&SrchMode=1&sid=1&Fmt=6&VInst=PROD&VType=PQD&RQT=309&VName=PQD&TS=1224509768&clientId=7750.

Morse, J. M. (2001). Toward a praxis of suffering. *Advances in Nursing Science, 24*(1), 47–59.

Murata, H. (2003). Spiritual pain and its care in patients with terminal cancer: Construction of a conceptual framework by philosophical approach. *Palliative and Supportive Care, 1,* 15–21.

Polit, D. F., & Beck, C. T. (2012) *Nursing research: Generating and assessing evidence for nursing practice* (9th ed.). Philadelphia, PA: Wolters Kluwer Lippincott Williams & Wilkins.

Robinson, J. H. (1995). Grief responses, coping processes, and social support of widows: Research with Roy's model. *Nursing Science Quarterly, 8*(4), 158–164.

Roy, S. C. (1988). An explication of the philosophical assumptions of the Roy adaptation model. *Nursing Science Quarterly, 1*(1), 26–34.

Roy, S. C. (1997). Future of the Roy model: Challenge to redefine adaptation. *Nursing Science Quarterly, 10*(1), 42–48.

Roy, S. C. (2009). *The Roy adaptation model* (3rd ed.). Upper Saddle River, NJ: Pearson Education.

Roy, S. C., & Andrews, H. A. (1999). *The Roy adaptation model* (2nd ed.). Stamford, CT: Appleton & Lange.

Sessanna, L., Finnell, D., & Jezewski, M. A. (2007). Spirituality in nursing and health-related literature. *Journal of Holistic Nursing, 25*(4), 252–262.

Short, J. K. (2004). *The lived experience of mothers coping with the birth of a stillborn infant.* Toledo, OH: Medical College of Ohio. Retrieved from http://proquest.umi.com/pqdweb?did=766854591&Fmt=6&clientId=7750&RQT=309&VName=PQD.

Smith, W. C., III. (2001). *Spousal grief in working men: A qualitative study.* Toledo, OH: Medical College of Ohio at Toledo. Retrieved from http://proquest.umi.com/pqdweb?index=58&did=727201391&SrchMode=1&sid=1&Fmt=6&VInst=PROD&VType=PQD&RQT=309&VName=PQD&TS=1224508512&clientId=7750.

Torges, C. M., Stewart, A. J., & Nolen-Hoeksma, S. (2008). Regret resolution, aging, and adapting to loss. *Psychology and Aging, 23*(1), 169–180.

Watson, S. A. (2006). *The lived experience of losing a loved one to a sudden traumatic death.* Toledo, OH: Medical College of Ohio. Retrieved from http://proquest.umi.com/pqdweb? did=1428837291&Fmt=6&clientId=7750&RQT=309&VName=PQD.

Yang, W., Staps, T., & Hijmans. E. (2010). Existential crisis and the awareness of dying: The role of meaning and spirituality. *Omega, 61*(1), 53–69.

10

Synthesis of Middle Range Theory of Adapting to Chronic Health Conditions: A Lifelong Process and a Common Journey

ELLEN B. BUCKNER AND SUSAN J. HAYDEN

In considering clusters of studies using the Roy adaptation model (RAM) to provide a basis for a middle range theory (MRT), a clear choice was studies that included persons dealing with chronic health conditions. Among the studies described in this project were those that provide research findings related to this important health challenge. Over 100 million Americans, approximately half of adults, have at least one chronic illness. Chronic illness is the number one cause of death worldwide and by 2020 is expected to account for 73% of all deaths and 60% of the global burden of disease (World Health Organization [WHO], Integrated chronic disease prevention and control, n.d.). Adaptation in chronic illness begins with changes in the stimuli for adaptation. Focal stimuli arise in the physiological domain indicating disequilibrium or disorder. The physiological changes associated with the underlying condition produce both physical and behavioral stimuli. Initial adaptation to emerging chronic conditions may be slow in onset or rapid. If there are warning signs or known risk factors, adaptation may take place in a situation of relative stability with opportunities for recognition, understanding, and choice. The initial adaptive response may include prevention or general health-promotion actions. In particular, initial recognition and adaptation can take place without the sense of fear or overwhelming devastation that may accompany the rapid onset.

Rapid onset of chronic health conditions, by contrast, comes not only with serious acute or life-threatening illness but also presents completely destabilizing experiences crossing all four adaptive modes, that is, physiologic, self-concept, role function, and interdependence. The sheer ability to comprehend the rapid onset and unexpected chronic condition is limited by the person's internal and external resources. The further ability to adapt across modes likewise demands a comprehensive human response that may be supported by a deliberative nursing care process.

Persons adapting to changes in chronic health conditions require both regulator and cognator coping processes. In adapting to chronic illness, the two types of processes are interrelated as engagement of the cognator results in higher effectiveness of self-management with benefits to overall physiological stability and enhanced adaptation through the regulator processes. Improved stability in the regulator reduces the affect of stimuli, making the condition more amenable to coping and adaptive responses.

Nursing intervention is a deliberate, directed process to facilitate a person's adaptive processing. Nursing is described in the RAM as the science and practice that expands adaptive abilities and enhances person and environment transformation (Roy, 2012). Nursing intervention may function as a coaching or educative process and as a means of building social support networks to include others who have developed coping strategies to the particular chronic health condition. The MRT of adapting in chronic health conditions draws on a body of both descriptive and intervention research from the studies reviewed in Part II. This chapter provides a brief background on chronic health conditions then uses the six-step process for generating MRT described in Chapters 2 and 7. That is, the studies are selected and described and the concepts and their relationships are derived. The MRT generated is depicted and implications for change in practice are recommended.

BACKGROUND

Chronic health conditions are the major contributor to health status. Both the WHO and the Centers for Disease Control (CDC) state that chronic disease is the leading cause of death and disability (CDC, 2012; WHO, n.d). Illnesses such as heart disease, cancer, and stroke, and lifestyle factors such as obesity, lack of exercise, smoking, and alcohol consumption add to the scope of the problem. As noted, over 100 million Americans, approximately one half of adults, have at least one chronic illness and many of these are caused or complicated by lifestyle factors. For example, obesity and the lifestyle factors associated with it are a major health concern. One quarter of those with chronic health conditions report daily activity limitations. Given the prevalence of chronic illness, it is of interest to note that four of the common causes of such conditions are modifiable. These causes are lack of physical activity, poor nutrition, tobacco use, and excessive alcohol consumption (CDC, 2012). According to the WHO, chronic diseases are diseases of prolonged duration and generally slow progression. Chronic diseases are by far the leading cause of mortality in the world, accounting for 63% of deaths. Out of the 36 million people worldwide who died from chronic disease in 2008, most were over age 60 and most deaths occurred in low- and middle-income countries (WHO, n.d.).

Nursing management of chronic illness occurs in numerous settings. Advance practice nurses are making a significant difference in access to care for chronic health conditions and nurse-led clinics provide services while building trust and rapport. "Navigating care" is a term for building communication, continuity, and trust between practitioners and patients that can be used in identifying suitable patients for practice of nurse-led care (Mahomed, St. John, & Patterson, 2012). This approach informs the practice and organization of nurse-led care to enhance patient satisfaction. Clinical nurse specialists function in acute care environments to provide high-quality and cost-effective care to patients with chronic diseases. Clinical nurse specialists have a significant impact on patient and family outcomes (Moore & McQuestion, 2012). The movement for nursing management is present in the United States and is growing around the world, providing a level of care commensurate with client needs for holistic assessment and management. Application of the RAM in chronic health conditions promises to link established grand nursing theory, MRT, and research with interventions to promote adaptive outcomes. The result will be the development of a body of knowledge supporting innovative middle range nursing theory applied in practice in settings uniquely relevant to patient transformations in chronic health conditions (Box 10.1).

BOX 10.1
KEY DESCRIPTIONS RELATED TO CHRONIC
HEALTH CONDITIONS

Chronic diseases—those of prolonged duration and generally slow progression

Slow onset—occurs with warning signs or known risk factors; takes place in a situation of relative stability with opportunities for recognition, understanding and choice, for example, diabetes

Rapid onset—occurs with serious acute or life-threatening illness; presents as a destabilizing experience with a sense of fear or overwhelming devastation, for example, some types of cancer

---

GENERATING MRT FOR ADAPTING TO CHRONIC HEALTH CONDITIONS

The purpose of this chapter is to present a MRT of adapting to chronic health conditions. The significance of MRT for knowledge development in nursing and how research can be used to develop such theory are described in Chapters 2 and 7. Following the six steps of creating a MRT described earlier, we clustered similar observations together and identified major concepts from a selection of studies. Major concepts (categories) of stimuli, adaptation processes, and outcomes emerge in relation to adapting to chronic health conditions. By using this approach, concepts identified within each major category describe adaptation within the MRT.

The specific health conditions may be major metabolic alterations such as diabetes, asthma, multiple sclerosis (MS), or kidney disease. They may be chronic conditions as sequelae to adaptation to a more acute process such as cancer. They may be characterized by or associated with major psychosocial alterations such as depression or attention deficit hyperactivity disorder (ADHD) as a primary or secondary effect of the health condition. All constitute stimuli requiring adaptation.

Adapting in chronic health conditions is *a lifelong process* (Hill, Weinert, & Cudney, 2006). In chronic health conditions there are identifiable stages. Just as human development has critical periods and stages or phases of growth and change, so chronic conditions require adaptation over a longitudinal course with varying degrees of severity of symptoms. Adaptation processing has been defined by Roy (2011) as the patterning of coping behaviors that take in, handle, and respond to stressors and are directed to survival, growth, reproduction, mastery, and transcendence. In chronic conditions, adaptation is a dynamic process across stages of the chronic health condition and may or may not require nursing intervention and treatment approaches. As with many experiences requiring adaptive energy and effort, the investment of the person will vary over time and with experiences. As circumstances change and the dynamic nature of physical adaptation unfolds, there will be times of greater or lesser stimuli. These changes require responses that include developing new and creative strategies for coping. The active engagement of the person will develop, change, and grow over time with all adaptive modes involved in these changing states.

Outcomes of adaptation may vary with the level of severity of the underlying health condition, ability of the human body to stabilize, and time of engagement in the adaptive processing. Outcomes vary over time with goals for adaptation changing with differing stages of health conditions and human responses. The outcomes of adaptation also offer guidance for further reassessment of the need for nursing intervention. Nursing intervention and self-management processes use evaluation to revise and modify treatment and support protocols and procedures. Outcomes of adaptation change across the stage of life and the adaptation responses.

As the MRT of adapting in chronic health conditions is developed below, the reader is asked to recognize that each person and supportive network for that person or group will have unique ways of adapting. The dynamic nature of adaptation, with the perspective of a changing chronic condition, will present varying demands and require varying actions by the person resulting in an individualized way of adapting. The nurse identifies the processes and effectiveness of adaptation with each individual and plans care accordingly. Nursing care may be structured, planned, and demonstrated through evidence. Nursing care is also sensitive, responsive, and creative within the interaction with the individual. These contrasting nursing care approaches—structured and responsive—characterize the nursing process in care of persons with chronic health conditions.

Studies Selected for MRT Development—Step 1

Twenty studies reporting research based on the RAM were chosen for the MRT of adapting in chronic health conditions. In each study what was being reported was a population experiencing long-term adaptation processes to physical or behavioral conditions. For adult adaptation to chronic health conditions (heart failure, diabetes, MS, HIV/AIDS, kidney disease, and cancer) the first-stage response involves stabilization with regulator and cognator mechanisms. Physiological adaptation is mediated by the regulator mechanism but is highly influenced by the cognator. Descriptive studies as well as multivariate designs detail the nature of the illness as a focal stimulus and the influence of the condition across all adaptive modes. Coping strategies and adaptive processing have emerged in response to stimuli. In the descriptive studies there were both qualitative data obtained from interviews and quantitative data obtained through questionnaires. The multivariate studies used multiple instruments, mainly in survey designs. Participants were described as individuals.

Descriptive and Multivariate Studies

Burns (2004) presented foundational work identifying the adaptation of individuals with end-stage renal disease (ESRD). Her work, done with 102 African Americans receiving hemodialysis, describes the pervasive influence of chronic conditions on adaptation. Findings were evident across all four adaptive modes and interaction among modes is clearly seen. Instruments included scales to measure stressors, coping, and adjustment. In Burns's study, participants noted numerous symptoms, or stimuli as factors influencing adaptation in all adaptive modes. In the physical domain, they described fatigue, muscle soreness, physical limitations, and other complaints. Participants also reported their physical appearance had changed, and they were sad, depressed, and/or anxious. Furthermore, participants described additional unpleasant and disturbing effects from the treatment itself (Burns, 2004). Hemodialysis and related therapies were the source of physical stressors in fluid limitations, food limitations, increased painful sticks, physical restrictions, and others. As will be noted later this finding led to the proposition that treatment procedures, though beneficial in overall physical adaptation, represent an additional major stressor in adapting to chronic conditions.

Thomas (2007) looked at adults with heart failure and reported work that centered on the self-concept mode. She specifically investigated the relationship between self-concept and adherence in the conceptual dimensions of self-concept identified by Roy (2009), that is, body image, body sensation, self-ideal, self-consistency, and moral–ethical–spiritual self. She differentiated stimuli as resulting in threat to self that produces anxiety and emotional-centered responses versus as a challenge that results in problem-solving responses. Three researcher-designed instruments were used to measure challenge and threat of lifestyle behaviors in each of the self-concept dimensions. There were significant inverse relationships between threat and adherence and significant positive relationships between challenge and adherence. The author concluded that the more regimens are perceived as a threat to the self-concept and its dimensions the more adaptation is compromised. Conversely, the extent to which requirements are perceived as challenges to be met, the more the adaptation process is enhanced. These findings also supported the role of the cognator as directing compensatory behavior through the self-concept mode and contributing to adaptation. This study exemplified a predictive design with statistically significant relationships.

In studies of living with MS, the Roy-based approach revealed that the meaning of illness described how persons make sense of the illness for themselves (Gagliardi, 2003; Gagliardi, Frederickson, & Shanley, 2002). Qualitative data were obtained using a naturalistic descriptive method. Participants ($n = 18$) were involved in three interviews conducted over a year. Interview questions captured changes in adaptation over time. Major themes for each of the adaptive modes were: "We are not completely the same" (physical), "How I view my future" and "let me tell you about my feelings" (self-concept), "How I see work" (role function), and "Let me tell you about my life" (interdependence). The assessment of adaptive modes was the basis for developing nursing approaches. More interrelation occurred among modes in this area, for example, feelings about sexuality described both self-concept and interdependence modes. These publications assist in explaining the processes and their interrelationships.

In studies of women's adjustment to diabetes, Willoughby, Kee, and Demi (2000) investigated a variety of psychosocial factors affecting adaptation. Instruments measured coping and adjustment among other variables. Diabetes was the focal stimulus, with the main contextual stimuli including social support and personal resources. Better adjustment, and hence adaptation, was associated with greater social support, more resources, and more effective coping. A stepwise regression linking various psychosocial factors found personal resources account for 43% of variance and social support another 4%. Authors noted in the discussion the importance of adjustment in metabolic control. Thus the physiologic adaptive mode and the regulator processes may also be influenced by adjustment, and adjustment is a function of self-concept, role function, and interdependence modes. Their study was another example of a predictive model.

Henderson, Fogel, and Edwards (2003) reported work with 86 African American women with breast cancer and compared these findings to previous work with Caucasian women. Measures described ways of coping and study participants reported positive reappraisal and seeking social support as the most frequently used strategies for coping and adaptation, with planful problem solving the next most frequent. In a study of self-concept and emotional indicators in children with HIV, a universal tool, human figure drawing, was effective as a screening tool in an orphanage school (Waweru, Reynolds, & Buckner, 2008). The focus on adaptation assessment and support for adaptation processing was a sensitive and feasible strategy for identifying children at risk for mental health problems. Thus continued work demonstrates the descriptive power of the model in unifying adaptive processes and modes.

LeMone (1995) initiated a pilot project using the Roy framework as a means to evaluate the adaptive modes in understanding the human response to diabetes, in particular in the area of sexuality. She incorporated anatomy and physiology, psychosocial, behavioral, and social factors, and developed an interview guide that assessed persons in all adaptive modes. Ten patients participated in the pilot and results indicated the tool was feasible in identifying client concerns in the area of sexuality. Because sexuality related to physical function, self-concept, role function, and interdependence, the tool was found to have relevance to the RAM and MRT.

Adolescents' responses to chronic behavioral conditions were the focus of a qualitative study of perceptions of ADHD (Knipp, 2006). Adolescents

($n = 15$) responded to an instrument specifically eliciting responses in the four adaptive modes. Responses included statements that with medications things were better with family and were not changed with friends. These responses demonstrated adaptation across modes and an integrated adaptive response to treatment adherence. The study again demonstrates richness and the descriptive power of the RAM.

In a study with 375 newly diagnosed cancer patients, Nuamah, Cooley, Fawcett, and McCorkle (1999) generated a structural equation model (SEM) of physical symptoms, affective status, and social/functional support. They found that severity of illness and cancer treatment had the strongest association with adaptive responses. They also found that initial responses were predictive of later responses, establishing a pattern for understanding longitudinal relationships. Likewise, in a study of 102 children with cancer, Yeh (2002) used SEM to relate severity of illness with stage of illness within the framework of the RAM. Their study supported the proposition that environmental stimuli influence biobehavioral responses.

In the authors' works above, specific relationships have been demonstrated through integration of conceptual and research findings. The stimuli for adaptation, adaptive modes, and regulator/cognator processes are included by a range of authors presenting support for a beginning cohesive adaptive MRT of adapting in chronic conditions.

Intervention Studies

Another set of studies has looked at interventions in efforts to determine approaches for nursing action and to demonstrate effectiveness in persons adapting to chronic illness. Several major types of interventions were introduced in the selected studies. Interventions included provision of knowledge resources in different formats, encouraging or providing social support, or participation in an exercise regimen.

Education and social support are integral to adaption across several modes. Intervention studies have chosen to enhance knowledge and social support through mailed information, computer-based instruction, telephone or in-person support groups (Hill et al., 2006; Samarel et al., 1998; Samarel, Tulman, & Fawcett, 2002; Zeigler, Smith, & Fawcett, 2004). The participants in the first study included women in rural areas who had a number of chronic health conditions whereas the last three studies included women with breast cancer. In these studies findings demonstrated relative successes and/or lack of effectiveness. The provision of information—mailed, by phone or in person—enhanced knowledge. Computer-delivered intervention made available to rural women was effective in an experimental group for increasing self-esteem, social support, and empowerment, compared to control group. Some positive changes also occurred in depression, loneliness, self-efficacy, and stress (Hill et al., 2006). The combination of information, emotional support, and social support was effective in community-based support groups in which qualitative data reflected all four adaptive modes of the Roy model, with participants sharing a *common journey* (Zeigler et al., 2004).

Bakan and Akyol (2008) demonstrated an integrated package of theory-guided intervention for use in the chronic condition of heart failure. Participants received information, an exercise program, and social support. The comprehensive, multimodal intervention was effective in increasing adaptation on a number of outcome measures. Participants demonstrated increased quality of life, increased functional capacity, and social support. This study provided evidence to support the role of the nursing intervention to enhance adaptation in multiple domains and stages for development of the action components of the MRT.

One study reported a cancer rehabilitation evaluation system as the intervention (Young-McCaughan et al., 2003). Investigators found positive effects of an intervention implemented through a Roy framework. Measures included an actigraph wrist monitor to measure duration and pattern of sleep, including daytime napping, and a quality-of-life measure for cancer patients. Participants in their study increased exercise tolerance, improved sleep patterns, and reported higher quality of life. In this study the intervention was conceptualized as facilitating adaptation to both the chronic condition and treatments. Improvements crossed all modes, indicating the goal of adaptation was met. The rehabilitation program in particular was interpreted as providing a safe and effective approach for restoring confidence after uncertainty and building normalcy during and after a significant health challenge.

Camp settings have served as places for healing and adaptation processing and provided a place for naturalistic interventions. A program for young teens with asthma combined the novel experience of camp with educational and self-management reinforcement (Buckner et al., 2007). Campers ($n = 34$) participated over 2 years having measurement of physiological function, knowledge, social and general self-efficacy, and asthma responsibility. Findings were that physiological stability was maintained or improved with better medication management in spite of natural triggers. Participants reported a new sense of normalcy as they interacted with age peers who shared a diagnosis and a common journey. In a study of adolescents with cancer who had attended their specialty camp, adaptive responses were noted in a Roy model–based interview guide (Ramini, Brown, & Buckner, 2008). Detailed case studies of five participants showed how they embraced changes associated with the condition and/or treatment and shared the bonds of friendship in the naturalistic setting.

In a school-based study Frame (2003) created a model of preadolescent empowerment as a means of increasing self-worth in preadolescents with ADHD. In her experimental intervention study, adolescents received an after-school empowerment support group curriculum called "Social Skills Training and Responsibilities for Students with ADHD" (STARS). The content covered aspects of ADHD and self-management. The support group concept included children helping children with the school nurse as a facilitator of the group process. Findings were significant for a positive change in self-worth.

The preceding descriptive qualitative and quantitative, multivariate, and interventional studies are an intentional body of nursing research linking theory to practice. Middle range theories can add significantly to these links; the one detailed below was generated from the concepts and relationships of the studies.

Concepts—Steps 2 and 3

The MRT of adapting in chronic conditions is developed as a longitudinal process with stimuli occurring over time, with adaptation processing and outcomes derived from the RAM. Thus the major concepts identified are congruent with the model concepts as noted in Step 2 described in Chapter 7 for the process of generating MRT. In the physiologic mode, the onset of the chronic condition is defined by a change in health status. The progression of that illness is dependent on physical manifestations of the particular illness and whether the initial experience of the condition has a slow or rapid onset.

Regulator mechanisms are at work both as severity changes and as the body responds to physical changes. Assumptions of the RAM include the presence of certain needs. In the self-concept mode, these are psychological and spiritual integrity with a sense of unity, meaning, and purposefulness in the universe (Roy, 2012). Role function is one of the primary motivators for individuals in their adaptation to chronic health conditions. In the social context of family, community, and society, persons take on roles of wife/husband/partner, mother/father, friend, worker, and member, among others. In the interdependence mode, adaptation requires individuals to engage with others in active ways. The others may include family and friends, caregivers, health care providers, and other key persons such as teachers or employers.

Concept 1—Stimuli

Focal Stimuli

Physical changes occur at the onset of a chronic illness. The severity of initial symptoms in chronic illness is the primary or focal stimulus confronting the person adapting to chronic health conditions. Looking at the three types of stimuli makes the concepts discrete and observable at the level of abstraction for an MRT, as noted in Step 3 of the process used. Physical changes adversely impact adaptive levels (Nuamah et al., 1999; Yeh, 2002). In the general MRT of adapting to chronic health conditions, the adaptive levels of integrated, compensatory, and compromised describe decreasing effectiveness and/or decreasing ability for the cognator and regulator processes to produce stability in the physiological processes. With increasing severity of illness, there are increasing changes in physical health and well-being (Nuamah et al., 1999; Yeh, 2002). Symptom control becomes a significant goal and both traditional treatment and alternative or complementary therapies may be sought (Burns, 2004). With intervention, there may be the opportunity for stabilization of the condition and prevention of health consequences. Treatment, either traditional or complementary, may function as a primary adaptive process in both the cognator and regulator subsystems. In this stage of primary adaptive response, treatment is curative and/or mediates the effects of illness. Secondarily, patients report that treatment is also a focal stimulus for the need for further adaptation. In this secondary adaptive response, treatment is a stressor with restrictions, inconveniences, and/or its own stressors of discomfort. Stressors from treatment require the individual to adapt to another set of stimuli. Treatment restrictions become a focal stimulus for another step in adaptation (Burns, 2004).

With the early experiences of manifestation of illness or the stage of diagnosis of the condition, initial cognator processes must process the changing physical status. Behavioral change can occur with treatment for emotional–mental health conditions supporting adaptation in role function of adolescents in school (Knipp, 2006). Perceptions of illness and treatment can be seen as a threat or challenge with differential effects on adaptation (Thomas, 2007). Frame (2003) likewise reported students participating in a STARS support group for adolescents with ADHD initially exhibited impulsivity and disorganization. In these examples an identity and set of behaviors emerged that reflect the self-concept adaptive mode for students in school settings.

Contextual Stimuli

Contextual stimuli are defined in the model as all other stimuli present that can contribute to the affect of the focal stimulus. Coping strategies are developed over time so onset of the chronic illness in youth or adulthood will profoundly influence this contextual stimulus. The meaning of illness is intricately tied to the person's adaptive capacity (Gagliardi, Frederickson, & Shanley, 2002). This in turn may be functionally related to culture, community, and spirituality. This perspective can be captured in a MRT with flexibility to encompass numerous theoretical and practical applications. Social support provides the context of care and development of coping and adaptive processes. Willoughby et al. (2000), working with women with diabetes, described the main contextual stimuli to include social support, and personal resources. Better adjustment, and hence adaptation, was associated with greater social support, more resources, and more effective coping.

Residual Stimuli

Residual stimuli are defined as those factors with uncertain contribution to the affect of the focal stimuli. Residual stimuli may include the patient's developmental stage and other individual factors. In the selected studies the residual stimuli included the influence of time, and the setting for adaptation as both community based (home, work, school) and health related (clinic, hospital, other). Time is essential for adaptation but also reflects periods of vulnerability as time for treatment/intervention implementation can result in frustration. Procedures, discomforts, and worsening illness decrease the sense of competence and confidence over time. Empowerment is challenged and self-efficacy may decline with time. The pivotal role of nursing in shifting the focus toward effective use of time to promote adaptive outcomes is the key to realizing adaptation. Residual stimuli have variable effects depending on the situation and stability of circumstances surrounding the adaptive imperative.

Concept 2—Coping Processes

Individual Adaptive Processes (Intrinsic)

Cognator. The cognator subsystem is engaged in all four cognitive–emotive channels: perceptual and information processing, learning, judgment, and emotion (Roy, 2012). Individuals must perceive changes in physical health, obtain information, and go through information processing. As the need for information grows, persons seek information through established formal and informal channels. Health care provides Internet-based sources for consumer or lay persons such as MEDLINE Plus®, and friends and family all contribute to the person's knowledge base. Information processing is needed for the patient to obtain a general understanding of the illness and its potential effects. The individual responds through learning, judgment, and emotion, acquiring new understandings, and employing judgment, with effects in the underlying emotions.

Planned problem solving. Planned problem solving is another adaptation process of the cognator subsystem. Planned problem solving presupposes a baseline level of physical stability, self-concept, self-management, role function, and social support. With changes in baseline, the individual recognizes a problem is occurring. This signifies the need for new strategies and efforts to make change and adapt in new ways. This recognition often results in health-care-seeking behavior and nurses and other health care providers are consulted. Given the toolkit of the provider, more or fewer tools may be available for planned problem solving. Tools for the next stage of adaptation may include new or higher level medications and/or treatments, reinforcements of current techniques, institution of new approaches or redoubling of efforts in implementation. Changes in reappraisal, self-management, and social support may all be required. An effective adaptation integrates techniques with a new normalcy that supports the integrity of the individual. Planned problem solving was identified as a positive coping strategy in African American women with breast cancer (Henderson et al., 2003).

Regulator. The regulator subsystem involves the neural, chemical, and endocrine systems (Roy, 2009). Through these mechanisms changes in one physical system or area initiate changes in other areas, either adaptive or ineffective related to the physical changes. However, adaptation is not merely a function of severity but also of coping strategies and skills in illness management. A reciprocal relationship exists whereby effective self-management can ameliorate manifestations of illness and coping and adaptation at higher levels can decrease severity level. Increased disease severity demands more active responses in the cognator processes. Regulator mechanisms for illness control may be insufficient as the disease progresses and even the best use of the cognator action may be insufficient. However, the person's adaptation level is responsive independent of the actual severity level of disease, and effective adaptation can produce an integrated response at every level of severity. Additional coping measures and cognator processes may become operative over time as persons adapt in varying ways to the stimuli of the chronic condition. Findings from Nuamah et al. (1999) supported that initial responses predicted later responses.

Self-management. Self-management is the process whereby the individual takes on the responsibility, tasks, and perspective necessary for effective implementation of health care practices. For each chronic illness the self-management implications are different and their interaction with personal lifestyles allows for both variability and flexibility in implementation. Self-management requires information that may come from several sources. The nurse functions as both a provider of health information and an interpreter of that information. In the educational interaction, the nurse works directly with the person to establish goals, select intervention strategies, and encourage implementation of these in the context of his or her life.

Responsibility taking and self-efficacy are sub concepts under the larger concept of self-management. Adaptive processing in chronic conditions incorporates the individual's taking on the responsibility of self-management. The initial stage of self-management is awareness and acceptance of the condition. This is followed by information seeking and information processing to create an awareness of the need for adaptation. In many chronic health conditions there are specific steps one can take to promote adaptation but readiness to take on those activities means the individual must have acquired a sense of responsibility. Self-efficacy is one route to individual responsibility and reflects the capacity to succeed or achieve a level of competence. Self-efficacy was measured in a study of adolescents transitioning to more active responsibility (Buckner et al., 2007). Adolescents also participated in active learning with reinforcement for responsibility taking.

Reappraisal. One MRT concept for adaptive processing is termed "reappraisal" (Henderson et al., 2003). In reappraisal, the individual obtains new information, processes the meaning of this for self and others, applies some level of judgment and decision making, and integrates emotion in to the response. Adaptation at this point may be adaptive or ineffective and nursing intervention may be required to assist the individual to his or her best adaptive response. In the MRT of adaptation to chronic illness being derived, reappraisal occurs repeatedly as changes take place within the more inclusive process.

Spirituality. In several studies, the primary coping strategy identified by participants was related to spirituality, faith, and trust in God (Burns, 2004). This coping strategy gave people hope, strength, and patience. It promoted trust in ways that were not immediately verifiable, supporting adaptation over time.

Additional influences may be noted in establishing self-management, including locus of control, spirituality, and degree of dependence. Degree of dependence occurs again in the discussion of the interdependence adaptive mode. Empowerment and self-efficacy are two measurable concepts in the self-concept mode. Adaptation is built on individual characteristics and activities. Readiness, knowledge, and learning styles all affect the quality and direction of reappraisal. With readiness the person is able to acknowledge the changes, take in manageable quantities of new knowledge, and integrate these with learning styles using judgment and positive emotion. For example, health care parameters of health literacy, maturity, and responsibility all affect reappraisal processing as it develops. Spirituality and faith in God were identified by participants as positive adaptive processes.

Engaging With Others for Adaptation (Extrinsic)

Health care seeking.   In several studies, coping and adaptive processing emerged from the interdependence mode. Health care providers were sought to give information and to provide treatment. Family and friends provided love, respect, and a sense of self-worth and value (LeMone, 1995). Breast cancer support groups provided information and facilitated emotional adaptation (Samarel et al., 1998; Zeigler et al., 2004).

Nursing interventions.   Interventions provided by nurses include assisting the individual to explore his or her purpose as an adapting person; identify resources and social support; and assist in the integration of knowledge, experience, and support to produce an adaptive response (Burns, 2004; LeMone, 1995). Nursing interventions may modify stimuli, facilitate adaptive processing, and influence outcomes.

Seeking social support.   Two major sub processes occur in the MRT. First, persons begin seeking social support. This may have been a consistent process in the person's life or a new one. It may follow familiar paths or forge new ones. Social support may be available from friends or specialized support groups. In the latter, relevant knowledge may be enhanced through sharing of information, perspectives, and common activities. Some level of social support is required in adapting to chronic conditions, however, the amount, type, and consistency of social support, both given and received, varies from person to person. The adaptive effect of social support also varies and the end result is a complex set of interrelationships, not just a presence or absence. Henderson et al. (2003) reported seeking social support as one of the most frequently used strategies for coping and adaptation.

Concept 3—Outcomes

Functional Ability

Functional outcomes are a direct result of adaptation processing and influence adaptation in all modes. In the physiological mode, adaptive responses include stabilization of the basic physiological equilibrium, with corresponding decreases in symptom severity. Increased functional ability may also emerge with improved physical function and modifications in lifestyle, demands, and resources to meet needs and balance one's activities. With integrated adaptation, functional ability can remain high, contributing positively to the new normalcy and consistency of the role over time. With ineffective adaptation, individuals' functional ability deteriorates, role performance declines, and life satisfaction is significantly altered. Therefore, one of the major goals of adaptation is maintenance of role function. Specific role functions that may be altered in adapting to chronic conditions are sexuality, independence, and economic/financial stability (Gagliardi, 2003; Gagliardi, Federickson, & Shanley, 2002; LeMone, 1995; Willoughby et al., 2000).

Normalcy

Normalcy is a key concept in adaptation in the self-concept mode. As adaptation to chronic illness proceeds, the person develops a new normalcy. This new status may be stable or unstable and may again require nursing for assistance in reaching a person's best adaptive response. Through reappraisal using all cognator processes, the new normalcy may be both effective and integrated. Examples of studies with findings of reappraisal and normalcy include that of Henderson et al. (2003), who interviewed African American women with breast cancer and found positive reappraisal was their primary coping mechanisms. In adolescents social support was part of a group experience in a specialty camp and participants asthma valued the opportunity for a sense of normalcy (Buckner et al., 2007). Specialty support groups provide innovations, such as play, identity validation, and support for emerging independence, which assist both with self-management of illness and further development as individuals.

Role Consistency

Role consistency is a stabilization of role function and interdependence as an outcome of adaptation. It is based on all the processes described as well as additional processes of use of information and use of support. Gagliardi, Frederickson, and Shanley (2002) identified statements that showed change in role reflected in the theme of "how I view work."

Empowerment was defined for the study by Frame (2003) as a power within an individual that cannot be controlled by others. The author noted that empowerment leads to the creation of power and the decrease of powerlessness. Findings showed that participants sometimes draw on helping forces such as interventions by the school nurse. Empowerment is a contributor to self-management and taking responsibility. Frame (2003) likewise reported students participating in a STARS support group for adolescents with ADHD experienced a sense of normalcy in the group meetings that helped them realize a personal identity. In these examples an outcome emerged that reflects the self-concept adaptive mode for students in school settings. Nursing intervention was effective in increasing their sense of empowerment (Frame, 2003).

Summary: Stages of Adaptation in Chronic Conditions

From the above discussion it is evident that adaptation occurs in all modes, through both regulator and cognator subsystems, and results in complex interactive processes. These processes converge in integrated adaptation to promote integrity of the individual in the context of family and society. When ineffective adaptation occurs, nursing care is needed and may be directed toward any of the processes of adapting in chronic conditions. The MRT depicted below is an example layout of processes which in reality are highly dynamic with overlapping, regression, and additional connections and pathways. Sequential stages of reappraisal, seeking support, and planned problem solving define progress throughout adapting to chronic health conditions.

Throughout adapting to chronic conditions, the regulator and cognator subsystems function to stabilize physiologic processes, regulate emotion, and promote functional ability. The RAM-based research cited has demonstrated evidence linking the subsystems, modes, and processes. Propositions for the MRT are generated from the concepts and relationships.

Propositions and Evidence—Steps 5 and 6

In constructing an MRT, relational statements or propositions form the basis of the theory as identified in Step 5 of the processes used in this project. The statements that follow list propositions that have their origin in the study observations, findings, inferences, and conclusions. Citing these origins provides the evidence noted in Step 6 of the MRT. Propositions were organized according to the clusters identified in Chapter 2. This MRT is focused on the individual; therefore propositions in group adaptation were not generated. Propositions are depicted in Table 10.1.

Internal Coping Processes—Individual

Proposition 1 states that perceptions change over time and reflect reappraisal/adaptive change resulting in normalcy or a "new normalcy." In two studies of persons with MS, authors noted changing perceptions with adaptation (Gagliardi, 2003; Gagliardi et al., 2002). In a study of

TABLE 10.1
Propositions of MRT of Adapting in Chronic Health Conditions

Internal Coping Processes—Individual

1. Perceptions change over time and reflect reappraisal/adaptation resulting in normalcy or a "new normalcy."
2. Adaptive processes in chronic health conditions include being empowered, embracing changes, seeking social support, problem solving, self-efficacy, and taking responsibility for self-management.
3. Cognator processes include information processing and learning about the chronic condition and may include personal spirituality in support of cognitive–emotional processing.
4. Regulator mechanisms are adaptive when treatments and lifestyle modifications are effective.
5. Self-management as adaptive processing requires both knowledge and application of that knowledge integrated with responsibility to transform the individual.

Adaptive Modes

6. All domains (physiologic, self-concept, role function, and interdependence) are affected in chronic health conditions, and all are integrated in adaptation.
7. Adaptation in chronic health conditions requires individuals to engage with others in the interdependence mode.
8. Greater adaptation is associated with greater social support, more resources, and more effective coping; lower adaptation is related to greater perceived problems.
9. Role function is a primary motivator for adaptation, with integrated adaptation contributing to the outcome of role consistency.

Stimuli—Internal and External

10. The onset of chronic illness and/or symptoms initiates the adaptive response.
11. Level of severity changes over time affecting adaptive processing and outcomes.
12. Treatments represent an additional major stressor in adapting to chronic conditions.
13. The meaning of illness/perception is a stimulus for initiation of adaptive processing and contributes to its character.
14. Threat and adherence are inversely related, whereas challenge and adherence are positively related.
15. Residual stimuli have variable influences on adaptation.

Nursing Process

16. Nursing intervention may function as a primary adaptive process with improved functional ability (stabilization, symptom control) as a major goal or outcome.
17. Nursing interventions of education and social support are integral to adaptation over several modes, building knowledge, self-esteem, and empowerment.
18. Empowerment is evidence of role consistency and self-integration in adaptation to chronic conditions.

coping by African American women with breast cancer, reappraisal was identified as a positive coping strategy (Henderson et al., 2003).

Proposition 2 states that adaptive processes in chronic health conditions include being empowered, embracing changes, problem solving, self-efficacy, taking responsibility for self-management, reappraisal, health care seeking, and seeking social support. Numerous authors in the selected set of studies have identified and described effects of adaptive processing. Frame (2003) described empowering of preadolescents with ADHD as an adaptive process. Ramini et al. (2008) described adolescence using the process of embracing changes to cope with changes from cancer and its treatment. Also, in the study of coping by African American women with breast cancer, seeking social support and planned problem solving were identified as positive coping strategies (Henderson et al., 2003). Buckner et al. (2007) measured changing self-efficacy as a process supporting development of self-management and reports the changing responsibility from parent to the adolescent with asthma.

Propositions 3 and 4 restate the linkages between the cognator and regulator mechanisms in the process of adapting to chronic health conditions. Cognator processes include information processing and learning about chronic conditions and may include personal spirituality in support of cognitive–emotional processing. Regulator mechanisms are adaptive when treatments and lifestyle modifications are effective.

Proposition 5 describes the significance of self-management across categories of concepts. Self-management as adaptive processing requires both knowledge and application of that knowledge integrated with responsibility to transform the individual. In addition, at this stage one uses self-efficacy and resources. Effective self-management can ameliorate effects of illness, supporting adaptation (Buckner et al., 2007; Knipp, 2006).

Adaptive Modes

Propositions 6 through 9 relate individual adaptive modes to outcomes. Proposition 6 states all domains, that is, physiologic, self-concept, role function, and interdependence adaptive modes are affected in chronic health conditions and all are integrated in adaptation. This proposition is reflected in all the studies selected in one or more ways. Nursing intervention programs incorporate a multimodal set of techniques that resulted in adaptation across multiple domains, including nursing interventions supporting discussion of purpose, meaning, and spirituality (Burns, 2004; LeMone, 1995).

Proposition 7 states that adaptation in chronic health conditions requires individuals to engage with others in the interdependence mode. Both descriptive and intervention studies acknowledge the importance of patients health-seeking behaviors, adherence to treatments, and willingness to participate in social support groups (Gallagher, 1998; Samarel et al., 1998; Thomas, 2007; Zeigler et al., 2004).

Proposition 8 states that greater adaptation is associated with greater social support, more resources, and more effective coping. This was supported by findings from women's psychosocial adjustment to diabetes in which personal resources and social support had the strongest association with positive adaptive outcomes (Willoughby et al., 2000). Proposition 8 also states that, in adapting to chronic health conditions, as perceived problems increase, outcomes are less positive. This is based on the finding of Burns (2004) with hemodialysis patients that problems were most associated with adaptation in role function and interdependence modes. Self-esteem was lower when problems were greater. Coping ability was not correlated significantly.

Propositions 9 specifically relates to the adaptive mode of role function. It states that role function is a primary motivator for adaptation with integrated adaptation contributing to the outcome of role consistency. Numerous studies include role function as a significant adaptive mode in the theoretical framework. One study of persons with MS describes specific role-function adaptations (Gagliardi et al., 2002). Adolescents participating in specialty camps described role functions relative to peers, which supported feelings of normalcy (Buckner et al., 2007; Ramini et al., 2008).

Stimuli—Internal and External

Propositions 10 through 15 refer to the stimuli for adaptation. The focal stimulus may be a physical change, the onset of a symptom, or a change in the personal meaning attached to one's health. These stimuli initiate a need to adapt. Proposition 10 states that the onset of chronic illness and/or symptoms initiates the adaptive response. In a study of African American patients with ESRD on hemodialysis, the authors reported participants identified significant problems with fatigue, muscle soreness, and other maladies (Burns, 2004). Coping and adaptive processing were reported in their study using multiple strategies, including trust in God. Proposition 11 states that the level of severity of illness and adaptive processing, which changes over time, affects the adaptive outcome. In one study biobehavioral responses were associated with changes in health-related quality of life (HRQOL), physical function, psychologic function, peer/school function, treatment/disease symptoms, and cognitive function (Yeh, 2002). Similarly, newly diagnosed cancer patients experienced symptom distress, depression, and changes in functional status, resulting in altered HRQOL (Nuamah et al., 1999). The relationship that initial adaptation was related to later responses was also supported (Nuamah et al., 1999). Proposition 11 states that the need to adapt increases as symptoms and distress increase, resulting in increased use of adaptive-processing strategies. For example, in a study by Gallagher (1998) in a sample of older women with urinary incontinence, urogenital distress was highly correlated with psychosocial impact ($r = .67$, $p < .01$) resulting in health seeking. Another investigator using the Roy model found that adaptation had a mediating effect between urinary incontinence and QOL (Toughill, 2001).

Proposition 12 states that treatment or intervention procedures, though beneficial in overall physical adaptation, represent an additional major stressor in adapting to chronic conditions. This comes from the work with hemodialysis patients who reported that the limitations and restrictions of therapy were most bothersome (Burns, 2004). This proposition recognizes the other side of therapy in chronic health conditions as an added stressor and stimulus for adaptation.

Proposition 13 identifies the meaning of illness/perception as both a stimulus and a means of adaptive processing. This was based on studies in adults with MS who were asked through a naturalistic methodology of interviews how they "make sense" of their illness (Gagliardi et al., 2002).

Proposition 14 gives direction for the MRT by framing the type of perception of health as a threat or challenge. It states that threat and adherence are inversely related, whereas challenge and adherence are positively related. These two possibilities relate the type of perceived stimuli to outcomes (Thomas, 2007). Based on the work of Thomas (2007), findings showed that when the changes were perceived as a challenge the person could adapt more positively.

In Proposition 15 we state that residual stimuli have variable influences on adaptation. Residual stimuli, defined as stimuli having undetermined affects, include developmental stage, time, culture, socioeconomic status and level of education or health literacy. These have variable influences on adaptation in different studies and are often uncontrolled variables. In some studies developmental level is a function of inclusion age but developmental level is seldom quantified.

Nursing Process

Propositions 16 through 18 describe relationships involving the nursing process, including interventions. Proposition 16 states that nursing intervention may function as an initial part of the adaptive process with improved functional ability, including stabilization and symptom control, as a major goal or outcome. In a study of HRQOL in patients with cancer, researchers found that severity of illness had the strongest association with biobehavioral responses (Nuamah et al., 1999). The need for symptom control was expressed by hemodialysis patients (Burns, 2004). Another example was the finding from qualitative findings from adolescents who described the effects of treatments for ADHD as "Medications are a hassle, but they work" (Knipp, 2006).

Proposition 17 states that nursing interventions of education and social support are integral to adaptation over several modes, acting through enhanced knowledge and self-esteem as mediators. One study demonstrated an integrated package of theory-guided interventions for use in the chronic condition of heart failure (Bakan & Akyol, 2008). Participants received information, a physical assessment tool, exercise program, and social support. Comprehensive, multimodal interventions were effective in increasing adaptation on a number of outcome measures in multiple studies (Hill et al., 2006; Young-McCaughan et al., 2003).

Proposition 18 states that empowerment is evidence of role consistency and self-integration in adaptation to chronic conditions. This is based on the work of Frame (2003), who demonstrated that nursing intervention in the form of a goal-oriented curriculum increased self-worth in preadolescents with ADHD.

In summary, propositions were generated for adaptation in chronic health conditions in areas of internal coping processes, stimuli, adaptive modes, nursing intervention, and outcomes. Findings from RAM-based research were used in the development of these propositions. Continued work is needed to confirm and further develop the structure.

Schema of MRT Derived From Statements—Step 5

The schematic of the MRT of adapting in chronic health conditions (Figure 10.1) details, Step 5 in the approach to generating MRT used in this project. The process begins with stimuli that require adaptation. Focal stimuli include the initial change, physical or behavioral, which identify an alteration in health status. The change may occur in slow or rapid onset. If slow, there may be opportunity to reduce risk or intervene to prevent onset. If rapid, a destabilization occurs in the health condition that contributes substantially to the initial perception of the chronic health condition. As the individual recognizes symptoms and links this to an understanding of the chronic illness, the individual begins adaptive processing. Focal stimuli also include the perception of the change in terms of its degree of threat or challenge. These perceptions set the tone for adaptive processing and have been linked to outcomes (Thomas, 2007). Finally, the effects of treatment, though potentially beneficial, are themselves focal stimuli as they may create additional unpleasant affects or limitations (Burns, 2004).

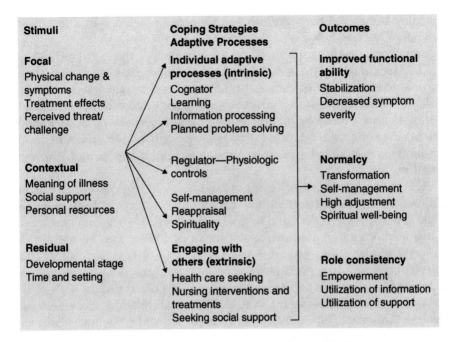

FIGURE 10.1 MRT of Adapting to Chronic Health Conditions

Contextual stimuli include the meaning of illness or the individual's ability to make sense of the condition and its changes (Gagliardi, 2003; Gagliardi et al., 2002). The context is governed by the presence and effectiveness of social support. Because chronic illness is a life-altering process, the availability of social support is paramount to adaptation. Social support contributes to meaning and can buffer the meaning of illness when compared to personal characteristics. Personal resources have been found to influence outcome in adults with diabetes (Willoughby et al., 2000).

Residual stimuli that have been demonstrated as having a variable affect are developmental stage (child, adolescent, adult, elder) and other factors (time, setting, culture, etc.). Differing manifestations of coping have been described in studies of children with HIV, adolescents with ADHD, and adults with MS (Gagliardi et al., 2002, Knipp, 2006; Waweru et al., 2008).

Coping and adapting processes are the instrumental forces that produce adaptation. In chronic health conditions, adaptive processes engage both cognator and regulator subsystems. The cognator is involved when information is processed and learning occurs. Information processing is required as the individual acquires knowledge about the chronic health condition and begins to apply this knowledge to experiences of illness.

Learning occurs as the person integrates new knowledge and treatments into his or her lifestyle.

In chronic health conditions the significance of the regulator subsystem is particularly important. Many chronic conditions, such as diabetes, are characterized by deficiencies in substances that regulate metabolism and functional abilities. Initial treatment targets these deficiencies, with corresponding outcomes of improved physiologic balance and function. The positive effects of adapting processes not only results in better coping but actually can result in better physiologic stabilization and improved function.

Self-management is a key concept linking several processes that are integral to forming adaptive relationships among concepts. Self-management is the ability for the individual to take responsibility for health care needs. It has been included within the construct of illness management along with self-efficacy and resource use (Weinert, Cudney, & Spring, 2008). Self-management functions both as an adaptive process and an outcome in the MRT. As an adaptive process it is the set of actions in both cognator and regulator subsystems that facilitate stabilization and integration into the person's lifestyle. Self-management is used to denote positive or adaptive processes, with effective self-management denoting a successful process. For the individual adapting to a chronic condition, the very establishment of a self-management plan or protocol is an effective outcome. It includes recognition of a change, assimilation of knowledge, and modification of lifestyle to incorporate activities essential to stabilization. The reappraisal process contributes to a new personal awareness that may include spirituality.

Additional adaptive processes require engaging beyond oneself and these can be facilitated by nursing intervention. Health care seeking in chronic health conditions usually results in a treatment plan and initiates a relationship with health care providers for planned problem solving. Seeking social support extends beyond the contextual stimulus by allowing the person to connect with others who have experienced the chronic illness. Support groups are a manifestation of the need for specialized social support networking (Samarel et al., 1998). Interventions provided by nurses include assisting the individual to explore his or her purpose as an adapting person; identify resources and social support; and assist in the integration of knowledge, experience, and support to produce an adaptive response.

Finally, adaptive outcomes cross all adaptive modes. In the physiologic mode an adaptive response is stabilization of the chronic condition with decreased symptom severity and increased functional ability. In the self-concept mode, a new sense of normalcy emerges. This includes the person experiencing transformation, managing his or her illness, and expressing a relatively high overall adjustment, often with a sense of spiritual well-being. In the role function and interdependence modes, the individual has added new roles characterized by information use and support use. Their new normalcy supports new ways of relating to others, with empowerment and personal role consistency as an outcome. These outcomes do not happen by chance but are an integrated, holistic response by the individual within one's own context.

TRANSLATIONS FOR PRACTICE AND POLICY

The MRT of adapting to chronic health conditions gives direction for development in practice and policy. Exemplars in practice and policy are derived from the new knowledge and described below.

Recommendations for Practice

Opportunities for practice parallel the stages of longitudinal progression of the chronic health condition. For example, in the initial stages of diabetes, there are physical changes associated with loss of glucose control. Symptoms may be subtle (thirst) or severe (coma). The nurse facilitates stabilization through both the regulator and cognator subsystems. In the regulator, medications fulfill deficits of insulin production in diabetes, restoring blood glucose to ranges needed for physiologic stability. The newly diagnosed person with diabetes requires information to develop self-management skills, such as blood-glucose monitoring and the ability to recognize and intervene in hypo- or hyperglycemia. This information must be incorporated through information processing as an adaptive process in the cognator subsystem. The individual's developing judgment adapts to the requirements of chronic health conditions. Adaptive processes in self-concept, role function, and interdependence modulate ongoing change. As the individual with diabetes realizes the new health status, he or she must go through a process of reappraisal to generate a new normalcy that incorporates treatments and lifestyle changes. The degree to which the outcome is achieved is the adaptation level. As severity of illness progresses over a lifetime, the person with diabetes may function in general or specialty settings with age-specific or health-specific peers. At each dynamic change, adaptive processes are needed to encourage growth, strengthen a social support network, and use knowledge to promote self-care, integrity, and unity.

One specific application to practice can be derived from the qualitative study of patients with MS in which themes emerged from participant quotes. Participants revealed five themes of (1) profound change, "We are not completely the same"; (2) shifting self-perceptions, "How I view my future"; (3) ways of interacting with others, "Let me tell you about my feelings"; (4) concern for role, "How I see work"; and (5) completeness of one's story, "Let me tell you about my life" (Gagliardi, 2003). The need to understand patients from these perspectives is supported by the studies in general and the derived theory. A recommendation for practice is that all nurses use cue questions to elicit in-depth responses as the nurse in any setting works with a person in a transition of a chronic health condition. Questions become "How do you feel you have changed?" and "How do you view your future?" or others. These engage the person in ways that show caring and can build rapport and trust. If the nurse–patient relationship lasts over time there is great potential for promoting adaptation throughout the lifelong process.

Encouraging the person to seek involvement in support groups or peer experiences relative to the chronic health condition opens another avenue for adaptation. In an intervention study of a cancer support group, 75% of participants had a more positive attitude after group experiences (Samarel et al., 1998). Participants reported benefits of utility of information received, utility of group for social support, lower anxiety, normalization, benefits of helping others, deliberate time to talk, knowing they were not alone, and burden lifted through sharing experiences. The "common journey" breast cancer support group was an effective intervention (Zeigler et al., 2004).

Future practice-based research is needed to develop instrumentation for perception of health. Such a scale (1–10) could be the basis for further assessment, especially if validated using a question such as "What does the number mean to you" (LeMone, 1995). Screening tools are needed to assess one's body (body image) and how one feels about oneself (self-concept). These must be specific and directive to identify alterations (LeMone, 1995). Instruments with universal reliability and validity and high feasibility and sensitivity can be used to describe adapting to chronic health conditions across cultures (Waweru et al., 2008). Additional studies are needed to explore adaptive processing in mental health conditions, such as post-traumatic stress disorder in returning veterans (Nayback, 2009).

Exemplar for Policy Change—Nurses in Community-Based Settings

The RAM-based research on adapting to chronic health conditions details numerous strategies for supporting adaptive processes through nursing support and intervention. In addition, these practices can also be the basis for policy changes. The exemplar for policy change based on this MRT is the role of nurses in community-based primary health-related settings. Three settings and the corresponding nursing role will be described— schools, camps, and community-based intervention agencies such as support groups and nurse-managed clinics. Each of these has the advantage of serving persons in a community-based environment where they live. In each setting the opportunity for longitudinal follow-up is possible, especially in ways that support long-term adaptation. These venues also facilitate relationship building with health care providers and with others who share the "common journey" of chronic health conditions. Effective use of nurses in community-based primary health care roles is a recommendation of the Institute of Medicine's Future of Nursing Report (Committee on the Robert Wood Johnson Foundation Initiative on the Future of Nursing, at the Institute of Medicine; Institute of Medicine, 2011). Legislation and economic development are needed to fulfill the promise of these emerging practice roles.

School Settings

Self-management in chronic health conditions can be facilitated by the presence of a school nurse (Frame, Kelly, & Bayley, 2003; Knipp, 2006). The school nurse is prepared for monitoring teen response following medication administration for ADHD or other chronic conditions. School nurses are uniquely positioned to facilitate communication among the student, parent, teacher, and health care provider. The studies showed that school nurses made a difference. Waweru et al. (2008) piloted tools for screening at-risk children in a school setting. This approach provided opportunity for follow up and interventions to promote emotional well-being in children experiencing both a chronic physiological illness (HIV) and the psychosocial devastation of being an orphan. Her application of the RAM focused on the self-concept mode and applied low-cost instruments (human figure drawing) to screen for emotional risk. This is an example of theory-based research in a school setting with universal tools applied to a significant chronic health need. Further, in school settings the National School Nurse Association recommends that nurses be present in every school or district. The presence of a professional nurse increases evidence-based practice to assure best practices for children.

Camp Setting

Camps for those with a given chronic health condition in a residential camp lasting 1 or more weeks are examples of immersion experiences for children and youth. Camps provide opportunities for developing a sense of normalcy, for active participation building physical capacity and self-confidence. In some camps specializing in chronic illness (e.g., asthma, diabetes, HIV) there are significant educational programs building knowledge and self-management skills. In addition there are deliberate program elements that facilitate the development of normalcy through reflection and shared experience. The common journey may wind through naturalistic environments, restoring a sense of environmental holism. Chief among these is the opportunity to relate to age peers who share the common journey of chronic health conditions. Adaptation has been linked to camp settings and developing normalcy in RAM-based studies (Buckner et al., 2007; Ramini et al., 2008). Additional concepts functioning within adaptive processes or outcomes are self-management, self-efficacy, and maturing responsibility. Ramini et al. (2008) described a positive strategy for adaptation, which included embracing changes, normalcy, uncontrolled side effects, immersion, and increased "freedom" or fewer restrictions.

Community-Based Intervention

Community-based intervention also includes development of support groups. For patients with cancer, studies of effectiveness of group participation demonstrated increased positive attitude across all four adaptive modes. These were based on the premise that cancer is a chronic disease (Zeigler et al., 2004). Multiple authors found that support group participation was effective for normalization (Samarel et al., 1998; Zeigler et al., 2004). Nurse-managed clinics may provide a holistic assessment and management of patients adapting to chronic health conditions.

The policy implication is to use all means available to establish nurses in these specific primary care roles in these settings—schools, camps, and communities. These are examples of effective and creative initiatives that provide meaningful opportunities for nurses to promote adapting to chronic illness, a need of great breadth and depth in our society. Every approach to advocacy will be used as school nurses are often cut when budgets tighten. Camps have been supported by statewide coalitions that recognize their value. Support groups are often supported by non-profit organization sponsors. Nurse-led clinics are emerging as a viable mechanism for community access to health care (Desborough, Forrest, & Parker, 2012).

CONCLUSION

Concepts and relationships described provide a view of the process of adapting with chronic health conditions. The initial focal stimulus is a change in physical health. This may be rapid or slow in onset with minimal change in comfort to life-threatening acute illness. Treatments, though beneficial, may present additional stressors serving as focal stimuli. Perceived health as threat or challenge sets the stage for negative or positive adaptation. Contextual stimuli include the meaning of illness and social support. Residual stimuli include developmental stages, time, culture, and others. All adaptive modes are integrated into the MRT and all modes function in interrelationships with each other and with the MRT as a whole. The central coping processes (cognator and regulator subsystems) of adaptation are reciprocal as actions taken in the cognator subsystem influence or engage the regulator subsystem. These processes are viewed as mutually integrated with responses in one initiating responses in the other. The general direction of adaptive responses toward integrated adaptation is set as the goal for outcomes.

REFERENCES

Bakan, G., & Akyol, A. (2008). Theory-guided interventions for adaptation to heart failure. *Journal of Advanced Nursing, 61*(6), 596–608.

Buckner, E., Simmons, S., Brakefield, J., Hawkins, A., Feeley, C., Kilgore, L., … Gibson, L. (2007). Maturing responsibility in young teens participating in an asthma camp: Adaptive mechanisms and outcomes. *Journal for Specialists in Pediatric Nursing, 12*(1), 24–36.

Burns, D. (2004). Physical and psychosocial adaptation of blacks on hemodialysis. *Applied Nursing Research, 17*(2), 116–124.

Centers for Disease Control [CDC]. (2012). *Chronic disease prevention and health promotion.* Retrieved from http://www.cdc.gov/chronicdisease/overview/index.htm.

Committee on the Robert Wood Johnson Foundation Initiative on the Future of Nursing, at the Institute of Medicine; Institute of Medicine. (2011). *The future of nursing: Leading change, advancing health.* Washington, DC: National Academies Press.

Desborough, J., Forrest, L., & Parker, R. (2012). Nurse-led primary healthcare walk-in centres: An integrative literature review. *Journal of Advanced Nursing, 68*(2), 248–263. doi:10.1111/j.1365-2648.2011.05798.x

Frame, K. (2003). Empowering preadolescents with ADHD: Demons or delights. *Advances in Nursing Science, 26*(2), 131–139.

Frame, K., Kelly, L., & Bayley, E. (2003). Clinical scholarship. Increasing perceptions of self-worth in preadolescents diagnosed with ADHD. *Journal of Nursing Scholarship, 35*(3), 225–229. doi:10.1111/j.1547-5069.2003.00225.x

Gagliardi, B. (2003). The experience of sexuality for individuals living with multiple sclerosis. *Journal of Clinical Nursing, 12*(4), 571–578. doi: 10.1046/j.1365-2702.2003.00739.x

Gagliardi, B., Frederickson, K., & Shanley, D. (2002). Living with multiple sclerosis: A Roy adaptation model-based study. *Nursing Science Quarterly, 15*(3), 230–236.

Gallagher, M. (1998). Urogenital distress and the psychosocial impact of urinary incontinence on elderly women...including commentary by Baggerly J. *Rehabilitation Nursing*, 23(4), 192–197.

Henderson, P., Fogel, J., & Edwards, Q. (2003). Coping strategies among African American women with breast cancer. *Southern Online Journal of Nursing Research*, 4(3), 20.

Hill, W., Weinert, C., & Cudney, S. (2006). Influence of a computer intervention on the psychological status of chronically ill rural women: Preliminary results. *Nursing Research*, 55(1), 34–42.

Knipp, D. (2006). Teens' perceptions about attention deficit/hyperactivity disorder and medications. *Journal of School Nursing*, 22(2), 120–125. doi:10.1177/105984050602200210

LeMone, P. (1995). Assessing psychosexual concerns in adults with diabetes: Pilot project using Roy's modes of adaptation. *Issues in Mental Health Nursing*, 16(1), 67–78.

Mahomed, R., St John, W., & Patterson, E. (2012). Understanding the process of patient satisfaction with nurse-led chronic disease management in general practice. *Journal of Advanced Nursing*, 68(11), 2538–2549. doi:10.1111/j.1365-2648.2012.05953.x

Moore, J., & McQuestion, M. (2012). The clinical nurse specialist in chronic diseases. *Clinical Nurse Specialist: The Journal for Advanced Nursing Practice*, 26(3), 149–163.

Nayback, A. (2009). PTSD in the combat veteran: Using Roy's adaptation model to examine the combat veteran as a human adaptive system. *Issues in Mental Health Nursing*, 30(5), 304–310. doi:10.1080/01612840902754404

Nuamah, I., Cooley, M., Fawcett, J., & McCorkle, R. (1999). Testing a theory for health-related quality of life in cancer patients: A structural equation approach. *Research in Nursing & Health*, 22(3), 231–242.

Ramini, S., Brown, R., & Buckner, E. (2008). Embracing changes: Adaptation by adolescents with cancer. *Pediatric Nursing*, 34(1), 72–79.

Roy, C. (2009). *The Roy adaptation model* (3rd ed.). Upper Saddle River, NJ: Prentice Hall.

Roy, C. (2011). Research based on the Roy adaptation model: Last 25 Years. *Nursing Science Quarterly*, 24(4), 312–320. doi:10.1177/0894318411419218

Roy, C. (2012). *Roy adaptation model: Key definitions*. Retrieved from http://www.bc.edu/content/bc/schools/son/faculty/featured/theorist/Roy_Adaptation_Model/Key_Definitions.html

Samarel, N., Fawcett, J., Krippendorf, K., Piacentino, J., Eliasof, B., Hughes, P., ... Ziegler, E. (1998). Women's perceptions of group support and adaptation to breast cancer. *Journal of Advanced Nursing*, 28(6), 1259–1268. doi:10.1046/j.1365-2648.1998.00831.x

Samarel, N., Tulman, L., & Fawcett, J. (2002). Effects of two types of social support and education on adaptation to early-stage breast cancer. *Research in Nursing & Health*, 25(6), 459–470.

Thomas, C. (2007). The influence of self-concept on adherence to recommended health regimens in adults with heart failure. *Journal of Cardiovascular Nursing*, 22(5), 405–416.

Toughill, E. (2001). *Quality of life: The impact of age, severity of urinary incontinence and adaptation.* New York, NY: New York University.

Waweru, S., Reynolds, A., & Buckner, E. (2008). Perceptions of children with HIV/AIDS from the USA and Kenya: Self-concept and emotional indicators. *Pediatric Nursing, 34*(2), 117–124.

Weinert, C., Cudney, S., & Spring, A. (2008). Evolution of a conceptual model for adaptation to chronic illness. *Journal of Nursing Scholarship, 40*(4), 364–372. doi:10.1111/j.1547-5069.2008.00241.x

Willoughby, D., Kee, C., & Demi, A. (2000). Women's psychosocial adjustment to diabetes. *Journal of Advanced Nursing, 32*(6), 1422–1430. doi:10.1046/j.1365-2648.2000.01620.x

World Health Organization [WHO]. (n.d.). *Integrated chronic disease prevention and control.* Retrieved from http://www.who.int/chp/about/integrated_cd/en/index.html

Yeh, C. (2002). Health-related quality of life in pediatric patients with cancer: A structural equation approach with the Roy adaptation model. *Cancer Nursing, 25*(1), 74–80.

Young-McCaughan, S., Mays, M., Arzola, S., Yoder, L., Dramiga, S., Leclerc, K., ... Nowlin, M. (2003). Change in exercise tolerance, activity and sleep patterns, and quality of life in patients with cancer participating in a structured exercise program... including commentary by Mock V. *Oncology Nursing Forum, 30*(3), 441–454. doi:10.1188/03.ONF.441-454

Zeigler, L., Smith, P., & Fawcett, J. (2004). Breast cancer: Evaluation of the Common Journey Breast Cancer Support Group. *Journal of Clinical Nursing, 13*(4), 467–478. doi:10.1046/j.1365-2702.2003.00893.x

11

Synthesis of Middle Range Theory of the Adapting Family

SUSAN J. HAYDEN AND ELLEN B. BUCKNER

Everyone belongs to a family, whether it is biological, by marriage, or by choice. The family has been considered the basic unit of our society (Treuthart, 1990), but with the changing times of the 21st century, the definition of family is altering. Since the early 1990s several authors (Belkin, 2011; Treuthart, 1990) have broadened the definition of "family" to include whoever the individual identifies as a member of the family.

The family of the 21st century is a dynamic group. It may be the traditional family of the past to include the biological nuclear family of mother–father–child, a blended family of multiple adults and children from different genetic backgrounds, a close-knit extended group living in close proximity, an expanded group separated by distance and characteristics, or a group of self-chosen persons with some common interest such as a work group or friendship cohort (Belkin, 2011). The family may be traditional or nontraditional, alternative, or a variety of any of the above. In some perspectives, a family is whatever one defines it to be, which is supported by Purnell and Paulenkia's (2008) definition of family as "two or more people who are emotionally connected" (p. 22). The family is an individual's most important primary group, acting as a resource, but often as a stressor as well (Freidman, Bowden, & Jones, 2003). The family has also been described as an adaptive system and a dynamic relational entity (Li & Shyu, 2007). Roy (2009) explained that families and groups proceed through transitions similar to individuals, with stimuli to deal with being influenced both by the family structure and its stage of transition. Different duties and responsibilities are seen in the various stages and structures.

The individual cannot be separated from the family; the family is the background for all assessments and interventions. The Roy adaptation model (RAM), with its four adaptive modes, provides a useful structure to examine these variations of family makeup and the ongoing pattern changes occurring as the family forms, develops, grows, and survives. The purpose of this chapter is to review research that has focused on families using the RAM as the conceptual framework, identify common concepts associated with the family, and construct a middle range theory (MRT) from these concepts.

GENERATING A MIDDLE RANGE THEORY

Following the steps identified in Chapter 2 and described further in Chapter 7, the selected studies will be briefly described. Common concepts will be identified and put in categories at the middle range level. Concepts will be interrelated to develop the propositions of a new MRT. These propositions are supported from the research findings of the studies included. A schematic of the MRT is presented and practice and policy changes are derived.

Studies Selected for Middle Range Theory Development—Step 1

Families were the focus of the studies selected and they explored family processes, interventions, and goals; coping methods through loss and rehabilitation; and adapting to disabilities, for both those affected and the caregiver. Thirteen studies were selected among the studies reviewed in Part II. All 13 studies met the criteria for research adequacy and were framed within the structure of the RAM described in Chapter 2. They all dealt with adapting families, and as the family is continuous throughout life even while changing, these studies covered a variety of aspects of family life.

A series of ethnographic studies followed a convenience sample of 23 Mexican American first-time mothers and fathers from the last trimester of pregnancy through the child's fourth year (Niska, 1999a, 1999b, 2001a, 2001b; Niska, Lia-Hoagberg, & Snyder, 1997). Data were collected through an ethnographic approach of living in the community, gathering contextual information, and then interviewing the participants. The interview process included returning to ask further questions once the initial responses were analyzed. Roy's (1983) early work described family adaptive processes as including nurturing, support, and socialization. In these studies the investigators identified that the families carried out the family adaptive processes using kinship, intimacy, storytelling, and ritualistic behaviors. Roy described families as adaptive systems with the goals of survival, continuity, and growth (Niska, 2001a). Survival was recognized as positive adaptation in the physical mode, that is, being healthy, having a reliable income, and being a united couple; whereas continuity was identified as accountability in role performance and function; and growth was obtained through effective communication, working together toward common goals, and planning ahead. These observations all coincide with Roy's (2009) current positive indicators of adaptation in group identity.

Niska et al. (1997) further explained that when health care providers used listening, appreciation, and welcoming, families were more likely to voice concerns and be actively involved in problem solving related to health care. Respect shown to the family assisted with adaptation. Family stories (Niska, 2001b) were found to be useful in adapting to new situations such as the child transitioning to school. Niska, Snyder, and Lia-Hoagberg (1999) explored the meaning of family health through their ethnographic study using the RAM with new Mexican American parents. The key findings of this analysis were that joint parenting was a key concept of having a healthy family, to include physical, emotional, social interactional, and spiritual integration of the new family unit. Unity, identified by the participants, coincides with Roy's theoretical formulation of family integration.

Other authors in the selected studies (Ciambelli, 1996; Domico, 1997; Kruszewski, 1999; Li & Shyu, 2007; Shyu, Liang, Lu, & Wu, 2004; Zbegner, 2003) addressed family adaptation to specific life events, either personally or as caregivers, with Tsai (2003) developing a MRT of caregiver stress. Two authors (Ciambelli, 1996; Zbegner, 2003) studied families with fertility problems from both the potential mother's and father's perspectives; and Kruszewski (1999) explored the experience of parents having to make the choice to terminate a pregnancy due to fetal anomalies. The final study (Hamilton & Bowers, 2007) explored the experience of genetic testing.

Adaptation to fertility issues was studied by two researchers using the RAM as a conceptual framework. To determine how families coped with infertility, Ciambelli (1996) studied 121 couples, seeking to determine whether gender, age, ethnicity or religion, socioeconomic status, educational level, or employment status affected coping strategies of effectiveness. A coping scale was used to collect self-report responses from both the potential parents. In this cross-sectional, exploratory model testing, findings indicated coping strategies and the level of coping effectiveness correlated to levels of physical demand, self-esteem, home and work functioning, and social support. Men were found to cope in a more optimistic way than the wives.

Although not addressing the family directly, Zbegner (2003) studied infertility, a family issue. The author conducted a retrospective exploratory study of 140 married women. A depressions inventory, a visual analog scale for energy, and scales for self-esteem, marital satisfaction, and parenthood motivation, and a demographic data form were all used to collect data related to the coping behaviors of infertile women. The investigator stated that the Roy model was not a good fit; however, that conclusion was based solely on its function in the resolution of fertility. In her study, Zbegner did find the adaptive modes to be interrelated, with one mode compensating for ineffective coping in other modes. This study found cost related to the fertility issues to be a focal stimulus. Explaining that even though the couple is affected, the woman is more emotionally invested, Zbegner did not specifically address the family. The author did, however, discuss communication between partners and marital satisfaction (family functioning) as contributing to the coping strategies and effectiveness for the woman.

Kruszewski (1999) developed a theory of psychosocial adaptation to termination of pregnancy due to fetal anomalies using the RAM as the theoretical framework. The purpose was to describe stressors and coping of the parents, and also to identify similarities and differences between the mothers and fathers related to stressors and coping processes. This was a qualitative, exploratory descriptive study using a purposive sample of 19 parents who had experienced the loss. Relationships were found among the focal and contextual stimuli, the coping processes, grief behavior, and health. Semi-structured interviews were used to discover focal and contextual stimuli and coping processes. The focal stimuli were identified as the responsibility for the well-being of the unborn as well as the regret and loss of the anticipated child. Although contextual stimuli included the gender of the parent (similar to Ciambelli), social thoughts related to abortion and disability, and the meaning of the anticipated new family member were also relevant. Relationships were found among the focal and contextual stimuli, the coping processes, grief behavior, and health. Coping processes used by this group included decision making, constructing a cause, transforming the relationship, reconstructing meaning, displacing blame, and what the investigator called "backgrounding," that is, shifting attention to other events and concerns or putting the event in the background.

Adapting to life events calls for adaption both in the individual and the family, as numerous authors have addressed. Two studies looked at the individual and then at caregivers in similar situations. The first of these, Shyu et al. (2004) tested a proposition from the RAM in a study of 87 elderly patients adapting to barriers of mobility after hip-fracture surgery. In a descriptive, correlational study the researchers tested the hypothesis that "subjective and objective environmental barriers have direct influences on hip-fractured elders' walking ability, ADLs (activities of daily living), and physical health-related role performance after controlling for pre-fracture self-care ability and health status" (p. 166). Data were collected through face-to-face interviews and home-environment assessments, using an activities of daily living index, an environmental barrier scale, a researcher-developed mobility scoring system, and sub scales of the Short-Form Health Survey (SF-36) to evaluate instrumental behaviors (ADLs and role limitations). With this purposive, convenience sample, focal stimuli were found to have a strong influence on the mobility of these individuals, with the cognator and regulator processes strongly predicting outcomes. These authors identified that, though Roy's model was developed in the Western culture, it is transferable to other settings.

In a later study, Li and Shyu (2007) expanded their study of adapting to hip-fracture surgery by studying the caregivers. This study used a grounded-theory method to investigate coping processes of the caregivers for eight discharged hip-surgery patients. This purposive sample included 12 caregivers and 8 care receivers, all interviewed, face to face, at 1 and 3 months postdischarge. Harmony within the interdependence mode was found to be a strong predictor of effective coping. This harmony was dependent on both internal and external factors. The internal factors included family composition, power distribution, autonomy, and communication patterns, whereas the external environments were the social network and cultural beliefs.

Domico (1997) used a descriptive correlational design to look at the impact of social support and the meaning and purpose in life on the quality of life of 104 spousal caregivers of persons with dementia. The author found that caregivers reported a moderately high perception of social support and quality of life. However, purpose and meaning of life were undifferentiated.

Another grounded-theory study (Hamilton & Bowers, 2007) examined genetic vulnerability in a purposive sample of 29 adults who had undergone predictive genetic testing (24 individuals) or decided against the testing (5 individuals). Face to face, e-mail, or phone interviews were conducted with validation of themes obtained by e-mail. Consistent with the grounded-theory method, interviews continued until data saturation was reached. This study led to a MRT declaring that the pooled effect of the focal (decision to have the testing and the results), contextual (family experience with the disease), and residual stimuli (state of science predicting the risk related to the genetic test) determined the level of adaptation.

The theory of genetic vulnerability that was developed from the data reinforced that the cognator coping processes are greatly influenced by people's perceptions and information processes.

In another study, Tsai (2003) developed a MRT to test the validity of the RAM in relation to caregiving. This theory identified the objective burden as the most important stimuli leading to caregiver stress and high levels of caregiver stress resulting in ineffective adaptation. Contextual stimuli included stress of life events, social support, and social role. Similar to other authors discussed previously, Tsai determined age, gender, and race as the residual stimuli affecting adaptation, and included the category of relationship with the caregiver. These inputs were found to produce responses in the four adaptive modes, leading to the outputs, or behaviors, in the physiologic, self-concept, role function, and interdependence modes. However, depression was an immediate outcome of perceived caregiver stress that intervened in the relationship between perceived caregiver stress and the adaptive modes measured as physical function, self-esteem/mastery, role enjoyment, and marital satisfaction.

These studies share common concepts. The common concepts make it possible to synthesize an MRT.

Concepts, Relationships, and Evidence—Steps 2, 3, 4, and 6

As with all of the Roy adaptation studies, the concepts that can be useful to generate an MRT include stimuli, coping strategies, and outcomes. Each of these concept groups was identified, categorized, and synthesized to complete step 2 of the process for generating a MRT decided on for this project. Many of the studies had similar concepts that were synthesized at the middle range level as indicated for step 3. The concepts are related in a schema depicted in Figure 11.1, as described in step 4 of the MRT development process. At the broad conceptual level, the focal, contextual, and residual stimuli relate to coping strategies that are conceptually connected to outcomes. As the related concepts are discussed, the findings of the studies providing evidence for relationships are listed, according to step 6 of the process for generating an MRT, as outlined by the team conducting this project.

Concept 1—Stimuli

Within the studies selected, the focal stimuli can be divided in two groups: family stage (Niska, 1999a, 1999b, 2001a, 2001b; Niska et al., 1997, 1999); and adapting to specific family events (Ciambelli, 1996; Domico, 1997; Hamilton & Bowers, 2007; Kruszeswki, 1999; Li & Shyu, 2007; Shyu et al.,

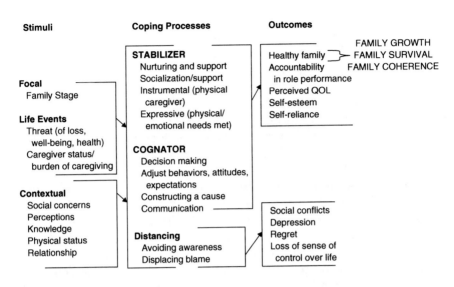

FIGURE 11.1   Schema of Middle Range Theory of Adaptation in Families

2004; Tsai, 2003; Zbegner, 2003). The major conceptual categories for this theory are listed in column 1 in Figure 11.1 and are described as follows:

- *Family stage* is the phase of family formation: beginning, childbearing, preschool children, school age, teenagers, launching, middle-aged, and retirement (Duvall, 1977); each stage faces different stressors that coincide with the developmental tasks associated with them.
- *Adapting to specific family events* occurs when families face specific occurrences, either planned or unexpected changes.

The five studies in the first category, *family stage*, include family processes and families in various developmental stages to include childbearing (three studies) and school age. Family processes of nurturing, support, and socialization (Niska, 1999a) were studied during early family formation (beginning and childbearing) time frames; those events studied during the childbearing stage included assessing acceptance of nursing interventions (Niska, 1999b), family survival, continuity, growth (Niska, 2001a), entry into public school for the oldest child (Niska, 2001b), defining family health (Niska et al., 1999), and identifying parental concerns for first-time parents (Niska et al., 1997). *Family events* occurring to family members included fertility concerns (Ciambelli, 1996; Zbegner, 2003), termination of pregnancy for fetal anomaly (Kruszewski, 1999), hip fractures (Li & Shyu, 2007; Shyu et al., 2004), genetic testing (Hamilton & Bowers, 2007), and dementia (Domico, 1997). Within this latter category, three studies (Domico, 1997; Li & Shyu, 2007; Tsai, 2003) specifically looked at the family member caregiver.

Focal stimuli are described by Roy (2009) as that "stimulus most immediately confronting the human system" (p. 31), or, in many of these studies, the cause of the need for adaptation. Along with the family stage as noted by Niska (1999a), the focal stimuli identified in these studies included the threat of a loss of a baby (Ciambelli, 1996; Kruszewski, 1999), health (Kruszewski, 1999), perceived wellness (Hamilton & Bowers, 2007), and caregiver status that included the burden of caregiving (Domico, 1997; Li & Shyu, 2007; Tsai, 2003).

Contextual stimuli, as described by Roy (2009), are all other stimuli present in the "situation that may contribute to the affect of the focal stimulus" (p. 31). These could be seen as the confounding variables in a research study, and included physical status, knowledge, social concerns, perceptions, and relationships. Stimuli in the physical-status group for the studies selected for this review included functional level (Ciambelli, 1996); physical health (Domico, 1997); physical energy level (Zbegner, 2003); level of physical demands (Ciambelli, 1996); and demographics to include age (Ciambelli, 1996; Domico, 1997; Tsai, 2003; Zbegner, 2003), gender (Domico, 1997; Tsai, 2003), race (Ciambelli, 1996; Tsai, 2003), education (Ciambelli, 1996; Hamilton & Bowers, 2007; Zbegner, 2003), and employment status (Ciambelli, 1996; Tsai, 2003; Zbegner, 2003).

The social concerns category included concerns, issues, characteristics, and the available social support network of both family and external family assistance (Ciambelli, 1996; Domico, 1997; Kruszewski, 1999; Li & Shyu, 2007; Tsai, 2003), self-esteem (Ciambelli, 1996; Zbegner, 2003), religiosity (Ciambelli, 1996), and purpose in life (Domico, 1997).

Included in the contextual stimuli categorized as family perceptions are specific perceptions (Hamilton & Bowers, 2007), social attitudes (Kruszewski, 1999), personal beliefs (Kruszewski, 1999), societal controversy (Kruszewski, 1999), personal meaning of the focal stimuli (Hamilton & Bowers, 2007; Kruszewski, 1999), and family experiences with the focal stimuli (Hamilton & Bowers, 2007). The knowledge stimuli found in the studies were knowledge related to the nature of the problem (Tsai, 2003) and state of the science related to the focal stimuli (Hamilton & Bowers, 2007). The last category of contextual stimuli is made up of relationships, to include relationship status (Li & Shyu, 2007; Tsai, 2003), devotion to other family members (Li & Shyu, 2007), and respect for authority (Li & Shyu, 2007).

Concept 2—Coping Strategies

Roy (2009) identified coping processes as the means an individual or group uses to establish adaptation. The stabilizer subsystem in the group correlates with the regulator for the individual, both acting to maintain equilibrium and growth potential. Although the regulator subsystem promotes adaptation through the neural, endocrine, and chemical systems working together, the stabilizer subsystem of family members works through structures, values, and daily activities to maintain the system. The cognator subsystem for the individual and the innovator subsystem for groups prepare for change through acquired means (Roy, 2009). For the individual, these coping strategies include processes of perception, information processing, learning, judgment, and emotion. The group responds to the stressors through processing information and developing strategies for change. The coping strategies used in the selected studies can be seen in the middle column of Figure 11.1 and are both positive and negative.

Positive coping strategies demonstrated in the selected studies included processes in both the stabilizer and cognator subsystems. Those stabilizing activities included nurturing (Ciambelli, 1996; Domico, 1997; Niska, 1999a; Zbegner, 2003), socialization (Niska, 1999a), and instrumental and expressive methods (Li & Shyu, 2007). Instrumental coping processes were seen as family members took the role of caregiver while showing minimal emotional attachment; physical care was the key factor in adapting to family changes. Expressive-style caregivers were more actively involved, adding affectionate interactions to the physical caregiving. The cognator processes included decision making (Kruszewski, 1999), constructing new ways of being (Kruszewski, 1999; Li & Shyu, 2007), and communication (Niska, 2001a). Constructing new ways included adjusting behaviors, attitudes, and expectations (Li & Shyu, 2007); defining a cause; and transforming and reconstructing moral codes and meanings (Kruszewski, 1999). In defining a cause, problem solving and information processing (Hamilton & Bowers, 2007) may be methods the family incorporates.

The negative coping strategies included distancing (Li & Shyu, 2007) and changing awareness (Ciambelli, 1996; Kruszewski, 1999). Distancing involved moving away from the stressors, either physically or emotionally. Changing awareness could be seen as avoidance (Ciambelli, 1996) or reducing awareness (Kruszewski, 1999) and displacing blame (Kruszewski, 1999). Although depression has been identified as a coping strategy (Tsai, 2003), others may see it as an outcome (Domico, 1997).

Concept 3—Outcomes

Roy defines outcomes as an adapted state in which the person is able to reach a higher level of wellness; the ideal outcome identified in the collected studies were coping processes that led to family growth, survival, and coherence (Roy, 2009). Two studies (Hamilton & Bowers, 2007; Kruszewski, 1999) did not address outcomes, as their purpose was to develop an MRT that would require testing at a later date. Of the remaining studies, the positive coping processes discussed previously led to positive outcomes that support family health, which was demonstrated through increased perceived quality of life, self-esteem, and self-reliance, along with accountability in role performance. Negative coping processes identified in these studies resulted in negative outcomes to include social conflicts, depression, and regret. These families verbalized feelings of a loss of control over their lives and decreased quality of life.

Physical-mode outcomes examined in the selected studies included physical functioning (Shyu et al., 2004; Tsai, 2003), energy level (Zbegner, 2003), self-care (Li & Shyu, 2007), and health of the family (Domico, 1997; Niska, 2001a); the self-concept mode was viewed through self-esteem and mastery (Tsai, 2003); the interdependence role was demonstrated through family unity (Niska et al., 1999), harmony within the family (Li & Shyu, 2007), marital satisfaction (Zbegner, 2003), and friend and family relationships and the social system (Tsai, 2003); and lastly, role function was considered role function in the family (Niska, 2001a), parenthood motivation (Zbegner, 2003), role enjoyment (Tsai, 2003), and changing family roles (Li & Shyu, 2007). Two authors addressed coping strategies across the four modes, with Ciambelli (1996) studying gender differences among adaptive modes and Domico (1997) examining quality of life across the four domains. In this section, the concepts have been identified. Within the framework, the concepts are synthesized at the middle range level. Finally, the interrelated concepts are depicted in a middle range schema of adapting families.

Propositions—Step 5

As described in previous chapters, a proposition is an abstract statement about the relationship between two variables, and although it is a part of the theory, it is not always directly observable. These statements, synthesized from specifics to somewhat more abstract ideas, are the propositions of the MRT of the adapting family. The propositions are listed in Table 11.1. Proposition 1 states that the family make-up is adaptive and dynamic. This particular type of system leads to Proposition 2: that the adequacy of cognator–regulator/stabilizer–innovator processes will affect adaptive processes leading to family growth, survival, and coherence. As the findings of many studies show, with effective coping, healthy families will prevail,

TABLE 11.1
Propositions of Middle Range Theory of the Adapting Family

1. The family is an adaptive, dynamic relational entity.
2. The adequacy of cognator–regulator/stabilizer–innovator processes will affect adaptive processes, leading to family growth, survival, and coherence.
3. Transitions, although inevitable, are particularly stressful times for families.
4. The nature and perception of the changes (focal stimuli) influence adaptation within the family.
5. Family nurturing, support, and socialization are relationally based.
6. Family coherence is demonstrated through love, respect, and loyalty and providing understanding and companionship.
7. Family growth, survival, and coherence (adaptation) are related to social support, communication, sharing, planning, and unity.
8. To achieve harmonious relationships within the family, behaviors, attitudes, and expectations must be adjusted (caregivers and care receivers).
9. Adaptive processes in all modes are interrelated and overlap thereby working together; one mode can compensate for ineffective coping in another mode within the family.
10. Age, physical health, social support, and purpose in life are predictors of quality of life and functioning of the family.
11. A disruption in relationship can lead to depression and interfere with adaptation in any individual's adaptive modes.
12. Nursing interventions respect family boundaries and address expressed concerns of the family.
13. Nursing interventions link families with community.

which is recognized as growth, survival, and coherence. Proposition 3 is also based on the dynamic nature of the family and identifies that families undergo frequent transitions that can be stressful. In other words, changes happen that include family structure and function with new members joining while others are leaving. These transitions can be the focal stimuli the family have to adapt to, and also influence the adapting ability. Proposition 4 states that the nature and perception of changes or focal stimuli influence adaptation within the family.

Propositions 5 through 8 relate to the interactions among the family members as they build relationships and deal with transitions that are inevitable. Proposition 5 notes that family nurturing, support, and socialization are relationally based. Proposition 6 spells out that family coherence is demonstrated through love, respect, and loyalty and by providing understanding and companionship. Roy (2009) used the family to show how family cohesion is a form of group identity within this adaptive mode of groups. Proposition 7 shows that family growth, survival, and coherence (adaptation) are related to social support, communication, sharing, planning, and unity. Social support, communication, and sharing dreams and expectations are seen across studies as essentials for effective coping. Proposition 8 acknowledges that, as shown in the studies of caregivers and care receivers, to achieve harmonious relationships within the family, behaviors, attitudes, and expectations must be continually adjusted.

The next propositions, 9 through 11, introduce the working of the adaptive processes in the family, identifying factors that enable, as well as block, effective coping and adaptation. Proposition 9 notes that adaptive processes in all adaptive modes are interrelated and overlap thereby working together; one mode can compensate for ineffective coping in another mode within the family. The studies used for this MRT have shown the four modes overlap, compensating for other modes if they fall short. Proposition 10 notes, based on the selected studies, that age, physical health, social support, and purpose in life are predictors of quality of life and functioning of the family. On the other hand, Proposition 11 recognizes that disruption in relationship can lead to depression and interfere with adaptation in any individual's adaptive modes. This was noted particularly in Domico's (1997) study of caregivers of spouses with Alzheimer's disease.

The final two proposals address how nurses can best meet the families' needs. Proposition 12 states that nursing interventions respect family boundaries and address expressed concerns of the family. To develop a trusting relationship, family boundaries must be respected. Family members will identify when they need help and what types of help they are open to. Their issues and concerns must be addressed; therefore, the nurses should include family members in the planning process. With increased family involvement in the planning of care, *noncompliance* may be a thing of the past. Finally, proposition 13 notes that nursing interventions link families with community. By introducing families to resources in the community, and opening the doors to available, appropriate health care partners, the nurse is more likely to facilitate compliance and encourage follow-up. Family members are likely to be the caregivers and having their confidence and trust is a major point of establishing an effective plan of care.

TRANSLATIONS FOR PRACTICE AND POLICY

Recommendation for Practice

Within the MRT of the adapting family, numerous coping strategies were identified as being effective within the family requiring adaptation. Nurses can learn from the findings that families want health care to provide interventions that will link them with the community (Niska, 1999b) in a meaningful way. Talk with and listen to the family members to determine what is needed and wanted, and what types of community connections will be most accepted. Health care providers must take the time to introduce the family unit to key individuals, identifying the help available, along with the expectations and means of participating. Health care providers must respect boundaries (Niska, 1999b) and provide nonjudgmental, respectful care–cultural differences may make the family hesitant to enter the system. Open communication with active listening will alert the provider to concerns, fears, superstitions, or other areas that must be addressed. Addressing the voiced (and often unvoiced) concerns (Niska et al., 1997; Niska, 2001b; Zbegner, 2003) of the family increases open communication and trust. All family units deserve nonjudgmental, respectful care; health care providers must go beyond cultural sensitivity and deliver culturally competent care. Every patient deserves that from all health care providers. Nurses can develop ways for the family to maintain ongoing contact with health care providers.

Three significant gaps were identified in the literature through this review of family-related research based on the RAM. First, there are minimal studies that examined the family as a unit; most of the included studies looked at the individuals within the family. No studies were found using the RAM that explored nontraditional families although these alternative family types are increasing in large numbers. The final area not found in the studies was the shared language within a family. To continue developing knowledge for practice, these gaps will need to be addressed. Recommendations for needed research include these areas as well as studies to test the middle range theories developed in these studies and in this chapter.

Examples From Practice

Case 1

Katie is a 10-year-old who has been admitted to the Pediatrics Unit following an open reduction of a fractured femur occurring after a fall from her horse. The horse determined the fence was too high to jump, but didn't relay that decision to Katie. As could be expected, Katie was scared to death when anyone even suggested she had to be moved or move herself. Mom and/or Dad stayed at the bedside all the time, with Dad going home to check on Katie's 15-year-old brother late each evening, to return shortly after breakfast. Katie's parents were protective and hesitant to allow the nurses and physical therapists to get her out of the bed. What if the rods were displaced with movement? Why did she have to move if it hurt so much? Why couldn't Katie keep getting the morphine so she wouldn't hurt? Night-shift nurses reported that Katie had used the bedpan and the urine had spilled in the bed because she wasn't able to lift up for it to be removed. They had replaced the draw sheet with Mom's help, but the linens were soiled and so was Katie.

The day nurse went into Katie's room, introduced herself to Mom and Katie, and sat down to discuss the plan of care. She asked Katie what her goals were for the day, and Katie just shrugged. The nurse next turned to Mom, asking the same question. Mom moved close to Katie and took hold of her hand, looking down at the floor, saying nothing. The nurse explained she would complete an assessment, and if everything was "normal" the plans should be to keep Katie as comfortable as possible (addressing concerns), but Katie needed to get up. The linens needed changing, but more important, Katie needed to move to prevent pneumonia, blood clots, and other complications. Mom and Katie asked numerous questions about the reasons for moving so soon after surgery, and the nurse gave basic explanations. Katie asked if she could get up herself. The nurse suggested Mom stand by the chair, and Katie and the nurse would work together. Each time Katie asked to wait, the nurse paused and let Katie and her Mom catch their breath. At one point, Katie requested the nurse step away from the bed and leave her alone. The nurse respected this boundary, stepping away for the decided-upon time. When Katie finally got settled in the chair, Mom said, "You must think we are awful, letting Katie make all the rules." The nurse told Mom that each family relates in ways that they have found effective, and that Katie's injury and surgery had certainly caused the family some added stress (non judgmental, respectful care). Each time Katie got up it was easier and much quicker. Mom and Katie thanked the day nurse for her patience and said they didn't know what they would do when they went home. The nurse made a social service consult for them to discuss community services available to them, as she remembered the need to link the family with the community.

Case 2

Mr. H., a 60-year-old, overweight male is being discharged from the hospital for the third time with hypertension and uncontrolled diabetes. Nurse Nunns brings in the discharge teaching packet and sets it on the bedside table. Mr. H. states, "There's no need to leave that there. I still have the packets I got on my last two visits." The nurse walks out, sputtering that "patients like him are a waste of time; they never do what they are told, and just keep coming back in with the same problems." Nurse Care hears her coworker and asks what the problem is. Nurse Nunn tells her what

Mr. H. said and Nurse Care asks if anyone had sat down with Mr. H. to see why he hadn't followed the discharge instructions. Nurse Nunn grumbles about being too busy. Nurse Care walks into Mr. H.'s room and asks how he is doing. When Mr. H. tells her he is headed home "again!" Nurse Care asks if he understands his discharge instructions and were there any that he thought he might have trouble following. Mr. H. laughs and says he isn't sure he could follow any of them as his wife does all the grocery shopping and cooking, and he just "eats what's served." Nurse Care asks if it would help if someone reviewed the diet with his wife, and Mr. H. replies that she works until 5:00 every day so can't come in while the dietician is in. Nurse Care contacts the dietician and sets up a visit for Mr. and Mrs. H. while Mr. H. is on the phone with his wife to confirm availability.

After that phone call, Mr. H. says, "Since you fixed that so easily, what about all these medicines? They must cost a ton of money. How am I supposed to get them every month?" Nurse Care inquires if he had checked with his insurance company to see what would be covered. Mr. H. responds, "Insurance cover medicine? Is that something new?" Nurse Care places a call to social services and they set up an appointment for when his wife will arrive to pick him up to discuss with them resources available and how to contact each. Mr. H. tells Nurse Care, "Things are so much easier when they work with my wife. I don't know about these things, and we sure don't know how to find these people you say are in the community to help us unless someone tells us they are there. We take care of our own, but no one has told us anyone else could help." With Mr. H.'s concerns addressed in a respectful, nonjudgmental way and links to the community made before discharge, Mr. H. followed up regularly in the clinic and controlled his diabetes and blood pressure without further admissions.

Exemplar for Practice-Policy Change

Although admission interviews ask for family history, *a change that nurses can help implement is to introduce a meaningful family history that is effectively used by all providers to plan care for adapting families.* In addition to the standard information on family health history and functional support, the health care provider needs to take the time to listen to the family, hearing their history and addressing their questions and concerns. Understanding the theory of adapting families helps to understand that families are unique and face challenges differently. Still they have many coping strategies that can be activated by the nurse to help them handle the health challenges they face. With this knowledge teaching can be more than a handout, but an actual time to discuss what the family needs to know to continue care. With more knowledgeable families, "non compliance" will decrease. Given the studies reviewed in this chapter and others, nurses can understand that a major cause of patients not following prescribed care is that they were not a part of the planning, and no one took the time to ask whether the plan would work for them and their families. Some providers, including nurses, may claim they are too busy, with heavy patient loads and increased computer work, to spend time with the patient and family. However, the time spent would not only build more trusting relationships, but also more effective family-centered care. One can readily assume that if time were well spent, time would be saved. New roles for nurses, such as case managers and patient navigators, can help coordinate care with community resources and policy implications to build a health care system responsive to the needs and responsibilities of families.

CONCLUSION

This chapter developed a new MRT of the adapting family using studies related to families based on the RAM. This knowledge includes propositional statements supported by the research that can be applied to practice. Practitioners can incorporate this new knowledge into their plan of care to deliver evidence-based care as well as conceptualize policy changes to improve holistic patient care.

REFERENCES

Belkin, L. (2011, February 24). Defining a family. *The New York Times Learning Network*. Retrieved from http://learning.blogs.nytimes.com/2011/02/24/how-do-you-define-family/?apage=1#comments

Ciambelli, M. (1996). Adaptation in marital partners with fertility problems: Testing a midrange theory derived from Roy's adaptation model (Doctoral dissertation, Wayne State University). *Dissertation Abstracts International, 57*(12B), 7448.

Domico, V. (1997). The impact of social support and meaning and purpose in life on quality of life of spousal caregivers of persons with dementia (Doctoral dissertation, University of Alabama at Birmingham). *Dissertation Abstracts International, 58*(12B), 6485.

Duvall, E. M. (1977). *Marriage and family development*. New York, NY: Lippincott.

Friedman, M. M., Bowden, V. R., & Jones, E. (2003). *Family nursing: Research, theory & practice*. Upper Saddle River, NJ: Prentice Hall.

Hamilton, R., & Bowers, B. (2007). The theory of genetic vulnerability: A Roy model exemplar. *Nursing Science Quarterly, 20*(3), 254–255.

Kruszewski, A. (1999). Psychosocial adaptation to termination of pregnancy for fetal anomaly (Doctoral dissertation, Wayne State University). *Dissertation Abstracts International, 61*(01B), 194.

Li, H.J., & Shyu, Y.L. (2007). Coping processes of Taiwanese families during the postdischarge period for an elderly family member with hip fracture. *Nursing Science Quarterly, 20*(3), 273–279.

Niska, K. (1999a). Mexican American family processes: Nurturing, support, and socialization. *Nursing Science Quarterly, 12*(2), 138–142.

Niska, K. (1999b). Family nursing interventions: Mexican American early family formation. *Nursing Science Quarterly, 12*(4), 335–340.

Niska, K. J. (2001a). Mexican American family survival, continuity, and growth: The parental perspective. *Nursing Science Quarterly, 14*(4), 322–329.

Niska, K. J. (2001b). Therapeutic use of parental stories to enhance Mexican American family socialization: Family transition to the community school system. *Public Health Nursing, 12*, 138–142.

Niska, K. J., Lia-Hoagberg, B., & Snyder, M. S. (1997). Parental concerns of Mexican American first time mothers and fathers. *Public Health Nursing, 14*(2), 111–117.

Niska, K. J., Snyder, M. S., & Lia-Hoagberg, B. (1999). The meaning of family health among Mexican American first time mothers and fathers. *Journal of Family Nursing, 5*, 218–233.

Purnell, L. N., & Paulanka, B. J. (Eds.). (2008). *Transcultural health care: A culturally competent approach* (2nd ed.). Philadelphia, PA: F.A. Davis.

Roy, S. C. (1983). Roy adaptation model. In R. Clements & F. Roberts (Eds.), *Family health: A theoretical approach to nursing care* (pp. 255–278). New York, NY: John Wiley.

Roy, S. C. (2009). *The Roy adaptation model* (3rd ed.). Upper Saddle River, NJ: Pearson Education.

Shyu, Y. I. L., Liang, J., Lu, J. F. R., & Wu, C. C. (2004). Environmental barriers and mobility in Taiwan: Is the Roy adaptation model applicable? *Nursing Science Quarterly, 17*(2), 165–170.

Treuthart, M. P. (1990–1991). Adopting a more realistic definition of "Family." *Gonzalas Law Review, 26*, 91.

Tsai, P. (2003). A middle range theory of caregiver stress. *Nursing Science Quarterly, 16*(2), 137–145.

Zbegner, D. K. (2003). *An exploratory retrospective study using the Roy adaptation model: The adaptive mode variables of physical energy level, self-esteem, marital satisfaction, and parenthood motivation as predictors of coping behaviors in infertile women* (Doctoral dissertation). Widener University School of Nursing, Chester, PA.

IV

Evidence-Based Practice: Redefined and Exemplified

Part IV is made up of the all-important Chapter 12 on evidence-based practice (EBP) and levels of readiness for practice. The work here responds to the issues raised in Chapter 1 about gaps between knowledge and practice. It derives its conclusions based on the processes carried out in this project. The processes for preparing the data of 172 studies were described in Part II in chapters on the qualitative studies and the quantitative studies, for which the description and evaluation of each study is reported in Chapters 3 to 6. The authors of Part III used this data for generating five middle range theories (MRT) on coping, adapting to life events, adapting to loss, adapting to chronic conditions, and the adapting family. Each of these MRTs follows the proposed six-step process and is described in Chapters 7 to 11. The author of Part IV uses this work to provide innovative applications of EBP that can be used emergently in practice.

All of the work done by the project team was aimed toward our central focus—to add to the current nursing research and provide evidence-based practice (EBP) to bridge knowledge and practice by using the research based on one theoretical framework as evidence. In this chapter the author takes the final step of integrating evidence into knowledge for nursing practice. The five MRTs are examined for commonalities in adapting of persons and families. The propositions from the MRT that support the general propositions of the RAM are identified. The evidence of the research-based

MRT is identified. The illustration of using the Roy adaptation model for EBP is shown by using the common concepts of the stimuli, coping processes, and adaptive outcomes and providing ways to implement this knowledge based on evidence for best practices across studies. A final application for nursing practice is provided by the author's creating a state of the art and science Nurse/Patient Alliance (NPA) Infrastructure and Portal for RAM Evidence.

12

Evidence-Based Practice Established
on the Levels of Readiness for Practice

CAROLYN PADOVANO

A major focus of this book is to use research to generate middle range theories (MRTs) that are supported by research findings. These findings can be used to exemplify Roy's redefinition of evidence for practice (Roy, 2009). Earlier in the movement, Ingersoll (2000) defined evidence-based practice (EBP) as the conscientious, explicit, and judicious use of theory-derived, research-based information for making decisions about care delivery and preferences. EBP in nursing claims to integrate the best evidence from research combined with clinical expertise, patient preferences, and existing resources—and to use this knowledge in clinical decision making. Proponents state that this method bridges the gap between nursing theory and knowledge and practice. The aim of this project was to add to the current work in nursing research and EBP to bridge knowledge and practice by using the research based on one theoretical framework as evidence for best practice. This chapter provides a background on EBP, both its history and models. The research reviewed in Part II and the MRTs generated in Part III from the studies are used to exemplify EBP based on Roy's (2009) definition of EBP. The usefulness of this distinctive vision of EBP is shown by exemplars for practice and policy.

BACKGROUND

History of Evidence-Based Practice

EBP began in medicine in the late 1980s; the aim was for practice to be grounded in quantitative research based primarily on randomized clinical trials (RCTs), meta-analysis, and/or outcome studies. The EBP movement was significant because it argued that evidence was vital to improving clinical practice. The methods proposed provided hard evidence on quality and cost-effective care while optimizing patient outcomes. Dluhy (2007) took a different perspective and in a compelling presentation asked nurses to consider the concerns and issues in using EBP quantitative methods in nursing. The issues she raised included:

1. Medical standards are used for the evidence, therefore, nurses are essentially used as medical technicians for medical outcomes.
2. One approach is used for all patients, however, in nursing practice, nurses shape customized interventions based on patients' needs and preferences.
3. Context-based interpretation of research really is not allowed, but the art of nursing involves the context that includes the beliefs and values of patients, caregivers, families, and communities.
4. In EBP, the use of qualitative research is unclear, however, nurses understand patients and their context using qualitative methods.
5. Certainty is imperative in EBP, but nurses know that their data are imperfect and patients do not respond predictably at all times.

For nurses the challenge and the solution is to expand their view of EBP to ensure patients receive care that is based on the strongest possible foundation of knowledge. Fawcett, Watson, Neuman, Walker, and Fitzpatrick (2001) and other authors have called for a broader view of EBP. In particular, these authors recommended that nurses should move from a focus on empirics to a focus on diverse patterns of knowing. They emphasized that nurses need theory-guided, evidence-based, holistic nursing practice where theory, inquiry, and evidence are inextricably linked in order to improve patient care. As noted, Baumann (2010) pointed out that nurses do not routinely discuss the limitations of EBP. The author provided a number of questions to consider, including whether EBP is able to be holistic, to provide for primary prevention and adequately contribute to development of theory and science.

Models of Evidence-Based Practice

As part of the movement to increase nursing's perspective and presence in this significant area, nurses have expanded their views on EBP.

Several nurses have developed systematic review processes that advocate for basing nursing practice on the best available evidence generated from a theoretical perspective. Pearson, Vaughan, and FitzGerald (2005) developed evidence-based guidelines to inform nursing practice and stated that the "core of evidence based practice is the systematic review of the literature on a particular condition, intervention, or issue" (p. 14).

Their method involves the following seven guidelines:

1. Develop a rigorous proposal or protocol subjected to peer review.
2. State the question or hypothesis that will be reviewed, and include the patients, settings, interventions, and outcomes to be studied.
3. Select the literature that identifies the participants of the primary studies, the interventions and outcomes, and the research methods.
4. Outline the strategy for the literature review, that is, the time frame, the search terms, and the databases that will be used.
5. Determine the inclusion and exclusion criteria of the studies based on their quality.
6. Explain how the data will be extracted from the research studies: the sample (the participants), the interventions, the outcome measures, and the results.
7. Plan how the extracted data will be aggregated, analyzed, and critically appraised for application into practice.

Similarly, 5 years later, Melnyk, Fineout-Overholt, Stillwell, and Williamson (2010) developed the seven steps of EBP for nursing and published their approach to improving care and patient outcomes in the *American Journal of Nursing* (*AJN*). The authors pointed out that most nurses' education predated EBP curricula and offered this simplified problem-solving method to the delivery of health care that integrates the best evidence from studies and patient-care data combined with clinician expertise, and patient preferences and values. The overview of the multi-step EBP includes:

1. Step Zero—cultivate a spirit of inquiry
2. Step One—ask questions in PICOT format (P = Patient population of interest, I = Intervention for area of interest, C = Comparison intervention or group, O = Outcome, and T = Time)
3. Step Two—search for the best evidence relevant to the clinical question
4. Step Three—critically appraise the evidence to determine the relevancy, validity, reliability, and applicability to the clinical question
5. Step Four—integrate the evidence with clinical expertise and patient preferences and values, as these variables are extremely important factors in customizing patient care

6. Step Five—evaluate the outcomes of the practice decisions or changes based on the evidence
7. Step Six—disseminate the EBP results to improve nursing practice and patient care

DISTINCTIVE DEFINITION OF EVIDENCE-BASED PRACTICE

Roy agreed with expanding the view of EBP and published her redefinition in 2009. The theorist's philosophy and model support this distinctive definition. The Roy adaptation model (RAM) is grounded in philosophy, values, and context – the beliefs of unity, diversity, self-identity, purposefulness of people, and people in society. These philosophical beliefs have been termed "veritivity" (Roy, 2009). The model supports seeking knowledge in all ways of knowing—personal, ethical (value based), esthetic, sociopolitical, as well as empiric. Roy also works toward all knowledge development that will improve nursing practice. Figure 12.1 depicts the relationship of beliefs and values in the process for integrating research findings into practice.

The description of EBP by Roy was developed from an earlier project of reviewing research based on the RAM (Boston-Based Adaptation in Research Nursing Society [BBARNS], 1999). In that project 163 studies were reviewed and 118 were used to describe contributions of the RAM to nursing science. Contributions included applications to practice. Based on propositions of the RAM tested in the research studies, applications to practice were evaluated for three levels of potential for implementation in practice. These levels were used to derive a redefinition of EBP. Roy offers one definition of EBP centered on theory-based research that can provide cumulative knowledge that is evaluated on levels of readiness for practice. Level 1 EBP is the level with the highest potential for implementation in practice. The four criteria for this level include: (1) proposition is supported by more than one study, (2) unequivocal support of hypotheses, (3) low risk, and (4) high clinical need. Level 2 EBP is described as the level that needs further clinical evaluation before implementation. The criteria in this level are as follows: (1) proposition supported, (2) generalizability is not clear, (3) risk is not clear, and (4) high clinical need. The studies, however, may be examined by advanced practice nurses with related expertise and a panel can determine readiness for practice by addressing areas that are unclear. Last, Roy identifies Level 3 EBP as that level that needs further testing before implementation. The criteria in this level include: (1) proposition has mixed support, (2) generalizability is unclear, (3) high risk, and (4) high clinical need. The criteria for each level are summarized in Table 12.1.

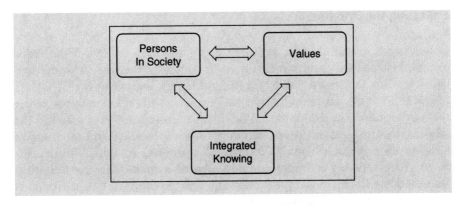

FIGURE 12.1   Applying the Roy Adaptation Model for EBP

TABLE 12.1
Criteria for Levels of Evidence-Based Practice

Level 1: High Potential for Implementation in Practice	Level 2: Needs Further Clinical Evaluation Before Implementation	Level 3: Needs Further Testing Before Implementation
(1) Proposition(s) is/are supported by more than one study	(1) Proposition(s) supported	(1) Proposition(s) has/have mixed support
(2) Unequivocal support of hypothesis(es)	(2) Generalizability is unclear	(2) Generalizability is unclear
(3) Low risk	(3) Risk is not clear	(3) High risk
(4) High clinical need	(4) High clinical need	(4) High clinical need

Source: Adapted from Roy (2009). *The Roy Adaptation Model (3rd edition)*. Upper Saddle River, NJ: Pearson.

THE ROY ADAPTATION ASSOCIATION SYSTEMATIC RESEARCH REVIEW

The Roy Adaptation Association (RAA) has sponsored reviews of this theory's research over several decades. As noted, project 1 of the first 25 years of research was published in 1999 (BBARNS). This is the second major review project published. For this book, 172 studies covering the years of 1995 to 2010 that used the RAM were examined. The review team followed a combination of the EBP guidelines and EBP described by Roy (2009) to evaluate the RAM studies. The processes used in the approach along with key definitions are discussed in Chapter 2.

Collecting the Evidence

Collecting the studies and evaluating the research followed the steps outlined earlier and summarized here. Specifically, the project team identified studies that were published in English, by searching the CINAHL, MEDLINE, PubMed, ProQuest, ERIC, and PsycINFO databases using the key words "Roy adaptation model" and "research." In reviewing the studies, the researchers used standard forms to extract and summarize a description of each study as follows: (1) author(s); (2) date; (3) purpose, research questions, or hypotheses—which also included how the studies tested the RAM; (4) sample; (5) design and methods; (6) measurements and/or instruments; and (7) findings.

Appraising the Evidence

The review team analyzed the quality of the research by applying specific criteria to both quantitative and qualitative studies. To summarize the criteria in general, for quantitative research, they examined: (1) *design—* efforts to control threats to external and internal validity; (2) *measurement* that included reliability and validity of instruments; (3) *data analysis* included appropriateness and precision; and (4) *interpretation of results* for accuracy of findings and consistency of conclusions. For qualitative research, they examined: (1) *method and design* for trustworthiness, credibility, transferability, dependability, and confirmability; (2) *audit trail,* which included analysis of raw data, data-reduction product, process notes, researcher intentions and dispositions, reflexive notes, instruments, and data reconstruction; (3) *data analysis* included appropriateness and precision; and (4) *interpretation of results* for accuracy of findings and consistency with conclusions (see Chapter 2 for definitions, and the process utilized).

For both quantitative and qualitative studies, the researchers closely evaluated the quality of the research that tested the RAM concepts. In addition, the team summarized the strengths and weaknesses of the research related to all criteria, and provided a final score of 1 to 5 for the overall quality of the research, in which number 1 was the lowest score and number 5 was the highest. The project team conducted interrater reliability testing to ensure that the team scored the quality of the research in the same manner and were in agreement. The scores for the raters were consistently over 90% in agreement. The one area of difference was settled by discussion to reach 100% agreement. The RAM studies selected to be included to contribute to building knowledge for practice had to obtain mainly quality scores of 4s and 5s and not more than one 3. This meant that at least 80% of criteria for the expected quality were met and the study could be included for further EBP development.

Of the 40 studies with qualitative designs using various approaches, reviews showed that scores ranged from the highest score of 20 ($n = 17$) to the lowest score of 16 ($n = 4$) so all studies were in the acceptable range. This meant that any of the qualitative studies could be selected to generate MRT and to provide evidence for practice. For the three types of quantitative designs, there were 126 studies evaluated. The reviewers reported scores that ranged from the highest score of 20 points ($n = 27$) to the lowest of 14 points ($n = 2$) and two studies received 15 points. The scores below the minimum points set resulted in four studies being removed from further consideration in generating knowledge. It should be noted that in the screening process 28 additional studies were deleted that did not clearly reflect either the use of the RAM or research. The description and evaluation of studies that were deemed research studies based on the RAM are described and evaluated in Chapters 3–6.

INTEGRATING EVIDENCE INTO KNOWLEDGE FOR NURSING PRACTICE

The project team used the highest quality research studies that could be rated for readiness for implementation based on the criteria described above. A key step in creating evidence for practice was generating MRT. The team members clustered studies together with similar research observations. Because the concepts of the model have been defined, described, and published over the past several decades, it was possible to identify studies with common concepts/variables, and with similar purposes and questions or hypotheses and related findings. The process of MRT development as described earlier was used to group concepts and results. The common content areas that emerged from this evaluation were built into middle range schemas for coping in general, adapting to life events, adapting to loss, adapting to chronic health conditions, and the adapting family. The findings from the studies provided the evidence for practice. Based on the evidence the team members then used study findings to generate MRTs. A total of 52 RAM research projects in the area of adapting/coping with life events, loss, chronic conditions, and within families were selected to generate MRTs. The findings from the studies had potential for implementation in practice and were selected to show how theory, based on the RAM, truly provides evidence for practice. For a summary of these studies, including their respective designs that were selected, refer to Table 12.2. The 6-step process for generating MRTs is accomplished in Chapters 7–11 in which the derivation of the five theories is described.

TABLE 12.2
Generating MRT: Selected Research and Designs for Evidence

Middle Range Theory	Studies Selected	Study Designs for Evidence
Coping—Chapter 7	Dunn (2005)	Explain–predict, structural equation modeling
	Flood and Scharer (2006)	Experimental pretest/posttest control group
	Raleigh, Robinson, Marold & Jamison (2006)	Mixed methods, quantitative and qualitative
	Levesque et al. (1998) and Ducharme et al. (1998) (5 studies each)	A posteriori theoretical modeling with structural equation analysis
	TOTAL: 5	
Coping with Life Events—Chapter 8	Cook, Green & Topp (2001)	Descriptive, exploratory
	Wright (2007)	Qualitative, phenomenological
	Hanna (2005)	Qualitative, modified phenomenological
	Polichnowski (2008)	Cross-sectional, predictive, correlational design using hierarchical multiple regression
	Woods and Isenberg (2001)	Predictive, series of regression equations
	Zhang (2004)	Explain–predict, causal modeling and path analysis
	Taylor (1997)	Descriptive correlational
	Martin (1995)	Descriptive survey
	Sparks (1999)	Intervention, 2 intervention groups and control group
	Lazenby (2001)	Phenomenological, descriptive
	Moore (2005)	Phenomenological, descriptive
	Clark (2001)	Phenomenological, descriptive
	TOTAL: 12	
Loss—Chapter 9	Martin (2003)	Phenomenological, descriptive
	Robinson (1995)	Descriptive, correlational
	Smith (2001)	Qualitative, phenomenological
	Short (2004)	Qualitative, phenomenological
	Watson (2006)	Qualitative, phenomenological
	Gandy (2003)	Qualitative, descriptive
	Dobratz (2002)	Grounded theory method, causal model
	Dobratz (2004)	Grounded theory
	TOTAL: 8	

Middle Range Theory	Studies Selected	Summary of Study Designs
Chronic conditions— Chapter 10	Burns (2004)	Explain, predict, path analysis
	Thomas (2007)	Descriptive correlational
	Gagliardi (2003)	Naturalistic study of cases
	Gagliardi, Frederickson & Shanley (2002)	Content analysis
	Willoughby, Kee & Demi (2000)	Descriptive correlational
	Henderson, Fogel & Edwards (2003)	Explain, predict, prescribe, regression analysis
	Waweru, Reynolds & Buckner (2008)	Mixed methods, qualitative and quantitative
	Lemone (1993, 1995)	Phenomenological descriptive
	Knipp (2006)	Phenomenological descriptive
	Hill, Weinert, & Cudney (2006)	Intervention, experimental with randomized groups, control group
	Samarel, Tulman, & Fawcett (2002)	Intervention, experimental
	Zeigler et al. (2004)	Intervention, single group pretest, posttest
	Bakan and Akyol (2008)	Intervention, experimental with secondary analysis
	Young-McCaughan et al. (2003)	Intervention, single group pretest and posttest
	Buckner et al. (2007)	Intervention, single group pretest and posttest
	Ramini, Brown & Buckner (2008)	Phenomenological descriptive
	TOTAL: 16	
Family—Chapter 11	Niska (1999a)	Ethnography
	Niska (1999b)	Ethnography
	Niska (2001)	Ethnography
	Ciambelli (1996)	Descriptive correlational
	Domico (1997)	Descriptive correlational
	Kruszewski (1999)	Phenomenological descriptive
	Li & Shyu (2007)	Content analysis, directed
	Shyu, Liang, Lu & Wu (2004)	Explain, predict, prescribe, regression analysis
	Zbegner (2003)	Explain, predict, prescribe, structural equation modeling
	Tsai (2003)	Explain, predict, prescribe, structural equation modeling
	Hamilton & Bowers (2007)	Grounded theory
	TOTAL: 11	

USING RAM FOR EBP: CONCEPTS AND OUTCOMES CITED FOR IMPLEMENTATION IN PRACTICE

All the research studies selected and the evidence used for the development of the five MRTs, that is, coping, adapting to life events, adapting to loss, adapting in to chronic health conditions, and the adapting family, presented in Part III, as noted are demonstrations of levels of EBP. Each individual MRT has high potential for implementation in practice; however, when reviewed collectively the evidence has stronger significance as it can be successfully applied across several different patient situations with varying conditions resulting in patient, family, community, and/or population adaptation. Whether coping or adapting to life events, such as normally occurring life changes, acute illnesses, chronic health conditions, and/or loss and death, several commonalities emerged. Nurses and patients can use these findings and results to promote health, prevent illnesses, improve disease conditions, speed recovery, and/or adapt to circumstances that cannot be changed to live fuller lives.

Stimuli Concepts

Each MRT identified that the focal stimuli—the internal or external changes confronting patients and/or families—were either expected, that is, changes in life that normally occur, or unexpected, that is, changes in life that are disruptive or disturbing. The authors explain that how patients and/or families react to the focal stimuli depends on the contextual stimuli or circumstances that surround the individual or family at that particular moment of life. The contextual stimuli influence how a patient or family perceives and thus reacts to the change that is the focal stimuli. The commonalities in contextual stimuli among these MRTs included: (1) the background and demographics of the participant, that is, who the person is, his or her identity defined by gender, age, race, ethnicity, religion, educational level, economic status, environment or residence, employment status, role in family and community; (2) the developmental stage and maturation or adjustment of the participant, that is, where the person is in his or her life progression such as infancy, early childhood, school age, adolescence, young adulthood, middle adulthood, and late adulthood; and (3) the personal characteristics, preferences, perspectives, dispositions, and attitudes of the participant, that is, what the person is about, the individual's perceptions, including values, beliefs, goals, and feelings. The authors also cited that the onset, intensity, severity, and duration of the focal stimuli influenced how participants adapted and coped; some authors labeled time and acuity factors as the residual stimuli.

Regulator and Cognator Subsystems Concepts and Adaptation Strategies

The middle range theorists also agreed that in order for patients and families to adapt to internal or external focal stimuli, either expected or unexpected, requires both stabilization with regulator activity and the promotion of cognator subsystem activity to meet the challenge. Some focal stimuli cited in the MRTs affected the patient physically, for example, acute illnesses and chronic conditions with varying diagnoses as well as the treatments and procedures endured. These experiences often involved the regulator subsystem, which included the neural, chemical, and endocrine systems. Other focal stimuli cited in the MRTs affected the patient personally, for example, verbal abuse, stress of illnesses or caregiving, or the death of a loved one. Dealing with these focal stimuli involved the individual's cognator subsystem activity, including perceptual and information processing, learning, judgment, and emotion. The authors concluded that the order of interventions prescribed for patients and families to reach adaptation depended on whether the stimuli invoked physical or personal changes, if these changes required immediate attention, and whether the changes were expected, such as changes in life that normally occur, or unexpected, that is, changes in life that are disruptive or disturbing.

Intervention and Outcome Concepts in Developmental Challenges

The MRTs that reviewed the developmental challenges show the relationships among the concepts of stimuli, regulator, and cognator processes as interventions aimed toward adaptive outcomes. Table 12.3 provides a summary of the commonalities among the concepts of the MRTs dealing with developmental challenges and then, looking at the rows across the columns in the table, illustrates the relationships.

The developmental events that were expected for families had predictive qualities that allowed patients and families to plan for change. In each of these situations the onset of the focal stimulus or change was known, such as managing responsibilities in the postpartum period and attitudes toward menopause. The intensity, severity, and the duration of the stimulus were somewhat limited, such as in the case of receiving immunizations and signing advanced directives. The interventions applied in practice depended on the contextual stimuli and focused on where the patient and family were physically, psychologically, and developmentally; how they felt about the change, including their self-concept, and their experiences dealing with change in the role function and interdependence modes. When families had experience with change, they were comfortable

TABLE 12.3

Summary of Commonalities Among Middle Range Theories: Adapting to Developmental Challenges

STIMULI: Focal, Contextual, Residual	INTERVENTION: Regulator and Cognator Subsytem	OUTCOME: Adaptative Modes
Expected Related to Internal or External Changes	Stabilize and Improve	Physiologic, Self Concept, Role Function, and Interdependence
Child—receiving immunizations	Change of input stimuli—soothing touch	Decrease pain sensation
Young adulthood—postpartum problems (managing chores/ child care, loss of income)	Direct action and/or selective attention	Effective transition to the role of mother
Middle adulthood—Attitudes toward menopause	Increase positive attitude and self-esteem	Decrease depression
Late adulthood—signing advanced directives	Systematically plan a head, use resources to make decisions	Decrease anxiety

with systematically planning ahead by obtaining information and using resources to direct decisions. They had used these approaches in the past in order to decrease anxiety about the change.

When the families understood how the change might affect them, but they had not actually dealt with that particular change before, effective nursing interventions included helping the patients to take direct action based on prescribed education and care plans. An example is nursing educational interventions aimed at improving physical and mental health by promoting positive attitudes and self-esteem thereby decreasing depression. These educational resources and plans of care also helped families choose where they needed to focus their attention when selective attention was needed for their immediate adaptation and coping. This was exemplified in the research dealing with women transitioning to the new role of mother. In some instances the most appropriate nursing intervention cited for other patients, such as preschoolers receiving immunization injections, was to change their input, that is, in this case receiving soothing touch. This approach was more effective than distraction in that it provided pleasant stimuli to replace the unpleasant needle insertion to decrease pain sensations and promote adaptation.

Intervention and Outcome Concepts in Situational Challenges

The MRTs that reviewed the situational challenges are presented in Table 12.4 in a summary of the common stimuli, interventions, and outcomes.

TABLE 12.4
Summary of Commonalities Among Middle Range Theories: Adapting to Situational Challenges

STIMULI: Focal, Contextual, Residual	INTERVENTION: Regulator and Cognator Subsytem	OUTCOME: Adaptative Modes
Unexpected Related to Disruptive/Disturbing Change	Stabilize and Improve	Physiologic, Self-Concept, Role Function, and Interdependence
• Chronic pain (adult, elders)	Improve functional status/performance Creativity/religion	Decrease pain intensity Decrease in depression life satisfaction/ purpose in life leads to successful aging
• Chronic illness (heart failure, diabetes, multiple sclerosis, kidney disease, HIV/AIDS, cancer)	Problem-solving techniques Education/use of computer Physical activity, nutrition Social support Religion/spirituality	Decrease pain and anxiety Decrease depression, loneliness, stress Decrease stress, increase self-esteem Effective coping, adaptation Trust in God, meaning and purpose of illness
• Stress of caregiving (families, professionals, elderly couples)	Hospice and social support Cognitive/emotive processing of environmental factors—includes active problem-solving techniques and an optimistic/confrontive approach	Increase ability and satisfaction in caring for others Decrease psychological distress
• Difficult work/school environments (physician verbal abuse, abortions, physical abuse, dating violence, traumatic stress)	Use knowledge/skills to deal with problem and behavior of others/spirituality Relate to others (emotional sharing) Get help from others (empathy)	Effective use of work/school team and your role Resolve moral distress Improve mental health

(continued)

TABLE 12.4
Summary of Commonalities Among Middle Range Theories: Adapting to Situational Challenges (*continued*)

STIMULI: Focal, Contextual, Residual	INTERVENTION: Regulator and Cognator Subsytem	OUTCOME: Adaptative Modes
Unexpected Related to Disruptive/Disturbing Change	Stabilize and Improve	Physiologic, Self-Concept, Role Function, and Interdependence
• Dealing with children in neonatal intensive care unit (cerebral palsy, cancer)	Social support Obtain information/ knowledge on disease Talk/bond with others	Increase supportive network Decrease anxiety and fear Return to normal
• Loss/death (spouse, infant, loved one, life itself)	Social support Spirituality/spiritual well-being Religion	Create memories Overcome loneliness Find meaning and strength Force self to move forward Learn new roles Form new relationships Connect to others and/or higher power
• Rehabilitation and disabilities (families)	Listening, appreciation, welcoming	More involved in problem solving

Adapting to situational challenges was unexpected for individuals and families and had disruptive or disturbing factors that they were required to deal with before being able to reach adaptation. If the onset of the focal stimulus or change was physiologic or disease related and disruptive (such as chronic pain, chronic illnesses, managing disease entities, and disabilities) and if the intensity, severity, and the duration of the stimulus was high or long term, nursing interventions always included decreasing the pain intensity first, and then working with individuals to improve their functional status and performance. When patients and families were stabilized, the next set of common nursing interventions included helping individuals and families obtain the right information and knowledge about the disease, condition, or disability that they now had to live with. Nurses also prescribed that individuals and families should connect with others dealing with the same condition. Talking and bonding with others, obtaining social support, and increasing this supportive network were cited as common interventions to help patients decrease anxiety and fear, so that even if they could not return to their prior condition, in being among others handling the same experiences, they were able to define a new normal.

When the onset of the focal stimulus or change was personal and/or disturbing, such as caregiver stress, difficult work or school environments, verbal abuse, traumatic stress, and death of a loved one, the intensity, severity, and the duration of the stimulus was typically described as high or long term. In these situations nursing interventions always included decreasing psychological/moral distress and depression by first stabilizing or helping the individual find balance. The nurse could then work with individuals to ultimately improve their overall mental health, including increasing positive self-concept. Common nursing interventions that emerged from the MRTs included teaching individuals and families about active problem-solving techniques and using optimistic and/or confrontive approaches. Another approach by nurses was using knowledge and skills to deal with the specific problems and/or the behavior of others, thus improving role function and interdependent behavior for the person. Other common nursing interventions used in these situational challenges included developing, using, and increasing social support networks in order to form new relationships, learn new roles, overcome loneliness and depression, and to force oneself to move forward and to create new memories. Relating to others by emotionally sharing, connecting to a higher power, and getting help from others were also cited as common interventions to alleviate anxiety thereby allowing individuals to find strength and meaning in their situation. Engaging in spiritual, religious, and creative activities was a significant coping strategy or intervention that both individuals and families used to clarify their purpose in life in order to increase life satisfaction, which in turn, led to the positive outcome of adapting as in successful aging, for example.

RAM PROPOSITIONS SUPPORTED BY THE MRT FOR IMPLEMENTATION IN PRACTICE

In the five MRTs, collective evidence also emerged supporting the generic propositions of the RAM, described in Chapter 2. A total of 62 propositions emerged from the five MRTs, as follows: the coping MRT included 12, the coping-with life events MRT contained 12, the adapting to loss MRT had 7, the adapting to chronic conditions MRT consisted of 18, and the adapting families MRT involved 13. In cluster one, the internal coping processes' propositions, all five MRTs had propositions supporting this cluster with a total of 15 statements. Similarly, in cluster two, the adaptive modes propositions, again all five MRTs had propositions supporting this cluster, which consisted of a total of 15 statements. Cluster Three, the internal and external stimuli propositions, included the highest number of propositional statements at 19, among all five of the MRTs. In contrast, cluster four, the group-adaptation propositions, contained five statements, the least number of statements. These were supported by only two of the five MRTs, that is, the coping-with-life events MRT and the adapting families MRT. Cluster five, the nursing-process propositions, again all five MRTs had supportive statements in this area for a total of 13. For a detailed summary of the MRT evidence supporting the individual propositions per cluster, see Table 12.5.

TABLE 12.5
Summary of Evidence From Middle Range Theories in Support of Roy's Propositions

RAM Propositions—Total Number of Supporting Statements Among All MRTs	MRT Propositions Supporting RAM Propositions
Cluster one: internal coping processes (15):	
1. The adequacy of cognator and regulator processes affect adaptive responses (1)	1. Coping (1)
2. Specific cognator processes that affect adaptive responses are: perception, information processing, learning, judgment, and emotion (10)	2. Coping (1), life events (4), chronic conditions (4), families (1)
3. Adaptation takes place over time as the regulator and cognator continue to process stimuli (4)	3. Life events (1), loss (2), chronic conditions (1)
Cluster two: observable behaviors in one or more adaptive modes (15):	
4. Adaptation in one mode is affected by adaptation in other modes *(8)*	4. Life events (2), loss (1), chronic conditions (5)
5. The adaptive modes change over time both during development and throughout life *(3)*	5. Life events (3)
6. Behavior in adaptive modes is classified as effective and ineffective to determine adaptation levels of integrated, compensatory, and compromised *(4)*	6. Coping (2), chronic conditions (1), families (1)
Cluster three: internal and external stimuli to the adaptive system (19):	
7. Internal and external stimuli influence cognator and regulator processes *(1)*	7. Loss (1)
8. Internal and external stimuli influence adaptive mode responses *(12)*	8. Coping (1), loss (1), chronic conditions (8), families (2)
9. The pooled effect of focal, contextual, and residual stimuli determines the adaptation level *(5)*	9. Coping (2), life events (1), loss (1), families (1)

(continued)

TABLE 12.5
Summary of Evidence From Middle Range Theories in Support of Roy's Propositions (*continued*)

RAM Propositions—Total Number of Supporting Statements Among All MRT	MRT Propositions Supporting RAM Propositions
10. Adaptation reflects the integration of the person with the environment *(1)*	10. Loss (1)
Cluster four: group adaptation (5):	
11. At the group level, stabilizer and innovator processes affect adaptation *(4)*	11. Life events (1), families (3)
12. Adaptation of groups takes place over time as the stabilizer and innovator continue to process stimuli *(1)*	12. Families (1)
Cluster five: nursing process (13):	
13. Nursing assessment and interventions relate to identifying and managing input to adaptive systems *(7)*	13. Coping (2), life events (1), chronic conditions (3), families (1)
14. Supporting and enhancing coping processes are interventions to promote adaptation *(6)*	14. Coping (2), loss (1), chronic conditions (1), families (2)

In a number of instances the individual propositions from the five MRTs could have matched more than one of the general propositions in the clusters. This is because each is a statement relating two major concepts and the concepts appear in different clusters. When a MRT propositional statement fit in with more than one general statement and cluster these propositions were counted more than once if the meaning matched up to more than one proposition. The level of generality versus complexity among the MRT statements varied. However, it is not surprising that cluster three, the internal and external stimuli to the adaptive system propositions, contained the most supportive statements (total = 19) because in all the MRTs, that is, coping, adapting to life events, chronic conditions, loss, or in family adaptation, both internal and external stimuli were identified to see what processes would lead to the adaptive mode outcomes. There were a total of 12 statements supporting propositions on adaptive modes. As stated in the previous section, all MRTs concluded that the onset of the stimulus, whether developmental or situational, the severity of the stimulus, and the cognition and perception of the stimulus are predictors for choosing the most appropriate interventions (treatment, education, direct action, social support, religion, spirituality, and so forth). Further, the order of their application again depends on that individuals' or families' circumstances in order to achieve healthy adaptive mode responses.

Similarly, all five MRTs in cluster one, propositions for internal coping processes, included the next most frequently occurring supportive propositions (total = 15). Four out of the five MRTs (coping, loss, chronic conditions, and adapting families) supported the propositional statement that *specific cognator processes that affect adaptive responses are: (a) perception, (b) information processing, (c) learning, (d) judgment, and (e) emotion.* There were a total of 10 individual statements from all MRTs that were related to these cognator activities. All MRTs supported the statement that all of the cognator processes affect adaptation; however, the majority of the MRTs emphasized perception and meaning as the key cognator process for individual and family adaptation, followed by the same number of statements about information processing and learning and experience, judgment and emotion, especially humor.

Likewise, all five MRTs in cluster two, observable behaviors in one or more adaptive-mode propositions, included a total of 15 supportive statements with three out of the five MRTs, that is, life events, loss, and chronic conditions, illustrating the supportive propositional statement: *adaptation in one mode is affected by adaptation in other modes* (total of eight individual statements). Whether the individual planned ahead or employed direct or selective action, by handling things systematically or by using resources and experience, his or her physiologic mode affected the degree of adaptation in his or her self-concept, role function, and interdependence modes and this affect was reciprocal. Another commonality among the MRT authors was that adaptive processes in all modes are basically interrelated, overlap, and thereby work together; some modes can compensate for others in order to achieve individual and/or family adaptation.

Another commonality among all five of the MRTs was in the supporting propositions of cluster five, the nursing-process propositions (total = 13). Both individual propositions: *nursing assessment and interventions relate to identifying and managing input to adaptive systems* (total = 7) and *supporting and enhancing coping processes are interventions to promote adaptation* (total = 6) were supported. All of the common interventions, coping processes/strategies, and outcomes relative to healthy adaptation were described in the previous sections and will not be repeated here. To review again, refer back to Tables 12.3 and 12.4.

Lastly, there were approximately seven propositions that related both to coping processes (cluster one) and interventions (cluster five) and basically support both clusters depending on whether the statement is instructive to the nurse or the individual and family. For the purpose of this review, if the statement was instructive to the individual or family it was either included in cluster one or four, and if the statement was instructive to the nurse it was included in cluster five. Further refinement and additions to Roy's propositions will be needed as the research studies and the evidence accumulates.

APPLICATION IN NURSING PRACTICE: INTEGRATING MIDDLE RANGE THEORIES

The commonalities of the five MRTs, that is, coping, coping with life events, adapting to loss, adapting to chronic health conditions, and the adapting family, help nurses to understand patients better when coping or adapting to life events, such as normally occurring life changes, acute illnesses, chronic health conditions, and with the loss of loved ones. This nursing knowledge derived from research based on the RAM has provided nurses with the necessary research findings to provide evidence to customize care and interventions for their patients based on their specific needs as identified by assessing the unique pattern of the focal, contextual, and residual stimuli. Focusing on individual patterns can result in improving outcomes, whether the goals are physiologic, self-concept, role function, and/or interdependence adaptation. Nursing knowledge has evolved and the valid evidence to enhance patient outcomes has grown significantly and accurately with the publication of this research book, the previous project (BBARNS, 1999), and other nursing research publications. As a result, this reliable evidence needs to be disseminated more widely and efficiently to nurses so that they can use this state-of-the-art and state-of-the-science information in their practice to improve their patients' care and quality of life. This evidence should also be packaged and disseminated for rapid access and direct use by individuals and families.

We live in a world where stress and demands plague us. The U.S. economic future is uncertain; unemployment rates have soared to an all-time high; the underinsured and the uninsured population keeps rising; the age of the population itself has increased substantially; and often several family members are relegated to being full-time caregivers. Nurses are in a position to help individuals, families, communities, and populations cope and adapt to the challenges listed above based on the evidence supporting these MRTs. Hence, with the increased use of mobile technologies, computers, and the Internet, nearly everyone has access to clinical information and social media and nursing should leverage these dissemination vehicles when working with colleagues and when caring for patients.

Developing the Nurse/Patient Alliance Infrastructure and Portal for RAM Evidence

The ability to implement the middle range nursing theories and the evidence for practice presented in this book requires a robust technical nursing infrastructure, platform, portal application, and database to support educational dissemination and social support needs of clinicians and patients. The author proposes the development of an evidenced-based nursing infrastructure and portal (see Figure 12.2) that applies best practice recommendations related to the evidence supporting significant RAM MRTs that have been generated to date. The knowledge will be available not only to nurses in the field who want to improve care for their patients but also to patients themselves who are looking for customized care depending on their developmental or situational changes and/or challenges.

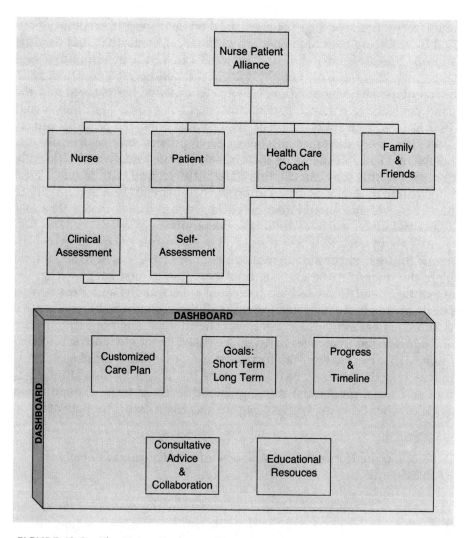

FIGURE 12.2   The Nurse/Patient Alliance Portal Infrastructure Based on RAM EBP

The Nurse/Patient Alliance (NPA) portal infrastructure would be developed using the same strategies employed by the Cochrane Collaboration, which allows patients and clinicians to browse on a database of the best practice evidence for a specific disease category (see http://www.cochrane.org/for more information). The NPA Database would be developed using the RAM MRTs. The database would contain the components of the MRTs and their associated data and the evidence (i.e., the effective treatments, interventions, strategies) that support adaptation and coping for acute or chronic conditions/diseases, and/or problems based on life events—like the new role of becoming a mother or a parent, dealing with the role of becoming a caregiver for a sick child or parent, or dealing with the loss of a loved one (bereavement) whether expected or not.

The NPA Home Page would contain four main areas—one area of the portal would be devoted to nurses, another would be dedicated to patients, and the last two areas would be designated as collaborative and consultative areas for the patients and the nurses to be able to work together in partnership with other health care providers (such as health care coaches), and the patient's family and friends. On this home page, the patients and nurses would be instructed to enter or click on their designated area in order to search on the focal stimuli (i.e., conditions, diseases, problems) confronting them or their patients at that particular time. The individual patient or nurse would then be prompted to describe the onset, intensity, severity, and duration of the stimuli, the characteristics of the main concepts of the MRT, that is, the conceptual and residual components of the focal stimuli.

The patients or the nurses then would be diverted to the main section/index of the NPA portal to complete an assessment (i.e., clinical or self-reported) that contained context specific questions to ascertain where the patient perceives himself or herself at this particular point in his or her life. This assessment or questionnaire would focus on the uniqueness of that individual and would be developed based on the evidence of the MRTs reviewed in this chapter. The assessment would include the following sections: (1) the background and demographics of the patient; (2) the developmental stage and maturation or adjustment of the patient; (3) the personal characteristics, preferences, perspectives, dispositions, and attitudes of the patient; and (4) the patient's health care goals based on his or her physiologic, self-concept, role function, and interdependence adaptation priorities. When the patients or the nurses finish completing this assessment, an automatic analysis would run (via the algorithms imbedded in the platform and application) and the results would generate a customized plan of care that would recommend the most effective interventions based on that specific patient's characteristics and goals in order to promote adaptation and coping using the RAM. This customized care plan would include dashboards and metrics, including short- and long-term measurable goals so that an individual nurse, his or her family/friends, or other health care coaching professionals could track the patient's progress via a timeline toward the overall health care objective of adaptation/ coping. The dashboard application would be available to patients, nurses, families and friends, or other health care coaching professionals via mobile devices, particularly cell phones and iPads so that they can set important alerts and reminders about the patient's care and share this information with others, such as appointment schedules, medication regimes, and time-sensitive interventions. The portal would also have the functionality to track and record the patient's progress via the dashboard, such as vital signs, blood test/procedure results, progress notes, and consult information. In developing this section of the portal, website exemplars such as My Optimal Health Club, which offers health care coaching and Caring Bridge, which offers online space for family, friends, and caregivers to connect with patients to manage and support their care will be modeled (see: http:// www.myoptimalhealthclub.org/positive-coping-with-health-conditions/ and http://www.caringbridge.org/about/ for more information).

The subsections/content of the NPA portal infrastructure would also contain and generate educational information specific to that patient's developmental or situational change or challenge, and would customize the education based on tailored interventions and on that individual's preferred learning style. The portal site would have the ability to host on-demand audio and video clips, live podcasts, and more traditional training, including conferences, workshops, seminars, resources, and tools. The Alliance would also host a collaborative space allowing patients the opportunity to find health care resources, support groups, and/or talk with other patients who had shared interests and challenges via e-mail, live chat, Skype, and blogs. Individuals would have the opportunity to consult with nurses in real-time for direct advice and they would have the ability to retain the nurse as a health care coach if they needed daily assistance in order to reach their adaptation goals. Similarly, nurses would be able to consult with nurse experts or other providers to manage complex and changing patient needs. Social-media tools would also be available at the Alliance, such as, Facebook, YouTube, and Twitter.

CONCLUSION

The key to implementing the MRTs and the EBP presented in this chapter requires nurses to align effective and meaningful interventions and quality health care with the needs of individuals and families. With new knowledge and the evidence behind it, nurses can meet the people where they are, at that moment of their lives. They can understand the context and meaning of the developmental or situational change or challenge for that particular person. This approach and the applications proposed can help to simplify interventions and care plans so that individuals feel as though promoting their health is part of their daily routine. This approach will most undoubtedly guarantee success in bridging the gap between nursing knowledge and practice.

REFERENCES

Baumann, S. (2010). The limitations of evidenced-based practice. *Nursing Science Quarterly, 23*(3), 226–230.

Boston-Based Adaptation Research in Nursing Society (BBARNS). (1999). *Roy adaptation model-based research: 25 years of contributions on nursing science.* Indianapolis, IN: Sigma Theta Tau International Center Nursing Press.

Dluhy, N. (2007). *Uncertainty, transparency, control: The allure of EBP.* Presented at Theory Research Interest Group Pre-Conference Workshop, Eastern Nursing Research Society, Providence, RI.

Fawcett, J., Watson, J., Neuman, B., Walker, P., & Fitzpatrick, J. (2001). On nursing theories and evidence. *Journal of Nursing Scholarship, 33*, 115–119.

Ingersoll, G. (2000). Evidence-based nursing: What it is and what it isn't. *Nursing Outlook, 48*, 151–152.

Melnyk, B., Fineout-Overholt, E., Stillwell, S., & Williamson, K. (2010). The seven steps of evidence-based practice. *American Journal of Nursing, 110*(1), 51–53.

Pearson, A., Vaughan, B., & FitzGerald, M. (2005). *Developing an evidence base for practice* (3rd ed.). London: Elsevier Limited.

Roy, C. (2009). *The Roy adaptation model* (3rd ed.). Upper Saddle River, NJ: Pearson Education.

V

Roy Adaptation Model–Based Research: Global View

*I*n this project we located, screened, described, evaluated, and used 172 studies based on the Roy adaptation model (RAM) to generate middle range theory for evidence-based practice. As a project team and the executive board of the Roy Adaptation Association, we are aware of knowledge development around the globe. We participate with members of our 6 international chapters in Japan, Colombia, Mexico, and Panama in projects related to research based on the RAM. From the beginning of the project we sought ways to address the global scope of RAM-based research, without taking away from the efforts to complete the main project. The theorist has visited each of the international chapters. However, one project member, Martha Whetsell, has spent more time in these countries as a consultant to the many implementation projects in research, education, and practice. She volunteered to survey the research and related issues in Latin America.

To fill out the global picture a brief survey of global key informants was carried out. The second author, Research Fellow Ann Harrington, worked with the theorist to conduct and analyze the global survey from selected countries. These two projects provided the content for Chapter 13 on the RAM-based global research. The authors combined their projects with the aim of reporting on: (1) research and RAM-based research in Latin America and (2) the estimate of research productivity and of theory-based research in selected countries around the globe.

13

Roy Adaptation Model–Based Research: Global View

MARTHA V. WHETSELL, ANN HARRINGTON, AND SISTER CALLISTA ROY

In a global society, progress in nursing in one part of the world affects nursing in other parts. Most societies around the globe face changing health issues that may differ from those of the United States but provide challenges to nurses just the same. The growth of nursing education experienced in the United States in the last century continues to take place in this country and in many others. For example, the International Network for Doctoral Education in Nursing (INDEN, 2013) reported doctoral programs located in 32 countries in 2013. The participating countries are listed in Box 13.1.

In Chapter 1 it was noted that with the growth of doctoral education, progress in nursing research occurred. The Roy Adaptation Association team was interested in nursing research around the globe and whether or not nursing theories and the Roy adaptation model (RAM) in particular were used as frameworks for research. In the review of English-speaking literature reported in Part II, a number of studies were noted that were conducted in other countries, some by scholars who studied in the United States. Given time constraints and language limitations, the project team, in lieu of a full research review, planned other approaches to survey research globally. One approach was to have a Spanish-speaking member of the team conduct a review with the assistance of the five chapters of the Roy Adaptation Association in Colombia, Mexico, and Panama. Second, the theorist directed a research fellow in conducting a survey of key informants in selected countries other than those already covered. The aims of

---

BOX 13.1
COUNTRIES WITH DOCTORAL PROGRAMS IN NURSING

Argentina	Greece	Poland
Australia	Hong Kong	South Africa
Belgium	India	Sweden
Brazil	Ireland	Switzerland
Canada	Japan	Taiwan
Chile	Korea	Thailand
Colombia	Mexico	The Netherlands
Czech Republic	Namibia	Turkey
Egypt	New Zealand	United Kingdom
Finland	Norway	United States
Germany	Philippines	

---

this chapter are to report on: (a) research and RAM-based research in Latin America and (b) the estimate of research productivity and of theory-based research in selected countries around the globe.

THEORY-BASED NURSING RESEARCH IN LATIN AMERICA

Background

There is no doubt that in the last decade, nursing education and nursing research in South America, Central America, and in Mexico underwent a significant change characterized by the application of theoretical nursing models. In many colleges of nursing educators articulated, supported, and provided direction for the development of research and integrated this development into nursing curricula. In this undertaking, colleges of nursing in other countries, like the ones in the United States, are comprised of self-organizing, continuous-learning centers. In evaluating their change we assessed their transformation without judgment, which turned out to be the key in identifying their progress and diversity.

Determining a need to assess the use of nursing theory in these countries was done considering that we have a large body of dissertations that were developed based on nursing conceptual frameworks. In order to analyze them we need to carry out a general assessment because this step precedes research analysis. The use and application of the theories also became an issue. The authors realized that the knowledge of scholars in these countries is prompted by the general information provided by texts and journals. In addition, being specialists themselves, every practitioner has many strata of knowledge useful for solving problems on the job. Knowledge for practice also is developed by experience and years of practice in the field.

In planning a general assessment, we considered several questions: (a) How, where, and by whom are nursing health concerns managed in these countries? (b) How do these health concerns reach a status of being serious and important, rather than exploratory and tangential for nursing? (c) What is the relative value of nursing research for evidence-based practice?

Results of Literature Review

A thorough review of the literature (from 2000 to 2011) was conducted on the subject of the use of nursing theory as a basis for the development of research in education and practice. The assessment taught us that different models were used in very different ways. Generally speaking, the search showed that what exists is a clear intention to meet the demands of the changes of health care systems all over South America, as well as to respond to demands emerging from education and practice. There was also a theme in the literature that education, curriculum development, and practice can benefit from the use of theoretical models.

The literature in Spanish-speaking journals and dissertations from 2000 to 2011 showed that the RAM was used as the conceptual framework in more than 180 studies conducted in Brazil, Chile, Colombia, Cuba, Granada, Mexico, Panama, and Peru. A previous literature review conducted in 2008 (Moreno & Alvarado, 2009) reported that the model had been used in the same countries with the exception of Chile, Cuba, and Granada After appraising the current literature, the first author realized that the analysis needed to address issues of consistency and methods in those studies. In the past researchers focused their aims on how the alteration of an adaptive mode affected the other adaptive modes and on how some stimuli affected the adaptation of individuals.

Analysis of Research and Contextual Questions

Fifty-six research publications using the RAM were chosen for the analysis. The analysis included focus of the research, relation to nursing education, instrument development, application to practice, and the substantive content. Research based on the Roy model in the early 2000s was descriptive in nature, as opposed to explanatory. With descriptive designs, the investigators frequently labeled and described some of the model concepts and categorized various elements of the adaptation process (Cavalcante, Olivera Lopes, & Araújo, 2005; Lopes Neto & Pagliuca, 2002). When reviewing those early studies we realized that it was not the use of the model that was the concern, but the way the model was used. In conducting this analysis, we did not critique nor judge the adoption of the model; rather, we assessed a generic approach to using the model. Our intention was to highlight how the use of the model guides the researchers' thinking. This thinking leads to a better use of evidence for the practice.

In the later 2000s studies were developed using quantitative designs. These studies were conducted for the analysis of the four adaptation modes, for the analysis of their relation to the coping processes, and for the development of nursing interventions to promote adaptation (Gonzalez, 2007). The majority of studies examined the adaptive modes of self-concept, role function, and interdependence and included subjects with chronic illnesses such as arthritis, cancer, and renal diseases. There were also studies that examined the adaptation of caregivers who take care of people with disabilities and with terminal illnesses.

In looking at the context of nursing research in these countries we can answer some questions raised. For the first question: How, where, and by whom are nursing health concerns managed in these countries? We found that some of the health concerns were managed by nurses and were investigated by nursing research. Further, the RAM-directed research occurred in hospital pediatric intensive care units (Monroy, 2003) and rehabilitation settings (Moreno, 2001). In addition, the RAM was the frame of reference for the curriculum of the school of nursing at La Sabana University, in Chia, Colombia. In answering the second question of how do these health concerns reach a status of being serious and important, rather than exploratory and tangential for nursing, we found out that mental health and mental disorders were not given the same degree of importance as physical health. One could speculate that nursing in Latin American countries must be understood within a context that physical pathology directs trends and issues in health care.

The third question raised was about the value of nursing research for evidence-based practice. We learned that various studies documented the important relationship between nursing intervention and health outcomes. This focus suggested an important connection between how research based on the RAM also served to direct the management of the workforce, which may be considered another form of evidence-based practice. Most reported studies are descriptive, using convenience samples of persons with chronic diseases. As noted, the majority of the researchers studied an alteration of an adaptive mode and how this alteration affected the other adaptive modes. Additionally, the research looked at how stimuli influenced the adaptation process of individuals. These investigators also indicated the implications of their findings for nursing practice.

Implications of Research Analysis

What is lacking in viewing the studies as a whole is the understanding that through the lens of the conceptual framework, a stronger and more well-defined methodology could be used. Well-articulated research grounded in theory yields powerful outcomes. On the other hand, we also were able to identify that health concerns and issues managed by nurses in these countries helped to formulate intellectual capital. This valuable asset encouraged their universities to develop nursing curricula based in theory. It also showed the need to deepen the understanding of the phenomenon of adaptation. Consolidating progress in the understanding of the RAM and valuing its implementation in research and practice can contribute to health and in this way perhaps positively affect a country's economy.

The education and regulation of nurses is diverse and varies in scope among the different countries. Despite these differences, some positive financial support allows nurses to seek higher education in masters' and doctoral programs. This has been a positive factor for nursing education and research. For example, the doctoral programs in Colombia, Panama, and Mexico are developing their research based on the RAM and therefore have facilitated student exchange among the countries and promoted multinational research. The RAM may help in an unparalleled opportunity to challenge the status quo in nursing and to contribute significantly to efforts to improve nursing practice for South Americans, Mexicans, and Central Americans. Such an effort requires the education of competent nurses functioning at all levels of health care systems. According to Roy (2009), basic nursing involves looking at individuals and groups as adaptive systems, centering on human processes and patterns. This view provides basic knowledge for the nursing profession. According to the RAM, nursing strives to understand the stability of adaptive patterns and the dynamics of evolving adaptation. The RAM model provides direction for exploring a specific contextual experience that acknowledges the development of the historic and current leadership role that nursing plays in Latin America. The nursing role will support the realization of important domestic, multinational, and cultural implications.

Directions for Future Research

Investigating the following four contextually based foci can provide specific direction for further research. This research can help to bridge the gap between assumptions and beliefs and real health issues.

1. Investigate the value of baccalaureate education in Latin America.
2. Investigate synchronization of nursing curricula by evaluating course content of undergraduate and graduate nursing curricula in Latin America.
3. Coordinate the linkage between quality doctoral nursing education and health outcomes, using as a pilot study in the three countries (Mexico, Colombia, and Panama) that have initiated new doctoral programs, and which would be a fertile ground for initiating synchronized doctoral curricula among different nations.
4. Evaluate course outcomes related to graduate clinical faculty expertise and leadership competencies.

The future of nursing in Latin America will benefit from investigating the contextual factors with heightened awareness of the need for baccalaureate education in nursing, providing the motivation to move toward the baccalaureate as the entry into practice credential. Given technologic and scientific advances, not only in the United States but also in developing countries, nursing practice requires that nurses be grounded in theory-based research and critical thinking. Evidence provided by research in the United States substantiates the usefulness of the RAM in the development of nursing education (Boston-Based Adaptation Research in Nursing Society [BBARNS], 1999). Based on the above premise, research will be conducted in the integration of new baccalaureate curricula throughout Latin America. Also, research will specifically investigate the relationships among adaptive processes. These advances will lead to increasing levels of knowledge. In response to globalization efforts, the ideal would be that the nursing education community in Latin America would promote sustainable theoretical knowledge networks. These networks can be used to determine theoretical bases for research and the empirical testing of nursing theory.

Future research can expand methods to move beyond description and correlations. In reviewing the 57 studies, the research was not directed toward testing explanations, predictions, or prescriptions. No research reviewed tested concept integrity or multivariate relationships. This type of research is necessary to understand the dynamics of the concept of adaptation and to plan effective interventions. Such methods are particularly important for individuals or families in transitions and over time during change. In early work Roy and Roberts (1981) noted that the adaptation model research implies multivariate and not nonlinear configurations. Roy stated that a simple linear, unidirectional, bivariate relationship will not capture the essence of the dynamics of evolving adaptation. It is research with multivariate designs and experimental interventions that produce the strongest evidence for practice. The study by González (2007) provided an example of testing an intervention based on understanding coping. The literature has been well documented, as noted in Chapter 12, indicating that the best and most economically adventitious results for patients are achieved when health professionals work together and produce evidence-based practice. Thus advancing methods in nursing research and working with other health professionals can strengthen the impact that nurses can have in these countries.

Summary of Theory and Research in Latin American

We witnessed much growth in nursing research in the Latin American countries and recognized the use of the RAM in education and research is making some contribution. Areas for future growth were identified. Examining the RAM in light of the philosophical assumption of veritivity can highlight the beliefs that the individual is viewed in the context of the purposefulness of human existence, the unity of purpose of humankind, responsibility for activity and creativity for the common good, and believing in value and meaning in life. These beliefs are supportive of creating meaning and purpose through research on behalf of a global society. Through current plans and projects for the future based on the RAM, we can consider the role of research, education, and practice in Latin America. As in any other part of the world there is a need to develop individual talents and intelligence. Further, the need is to develop responsible professionals in nursing whose efforts in practice and research advance the common good and give value and meaning to life.

THEORY-BASED RESEARCH REPORTED FROM A SELECTIVE GLOBAL SURVEY

As in Latin American, this is a time of rapid development of nursing research around the rest of the globe. In this text we have noted the connections of theory and research in the process of developing knowledge (Fawcett, 1978, 2010). There is little information on whether or not theory is used to guide research internationally, outside the Latin American countries already discussed. An eight-item survey was developed and entered into an electronic survey program. The theorist made a list of countries and identified contacts in each one who could be considered key informants. These persons were judged to be knowledgeable about research publications and nursing theory. Surveys were sent by e-mail to 40 key informants among the international contacts.

Results of Survey

Initially 27 respondents (68%) began the survey, however, a smaller number completed all the questions. The sample included key informants from 16 countries and territories including: Virgin Islands, Canada, Ireland, Sweden, Spain, Switzerland, Turkey ($n = 2$), Palestinian Jerusalem, Jordan, Thailand, South Korea, Taiwan, Philippines, Japan, and Nigeria. The respondents were asked to identify their positions and the positions of most researchers in their countries. The responses on positions of the respondents were: nursing education faculty, 83%; clinical practice, 11%; research institute professionals, 11%; and other, 17%. The category "other" included: adjunct faculty, student, or dean. The reports of positions of most researchers was similar, with slightly fewer working in research institutes, the category of "other" was not used and dual positions were not reported for researchers in general from these countries.

When asked to provide an approximate number of nursing research publications per year by researchers in their country, the respondents reported as follows: more than 300 = 29%; 101 to 300 = 24%; 26 to 100 = 29%; and less than 25 = 18%. In describing types of research conducted, the respondents estimated percentages of qualitative studies, quantitative studies using correlational or multivariate analysis, or intervention designs and randomized controlled clinical trials. In summary, the respondents from all countries reported the use of all the types of research, both qualitative and each type of quantitative designs. One respondent reported 80% of studies were qualitative in that country yet five respondents reported 10% of studies were qualitative in their countries. In the first quantitative category of correlational or multivariate studies, one respondent reported that 70% of studies are of this type and four respondents reported 40% and four reported 30%. For intervention research the highest number was one respondent reporting 40% and there were seven responses of 20%, but six responses of 10%. Finally, for randomized controlled clinical trials, one respondent reported 70% of studies in that country were of this type; one response was 40% and two responses were 20%.

In relation to the use of theory in published research, the respondents had four choices. The percentage of responses to each choice is listed in

Box 13.2. The responses are split in a way that might be expected, with about one third of responses indicating that the use of nursing theories and frameworks depends on the researcher. A little more than a third indicate that frameworks for nursing research are based on nursing theories or synthesize the variable of the study at the middle range level. In addition to the numerical responses, one of the write-in responses included: "Unfortunately currently too little attention is given to frameworks and nursing models. These should get more attention in research classes again!!"

Respondents also reported on the use of particular nursing theories as frameworks for published research in their countries. Table 13.1 reports the percentage reported for each theorist listed. The four theorists from the United States, Rogers, Orem, Roy, and Watson, were used for research to various extents. The respondents also wrote in the other theories used and

---

BOX 13.2
RESPONSE TO QUESTION OF USE OF THEORY IN RESEARCH

1. Frameworks for research are based on nursing theories — 11%

2. Frameworks for research synthesize the variable of the study at the middle range level — 28%

3. The use of nursing theories and frameworks depends on the researcher — 33%

4. There are no frameworks used in nursing research — 17%

5. Other — 11%

TABLE 13.1
Theorists Used in Nursing Research Reported by Respondents

	10%	20%	30%	40%	50%	60%
Martha Rogers	6*	0	0	0	0	1
Dorethea Orem	3	2	4	3	2	1
Callista Roy	1	7	1	3	2	1
Jean Watson	8	3	0	1	0	0

*Number of responses reporting percentage of studies using a given theory.

these included grand theories from the United States (Leininger, Neuman, Peplau, and Benner); middle range theories from the United States (Dodd, symptom management; Michel, uncertainty); education/psychological and health belief model; and theorists from other countries (Monika Krohwinkell, Katie Eriksson and Kari Martinsen, and McGill Model).

Implications of Survey

In this survey the range of development of research and theory-based research is apparent from some responses. The numbers of studies published each year in the countries reported on vary from 29% reporting more than 300 studies and 18% reporting fewer than 25 each year. The use of theories also varies, with 39% referring to theory at some level and 17% reporting that frameworks are not used in nursing research. If theory and research are important to knowledge development it may be considered that greater attention could be dedicated to theory-based research. Im and Chang (2012) conducted a 10-year review of current trends in nursing theories and concluded that greater efforts to link research to nursing practice and theory are needed in the United States as well as globally. Knowledge surrounding theory-based research needs to accompany the significant trend toward nursing research.

The authors acknowledge the limitations of the survey method used, in particular that the key informants were selected from a theorist's list of contacts. This approach was used based on previous experience in trying to obtain an international sample and getting minimal response. The responses will be considered in the context of this limitation. Still some indication of research and theory is represented. Future work can focus on efforts to get representative samples to validate the findings.

CONCLUSION

The reports of global theory-based research indicate that nursing research varies in quantity and type among countries. In addition there seems to be a growing use of nursing models in Latin American countries and this includes education and research. This was interpreted as a potential for positive effects on health care in these countries. In general it seems that understanding the role of theory in research can be enhanced. This connection may be looked at as a passing era in knowledge development in the United States. However, with better use of theory in research, it can be recognized that this link is the time-honored way of thinking promoted by philosophers of science and used by scholars in all disciplines.

REFERENCES

Boston-Based Adaptation Research in Nursing Society. (1999). *Roy adaptation model–based research: 25 years of contributions to nursing science.* Indianapolis, IN: Sigma Theta Tau International Center Nursing Press.

Cavalcante, M. V., Olivera Lopes M.V., Araujo, T. (2005) Study of the evidence for the concept of group in the Roy adaptation model. *Cultura de los Cuidados, 17,* 82–87.

Fawcett, J. (1978). The relationship between theory and research: A double helix. *Advances in Nursing Science, 1*(1), 49–62.

Fawcett, J. (2010). Theory testing and theory evaluation. In J. Butts & K. Rich (Eds.), *Philosophies and theories for advanced nursing practice* (pp. 605–623). Sudbury, MA: Jones & Bartlett Learning.

González, Y. M. (2007). Efficacy of two interventions based on the theory of coping and adaptation processing. *Roy Adaptation Association Review, 11*(1), 4.

Im, E., & Chang, S. (2012). Current trends in nursing theories. *Journal of Nursing Scholarship 44*(2), 156–164.

International Network for Doctoral Education in Nursing. (2012). Retrieved January 20, 2013 from www.nursing.jhu.edu. Directory of International Programs.

Lopes Neto, D., Pagliuca, L. M. F. (2002). Holistic approach of the term person in an empiric study: A critical analysis. *Revista Latino-Americana De Enfermagem, 10,* 825–830.

Monroy, P. (2003). Approximation to the experience of application of the Roy adaptation model in the pediatric intensive care unit. *Enfermeria Hoy, 1,* 17–20.

Moreno, M. E. (2001). Application of the model of adaptation in an outpatient rehabilitation service. *Aquichan, 1,* 14–17.

Moreno, M. E., & Alvarado, A. (2009). Application of Callista Roy adaptation model in Latin America. *Aquichan, 9,* 62–72.

Roy, C. (2009). *The Roy adaptation model* (3rd ed.). Upper Saddle River, NJ: Pearson Education.

Roy, C., & Roberts, S. (1981). *Theory construction in nursing: An adaptation model.* Englewood Cliffs, NJ: Prentice-Hall.

Appendix

Instruments Used in Roy
Model–Based Studies 1995 to 2010

KEVILLE FREDERICKSON, ALEXANDRA
BENNETT-ROACH, AND MARTHA V. WHETSELL

Measuring concepts of the Roy adaptation model (RAM) is a key issue in designing research that can be used for further knowledge development as in the project of developing middle range theory and evidence for practice. With the wealth of studies analyzed, the authors felt we could provide a real service to our readers by listing the instruments used in studies included in this review (Table A). Of the 172 studies in the accepted pool, 126 used quantitative designs and 40 used qualitative designs. Some were specifically aimed at instrument development. The information provided in this appendix focuses on the measurement strategies used in the 126 quantitative studies.

Step one was to come up with a list of all instruments or measurements used by the investigators. To make this useful we listed the studies in categories of the major concepts of the Roy adaptation model. The total number of instruments or measurement strategies was 242. This includes well-known tools as well as those developed by individual researchers for use in that study. This approach of providing the list is seen as a first step in an ongoing effort to continue to improve the quality of theory-based research for building knowledge for impacting change in practice.

We foresee the possibility of selecting the most frequently used instruments and examining their validity and reliability. The criteria for analysis of the instruments could be based on evaluation of the relationship of the instrument to the model concepts and the psychometric adequacy of the instrument. Based on this further evaluation, we can make recommendations for future use of instruments.

Based on our work in identifying and organizing the instruments and measurements, we can make some brief observations about measurement in research based on the RAM. In this 15-year review of RAM, 172 studies from 1995–2010, many more instruments were used for research than in the previous 25-year RAM research analyses of 163 studies from 1970 to 1994. There are a number of factors that may be contributing to this phenomenon. Of note is the increasing use of multivariate studies and related analyses. As a result, researchers are including more variables in their studies, which then require more instruments. This trend is encouraging as human behavior is multifactorial. The variety of instruments was much greater, however; disappointingly, there were fewer instruments used repeatedly. By using a wider variety of instruments, one must question the adequacy of the instruments to reflect the model concepts. Likewise, it is very difficult to establish instruments that have validity and correlation with model concepts and constructs.

From this review of instruments, it is clear that there is a great need to develop and use instruments that have been specifically derived from the model. Instruments that were reported in the literature as unsuited for the model were still used, in particular, the Rosenberg Self-Esteem instrument. Rosenberg's scale has consistently been demonstrated to have little validity when used with the model and very low methodological value, that is, low variation among scores and a conceptual base derived from and normed on adolescent/young college-age students. Rosenberg's scale is used often as a measure of self-concept because it is very short, 10 items. Yet instruments were developed based on the RAM with acceptable psychometric properties such as Zhan's Self-Consistency instrument and Coping and Adaptation Processing Scale (CAPS) by Roy have not been used frequently. Given the use of so many different instruments for RAM research, analysis needs to be done on these to determine the congruency of each item and the total instrument with the constructs and concepts of the model. Likewise, there needs to be evaluation of instrument clarity and readability, including literacy level. There needs to be greater utilization and evaluation of the known instruments derived from the model.

The authors plan to extend and publish this review of instruments to include making recommendations for use of instruments to measure concepts of the RAM. In addition efforts will be made through the Roy Adaptation Association (RAA) to have open access to instruments specifically developed based on the model.

TABLE A
Instruments Used in RAM-Based Research by Categories of Major Concepts

Self-Concept

- General self-concept measurements
  - Self-Confidence in Self-Monitoring Scale (SCSMS) (author)
  - Profile of Mood States (POMS)
  - Visual Analog Scale—Worry (VAS-W)
  - Harter's Self-Perception Profile for Children (Harter, 1985)
  - Symptom Experience Scale (SES)
  - Verbal Abuse Scale
  - Abuse Assessment Screen (modified) (Parker & McFarlane, 1991)
  - Researcher-developed tool adapted from The Verbal Abuse Scale (Manderino & Banton, 1994)
  - Health Related Powerless Scale (HRPS)
  - Nighttime Infant Care Index
  - Personal Meaning Index Subscale of the Life Attitude Profile—Revised
  - Anger Expression (AX) Scale
  - Job Satisfaction Scale
  - The Sexual Awareness Scale (SAS) designed by Snell (1991)
  - Danger Assessment (DA)
  - Silencing the Self Scale
  - Psychological Observation Weaning Evaluation Rating Scale (POWERS)
  - Arab-Speaking Patients' Acculturation Scale
  - Nurses' Spirituality and Delivery of Spiritual Care (NSDSC)
  - The Adherence Questionnaire
- Specific Components of Self-Concept
  - Anxiety
    - State Trait Anxiety Inventory (STAI)
    - Spielberger State-Trait Anxiety Inventory (STAI)
    - Anxiety subscale of the SCL-90R
  - Grief
    - Grief Experience Inventory Subscales (Sanders, Mauger, & Strong, 1985)
  - Stress
    - Perceived Stress Scale (PSS) (Cohen, Kamarck, & Mermelstein, 1983)
    - Nursing Stress Scale (Factor 1)
    - Symptom Distress Scale
    - Elderly Daily Stress Scale
    - Expanded Nurse Stress Scale
    - Parenting Stress Index/Short Form (PSI/SF)
  - Depression
    - Zung Self-Rating Depression Scale (SDS) (Zung, 1965, 1972)
    - Geriatric Depression Scale (Yesavage, Brink, & Rose, 1983)
    - BPI: Brief Pain Children's Depression Inventory (CDI) Inventory
    - Center for Epidemiological Studies—Depression (CES-D)

(continued)

TABLE A
Instruments Used in RAM-Based Research by Categories of Major Concepts (*continued*)

Self-Concept

- ○ Symptoms of Posttraumatic Stress Depression Scale
- ○ Hayes & Lohse Depression
- ○ Beck Depression Inventory
- Loneliness
  - ○ UCLA Loneliness Scale (Russell, 1996)
  - ○ University of CA Los Angeles, Loneliness Scale—version 3 (UCLA-3)
- Abuse
  - ○ Verbal Abuse Scale
  - ○ Abuse Assessment Screen (modified) (Parker & McFarlane, 1991)
  - ○ Researcher-developed tool adapted from The Verbal Abuse Scale (Manderino & Banton, 1994)
  - ○ Index of Spouse Abuse (ISA)
- Self-Esteem
  - ○ Rosenberg Self-Esteem Scale

- Combined
  - Functional Assessment and Cancer Therapy Scale (Fact-B)
  - Hospital Anxiety & Depression Scale
  - Study of Aging, Status and Sense of Control (ASOC), data collected by Mirowsky and Ross

Coping and Adaptation

- Self-control (CSQ COP) and Catastrophizing (CSQ CAT) subscales from the Coping Strategies Questionnaire
- The Self-Efficacy Scale (SES) (Sherer and colleagues, 1982)
- Thai Coping and Adaptation Processing Scale (TCAP)
- Coping and Adaptation Processing Scale (CAPS) (Roy, 2004, 2012)
- COPD Self-Efficacy Scale (CSES) (Wigal et al., 1991)
- Adaptation to Spinal Cord Injury Interview Schedule (ASCIIS)
- Non Religious Pain Coping Scale: (Lin, 1995)
- Religious Problem-Solving Scale (RPS) Short Form (Pargamet et al.,1988)
- Religious Coping Scale (R-COPE)
- Ways of Coping Questionnaire (WCQ)
- Diabetes Empowerment Scale (Anderson et al., 2000)
- PAIS: Psychosocial adjustment to illness scale
- Derogatis and Derogatis' Psychosocial Adjustment to Illness Scale-Self-Report Bereavement Interview
- Indices of Coping Responses
- F-Copes
- BriefRCOPE
- Jalowiec Coping Scale (Jalowiec, 1984)
- Parental Coping Strategies Inventory (PCSI)

Physiological

- General physiological measurements
  - Weight loss in the preceding 6 months was calculated, using a detailed weight-history report
  - Intervention—Therapeutic Biking Program (the Easy Rider Program), 1 hour a day, 5 days a week, for 2 weeks using a Duet bike
  - Arthritis Impact Management Scale Short Form (AIMS)
  - Chronic Conditions Questionnaire
  - Severity of Side Effects Questionnaire
  - Preoxygenation and tracheal suctioning practices survey (self-made-expert panel, pretested)
  - Coping with Urinary Incontinence
  - Extended Glasgow Outcome Scale (GOSE)
  - Karnofsky Performance Scale (KPS)
  - Common Toxicity Criteria scoring scale
  - Mini Mental Status Examination (MMSE)
  - Modified Functional Independence Measure (FIM)

- Specific components of physiological
  - Pain
    - Brief Pain Inventory
    - Pain Management Index
    - Short-Form McGill Pain Questionnaire (Melzack, 1987)
    - Satisfaction Question With Regard to Education (i.e., on a scale of 0 to 10—how valuable was the information you received to manage your pain?)
    - Medical Outcomes Study Patient Assessment Questionnaire (MOSPAQ) subscales:
    - Fatigue
    - Pain severity
    - Pain: presence assessed using a dichotomous scale
    - Years of pain = number of months
    - Body location(s) were identified by placing an X on a pain map and circling the most painful site
    - McGill Pain Questionnaire
    - Descriptor Scale (Herr & Mobily, 1991) assessed the level of pain intensity in the last week
  - Sleep
    - The General Sleep Disturbance Scale (GSDS)
    - Pittsburgh Sleep Quality Index
    - Modified Stanford Sleepiness Scale (SSS)
    - Epworth Sleepiness Scale (ESS)
    - Sleep Quality (SQ)
  - Oral health
    - Geriatric Oral Health Assessment Index (GOHAI) (Atchison & Dolan, 1990)
    - Brief Oral Health State Examination (BOHSE) (Kayser-Jones, Bird, Paul, Long, & Schell, 1995)
    - Count of number of teeth

(*continued*)

TABLE A
Instruments Used in RAM-Based Research by Categories of Major Concepts (*continued*)

Physiological

- Heart
  - Riegel, Heo et al.'s Minnesota Living with Heart Failure Questionnaire (MLWHF)
  - Cognitive Perception of Cardiovascular Healthy Lifestyles
  - The Preeclampsia/Gestational Hypertension Checklist (author)
- Fatigue
  - Functional Assessment of Chronic Illness Therapy-Fatigue Version IV (FACIT-F)
  - Chalder Fatigue Scale (14 items)
  - Revised Piper Fatigue Scale (PFS)
  - Myesthenia Gravis Fatigue Scale (Grohar-Murray, Sears, Hubsky, & Becker, 1994)
- Diabetes
  - The Problem Areas in Diabetes Questionnaire
  - The Diabetes Questionnaire
  - Diabetes Basic Knowledge Test (DBKT)
  - Diabetes Self-Report Test (DSRT)
- Symptoms
  - PTSD CheckList—Military Version (PCL-M)
  - SCL-PTSD scale
  - Rotterdam Symptom Checklist (RSCL)
  - Brief Symptom Inventory, French-validated version
  - Psychiatric Symptoms Index
  - Symptoms Questionnaire, CES-D
  - Self-Care Behavior Responses to Symptoms Questionnaire
  - Symptom Checklist-90-R
  - Symptom Checklist 35-Revised (SCL-35-R)
- Comorbidity
  - Charlson Comorbidity Index (CCI) (Charlson, Pompei, Ales, & MacKenzie, 1987)
  - Comorbidity Checklist (Guralnik, 1989)
- General health
  - Health Status SF-36
  - General Health Subscale of the Short Form 36 Health Survey, version 2
  - Scales Derived from the Medical Outcomes Study 36-item Short-Form Health Survey (SF-36):
  - Activity (ACT)
  - Health Perception (HP)
  - Self-Assessed Health Questionnaire
  - Physical Function subscale of Functional Status Questionnaire
  - Health Promoting Behavior Questionnaire
  - Perceived Health Competence Scale (PHCS)
  - Personal Health Questionnaire (PHQ)

Physiological

- o Medical Outcome Study 36
- o BP standardized protocol—two times, 1 month apart
- o BMI
- o Acute physiological and chronic health evaluation (APACHE III)
- o Environmental barriers (Shyu, Liang, Lu, & Wu, 2004)
- o Blood sugars, selected from range of the one most closely reflective of home-monitoring results for past month or last laboratory result
- o Energy Level-Visual analogue scale
- Mobility
  - o 6-Minute Walking Test
  - o Physical therapy assessment of range of motion, strength, and upper extremity girth
  - o Physical Activity Scale for the Elderly (PASE)
  - o Mobility, prefracture self-care ability and health status (Shyu, Liang, Lu, & Wu, 2004)
  - o Exercise Tolerance Test
- Pulmonary
  - o Interdependence: The Asthma Responsibility Questionnaire (ARQ) (McQuaid, Penza-Clyve, Nassau, & Fritz, 2001)
  - o Physiologic: Peak expiratory flow
  - o Numeric rating scale to measure dyspnea
  - o Physiologic status/disease severity measured using a Microlab 3100 portable spirometer
  - o Pulmonary Functional Status Scale (PFSS) (Weaver, Narsavage, & Guilfoyle, 1998)
  - o Weaning Readiness Assessment Scale (WRAS)
- Elimination
  - o Urogenital Distress Inventory (UDI)
  - o Incontinence Impact Questionnaire (IIQ)
  - o Cantril Self Anchoring Striving Scale: severity of urinary incontinence
- Nutrition
  - o Mini-Nutritional Assessment (MNA) (Guigoz, Vellas, & Garry, 1996)
- Gastro
  - o Morrow Assessment of Nausea and Emesis (MANE)
- Memory
  - o Revised Memory and Behavior Problems Checklist, French-validated version

Quality of Life and Well-Being

- Quality of Life Index
- Quality of Life in Epilepsy 89
- Quality of Life for Children with Cancer (QOLCC)
- Index of Well-Being (IWB) (Campbell, Converse, & Rodgers, 1976)
- Spiritual Well-Being Scale
- Existential Well-Being Scale, subscale of the Spirituality Well-Being Scale
- JAREL Spiritual Well-Being Scale (Hungelmann, Kenkel-Rossi, Klassen, & Stollenwerk, 1996)

(continued)

TABLE A
Instruments Used in RAM-Based Research by Categories of Major Concepts
(continued)

Quality of Life and Well-Being

- Life Satisfaction Index A (LSI-A)
- Life Satisfaction Index-Z
- Purpose in Life Test (PIL)
- Sickness Impact Profile (SIP) subscales:
  - Body Care & Movement
  - Home Management
  - Social Interaction
  - Recreation and Pastime
  - Work (if applicable)
- Short-Form-12 H-R QOL

Interdependence

- PRQ
  - Personal Resource Questionnaire
  - Personal Resources Scale adapted from the Family Resource Scale
- Owen's Interpersonal Support Evaluation List (ISEL)
- Interpersonal Support Evaluation Checklist (ISEL) (Cohen, Mermelstein, Kamarck, & Hoberman, 1985)
- Enforced Social Dependency Scale (Benoliel, McCorkle, & Young, 1980)—2
- Social Support Questionnaire—Short Form (SSQ-SF) (Sarason, Sarason, Shearin, & Pierce, 1987)
- Relationship Change Scale (RCS)
- Geriatric Social Readjustment Rating
- Interpersonal Relationship Inventory
- Work Relationship Index
- Hospitalized Patient Visiting Preference Questionnaire
- The Perceived Social Support scale
- Multidimensional scales of perceived social support
- Hospice Social Support Questionnaire (Adapted from Norbeck, 1981)
- The Modified Diabetes Social Support Questionnaire—Friends version

Group

- ENA Family Presence and Support Staff Assessment tool, modified by author
- Family Perception Inventory (FRI) (Hymovich, 1992)
- Coping, Spouse Coping, Concerns, Spouse Concerns Subscales of the Family Perception Inventory (FPI) (Hymovich, 1992)
- Mayer-Salovey-Caruso Emotional Intelligence Test (MSCEIT)
- Family needs Inventory Guide
- Children and Family Characteristics Questionnaire
- Family Coping Estimate (FCE)
- Spielberger State Trait Anxiety Inventory STAI
- Conflict Tactic Family Violence Scale
- Family APGAR Questionnaire
- The Modified Diabetes Family Behavioral Checklist-II
- Index of Marital Satisfaction-Hudson (1982)

Role

- Inventory of Functional Status After Childbirth (IFSAC)
- Inventory of Functional Status in the Elderly (IFSITE)
- Inventory of Functional Status—Caregiver of a Child in a Body Cast (IFSCCBC)
- Inventory of Functional Status Dialysis (IFS-D)
- Modified Inventory of Functional Status
- Functional Status Index: (FSI) (Jette,1987)
- Postpartum Self-Evaluation Questionnaire (Lederman, Weingarden, & Lederman, 1981)
- Job Satisfaction Survey
- Midlife Developmental Inventory (MIDI, 2000)
- Maton and Teti's School Status Questionnaire (Stevenson, Maton, & Teti, 1998)
- Social Activity Subscale on the Functional Status Questionnaire (FSQ)
- Prenatal Maternal Adaptation Questionnaire
- Postpartum Maternal Adaptation Questionnaire
- Hollingshead Index of Social Status
- Social Behavior Assessment Scale
- Social Functioning (SF)
- Role Limitation Emotional (RE)
- Scales Derived from Individual Traditional–Modernity Scale: Modernity Orientation (MO)
  • Student Role Expectation (SRE)
  • Maternal Role Expectation (MRE)
  • Student Role Involvement Questionnaire (SRIQ)
  • Maternal Role Involvement Questionnaire (MRIQ)
  • Social Support Scale (SS)
  • Role Strain (RS)
  • Role Gratification (RG)
- Lederman's prenatal and postpartum self-evaluation questionnaires
- Maternal Identity Scale (Kho, 1996)
- Social Support Scale (Bai, 1996)
- Maternal Sensitivity Scale (Han, 2002)
- Maternal–Fetal Attachment Scale (Cranley, 1981; translated and tested by Kim, 2000)
- Role Adaptation Questionnaire
- Two Factor Index of Social Position (TFISP)
- Parenthood Motivation List (van Balen & Trimbos-Kemper, 1995)
- Caregiving Hassles Scale
- Single-item scale: 0–10 regarding the extent to which they can perform their usual activities

Stimuli

- Quality of life—Functional Assessment of Cancer Therapy—Lung (FACT-L) (Cella, 1994)
- Inventory of Cancer
- Stage of cancer treatment and lab data from chart
- Cancer Rehabilitation Evaluation System SF (CARES-SF)
- Polypharmacy, operationally defined as the number of medications taken

(continued)

TABLE A
Instruments Used in RAM-Based Research by Categories of Major Concepts
(*continued*)

Stimuli
- The Grindler Body Attitudes Scale, variables such as age, gender, education level, diagnosis, number of years respondent has had ostomy, marital status, comorbid conditions, and medication use
- AUDIT, an alcohol measurement scale—The Alcohol Use Disorders Identification Test is a simple 10-question test developed by the World Health Organization to determine whether a person's alcohol consumption may be harmful

Researcher Designed to Measure More Than One RAM Concept
- Barriers Questionnaire-II—To examine the relationships among cancer pain, coping strategies, and quality of life among Arab American adults with cancer, and to test the Adaptation to Cancer Pain (ACP) model (Al-Atiyyat, 2009)
- Similes Preferences Inventory (SPI)—Examines the relationships between creativity, functional performance, and successful aging in the context of the RAM (Flood & Scharer, 2006)
- CES-D (Devine & Orme, 1985)—Purpose of study was to examine the effects of a computer-delivered intervention on measures of psychosocial health (social support, self-esteem, empowerment, self-efficacy, depression, loneliness, and stress) in chronically ill rural women
- Global health status questionnaire; health status, functional status, self-esteem, satisfaction with interpersonal relations (Sabatini, 2003)
- The Modified Patient Reactions Assessment: personal, psychological, and health care system factors that contribute to integrating lifestyle in Thai women with type 2 diabetes (Siripitayakunkit, Hanucharurnkul, Melkus, Vorapongsathorn, Rattarasarn, & Arpanantikul, 2008)
- Omaha System Intervention Scheme: women's physical, emotional, functional, and social adaptation; postpartum concerns; and learning needs during the first 2 weeks following caesarean birth and to identify relevant nursing interventions (Weiss, Fawcett, & Aber, 2009)

Total: 242 measurements

REFERENCES

Rosenberg, M. (1979). *Conceiving the self.* New York: Basic Books.

Roy, S. C. (2011). Research based on the Roy adaptation model: Last 25 years. *Nursing Science Quarterly, 24*(4), 312–320.

Zhan, L. (2000). Cognitive adaptation and self-consistency in hearing-impaired older persons: Testing Roy's adaptation model. *Nursing Science Quarterly, 13*(2), 158–165.

Index